DR DAVID COLLISON is a Fellow of the Royal Australasian College of Physicians and a consultant physician with a special interest in environmental health, hypnotherapy and psychiatric problems. Acknowledged internationally as one of the foremost authorities in his field, he is a founding member of the Australian Society of Clinical Ecology, now the Australian Society of Environmental Health, and currently its vice-president. He is also the immediate past-president of the International Society of Hypnosis.

TIMOTHY HALL has specialised in investigative writing, and this is his fiftieth book. A former correspondent for the London *Observer* and the BBC, he has also written extensively for the Sydney *Bulletin* and the *Reader's Digest*.

WHY DO I FEEL SO AWFUL?

DR DAVID R. COLLISON MB BS FRACP
with TIMOTHY HALL

ANGUS
& ROBERTSON
PUBLISHERS

ANGUS & ROBERTSON PUBLISHERS

Unit 4, Eden Park, 31 Waterloo Road,
North Ryde, NSW, Australia 2113;
16 Golden Square, London W1R 4BN,
United Kingdom

First published in Australia
by Angus & Robertson Publishers in 1989
Reprinted in 1989

Copyright © David R. Collison and Timothy Hall 1989

National Library of Australia
Cataloguing-in-publication data.

Collison, David R., 1937-
  Why do I feel so awful?

  Includes index.
  ISBN 0 207 15731 6.

  1. Environmentally induced diseases.
  2. Allergy. I. Hall, Timothy, 1938-
  II. Title.

616.97

Typeset in 11pt Garamond by Best-set Typesetter
Printed in Australia

Confusion now hath made his masterpiece

MACBETH, II, iii, 72

The wise gods make us admire our errors;
laugh at us while we strut to our confusion

ANTONY AND CLEOPATRA, III, xi, 82

I will not wait until the men in white coats with their white rats tell me
what I can see every day to be the truth.

DR RICHARD MACKARNESS MB BS DPM
NOT ALL IN THE MIND

Contents |

Introduction I

Good health is the most fundamental of rights. Implicit in that is that each of us has the right to expect that medicine will provide us with the means to get better when we are sick and to remain in good health when we are well. So why is it that perhaps 50 per cent of patients who go to their family doctor looking for a cure for their ills find that he or she can offer them nothing but pills and potions, which as often as not leave them feeling worse than before? What other profession could live with a failure rate of one in two?

Clearly, there is something very basic missing from the doctor's armoury, something that we were not taught at medical school, something that could explain this abject failure rate. I believe that we have found it and in the most logical place of all — in the food that we eat and the myriad chemicals that beset us. But not in a straightforward way that we could have seen at any time simply by opening our eyes.

This was a brilliant discovery — brilliant because it *wasn't* obvious, brilliant because the increasing numbers of doctors who now practise it believe that up to 80 per cent of all those symptoms and illnesses that at present get no help from orthodox medicine can now be properly treated. And brilliant because, although it is a revolutionary new tool for the doctor, it is also a means by which we can all safely and responsibly heal ourselves and then remain at the peak of good health.

This extraordinary new approach to medicine is called clinical ecology, an odd name which bothered my colleagues in America so much that they changed the name to environmental health. Whatever its name, I think you will agree when you have read this book that we have waited much too long for an approach that offers every one of us, doctors and patients alike, so much.

PART ONE

The Promise of Clinical Ecology

WESTERNERS —
VERY UNHEALTHY CREATURES ∎

One of the most depressing facts that family doctors have to come to terms with is that so many of their patients have illnesses and symptoms that cannot even be diagnosed properly, let alone treated.

Medicine has concentrated almost exclusively on microbes over the last hundred years or so, since Pasteur discovered that infectious diseases are caused by toxins, or poisons, which in turn are produced by bacteria, minute living organisms. The reward has been that most of the devastating epidemics of past centuries, such as typhoid, cholera and tuberculosis, are today a thing of the past throughout much of the world. But all this expertise has in no way meant that people living in Western countries are now healthy, or indeed, on average, are living any longer once they have survived infancy and early childhood. Medical science may have eliminated smallpox and most of the dangers of bacterial infections, but it has done little for the millions in those so-called advanced nations that are still afflicted with what we know as the diseases of degeneration, many of them quite unknown in undeveloped countries.

THE UNNATURAL DISEASES ∎

Almost without exception, these are diseases for which orthodox medicine, as we practise it, has no cure. They are all unnatural in that they never (or virtually never) occur among primates in the wild and rarely to people in undeveloped countries. They include heart disease, arthritis, diabetes, high blood pressure, gall stones, glaucoma, cataract and cancer in many of its forms. Patients suffering from these diseases can have their symptoms alleviated, to a greater or lesser degree, but only in rare cases does conventional medical therapy actually get down to the vital issue of establishing what is causing the disease in the first place, so that it can be prevented from recurring.

In addition to these life-threatening diseases, which shorten the lives of an estimated 60 per cent of the population, there are the far more numerous disorders and illnesses that plague modern society without actually killing people. Migraine is a painful example. It may not kill anyone (though it is quite capable of hospitalising its victims and leaving them wishing they *were* dead), but some 10 per cent of all people in Western countries are known to suffer either from migraine itself, or from headaches so painful that the sufferer considers them to be migraine. In Australia that means there are one and a half million people, not to mention their families who usually have to suffer with them, who would swear any oath that their lives are exquisitely and painfully spoilt by their headaches. The cost in lost productivity and government-subsidised drugs to control the pain, quite apart from the suffering, is immeasurable.

"YOU'RE NOT ILL — YOU'RE JUST PRETENDING" ■

It sometimes seems that almost every one of us is living and functioning at less than par. Headaches, migraines, fatigue, aches and pains, arthritis, depression and anxiety, and a host of other symptoms are taken so much for granted that many of us have come to regard them as an almost inseparable part of modern life. Even when we do take ourselves to the doctor, he or she often does nothing but prescribe drugs for the symptoms, whose side effects leave us feeling even worse than before.

As well as finding nothing wrong, the doctor is likely to leave you in no doubt, after a few visits for the same problem, that he or she thinks it is all in your mind and that the best thing you can do is go back home, or to work, pull yourself together and stop being a nuisance when there are genuinely ill patients waiting to be seen. It is a scenario that is so familiar that there is no need even to caricature it.

You *know* there is something wrong with you! You feel terrible, your head hurts. You force yourself out of bed, drag yourself to work, struggle through the day and then home again at night, exhausted, only to have a few hours restless sleep and wake feeling as tired as when you went to bed. Then you go through the whole sorry sequence all over again.

With no idea what causes many of the illnesses they are asked to treat and cure, doctors usually stall and order a barrage of expensive pathological tests, often repeated X-rays, CAT scans, and second, third and fourth opinions. In terms of sheer monetary cost, the price is enormous.

If it resulted in a cure more often than not, there might be some justification for persisting with this highly inefficient approach to medicine, but it doesn't. Even before writing referrals, general practitioners know — if they are truthful to themselves (they are rarely truthful to their patients, who have no wish to be told that their doctors have nothing useful to offer) — that none of the specialists is likely to be of any significant help. Only those patients suffering from diseases that are clearly diagnosable — fractures, gastrointestinal obstructions, infections and so on — can hope to receive worthwhile treatment.

DRUGS THAT MAKE THINGS WORSE ■

True, the pharmaceutical manufacturers have an arsenal of pills and potions for treating every imaginable symptom. But the basic fault of pharmaceutical drugs, with the obvious exceptions, is that they have little known connection with the disease process itself. (The exceptions are notably antibiotics, which are specific to acute infections and to chronic diseases like tuberculosis.) No matter how they go about achieving their ends, they work in a way that is wholly unrelated to nature's own methods of fighting disease. They often mask the problem rather than eliminate it; they rarely come without side effects; often, and most seriously, they frequently complicate the physician's job by erasing valuable clues to the real cause of the trouble.

Sometimes doctors pick drugs that will suppress symptoms non-specifically, like the broad-spectrum antibiotics, an approach that works on the wishful and quite erroneous assumption that you are sure to hit one of the symptoms if you scatter the shot widely enough. Sometimes they select the symptoms that seem to predominate (which can be very tricky when many patients present at the surgery with a catalogue of symptoms), and they write prescriptions for drugs about whose method of working they probably know little and their patients nothing at all. The prescribing doctor simply accepts the manufacturer's indications for prescribing, and its assurances that the drug is safe and that if there are any side effects, they will not be serious. In fact, if note were taken of the list of cautions and potential side effects, as they are set out in the package insert (the leaflet that is sometimes included in the packet with the drug and is usually removed by the pharmacist so that it won't be read by the patient), the doctor would rarely prescribe the drug and the patient would never take it.

BEWARE THE HIDDEN DANGERS OF THE "SAFE" DRUGS! ■

Finding a typical example of what I mean is easy enough. Very many drugs qualify and the one I have chosen, amitriptyline, was selected mainly because it *is* so commonly prescribed.

Amitriptyline is the generic, pharmaceutical name of an effective and very widely prescribed antidepressant. It is marketed under a series of trade names including Tryptanol, the original trade name. As well as being routinely used for the relief of depression, it is sometimes also prescribed for enuretics, or bedwetters. One glance at the known side effects would be enough to depress anyone — except that patients are rarely given an opportunity to see them.

Tryptanol has, of course, been passed as a drug that can safely be administered to humans and has been used for more than twenty years. Certainly most patients (and probably the majority of doctors) would assume that this means that it is completely safe as long as it is taken at no more than the recommended dosage. But what is the reality?

Charles E. Frosst, a marketing subsidiary of Merck, Sharp and Dohme (the company that first discovered and synthesised amitriptyline), markets Tryptanol and itself lists a string of precautions and dangers that are truly chilling. Caution must be used, it warns, in patients with a history of seizures, impaired liver function, urinary retention, glaucoma and cardiovascular disorders; or in those receiving thyroid medication. If schizophrenics receive the drug for the depressive component of their illness, their psychotic symptoms may be aggravated; if manic depressives are given it, it may make them more manic. Paranoid delusions may be exaggerated, sometimes with hostility. And all this before Frosst even gets to the known adverse reactions!

The safety of Tryptanol for pregnant and lactating women has not been established, Frosst goes on, and even though it is prescribed for enuresis (bed-wetting) in children, it is specifically not to be used for the treatment of depression in anyone under the age of 12.

The known adverse reactions include a list of cardiovascular problems, from high blood pressure and low blood pressure, to arrhythmia, heart block and stroke; numerous central nervous system and neuromuscular symptoms including disorientation, delusions, hallucinations, insomnia, nightmares, ataxia or unsteady gait, tinnitus (ringing in the ears) and seizures; and a host of other symptoms ranging from blurred vision, constipation, bone marrow depression, nausea, anorexia, vomiting, breast enlargement, testicular swelling in males, both increase and decrease in libido, elevated blood glucose levels, dizziness, weakness, fatigue, headache, weight gain and loss, swelling of the face and tongue, and various skin rashes. And still we haven't left the symptoms that may be experienced at the *recommended* dosage!

There is another long list dealing with overdosage symptoms which ends with the ultimate cautionary note that "deaths by deliberate or accidental overdosage have occurred with this class of drugs".

The manufacturer correctly points to the fact that these symptoms are only rarely encountered, but what is absolutely certain is that if they had *not* been encountered, the manufacturer would not be listing them. Except, of course, that the world doesn't see them, because the dispensing pharmacist removes the evidence before it gets to the patient, and many doctors recall, or prefer to remember, only that the drug is a useful antidepressant.

As a highly undesirable way of economising, most manufacturers have even stopped including the literature in the original package, which at least was available on demand. Dispensing pharmacists maintain that only about one drug in ten now contains this literature. An increasing number of responsible pharmacists include brief computer-printed notes on the drugs that they dispense, but apart from warnings about overconsumption, avoiding alcohol and drowsiness, they rarely list any of the potentially serious side effects.

However rare these undesirable side effects may be, the one thing that is surely indisputable is that by no stretch of the imagination can Tryptanol, or any of the other five trade names under which amitriptyline is marketed (or indeed most other routinely prescribed drugs), be described as harmless. They may be the preferred method of treatment, but they are certainly not safe.

CAUTION — DOCTOR AT WORK! ■

Before we leave the question of consumer protection, we ought to be deeply disturbed by findings such as those of the US Department of Health which recently reported that one in five patients in the major teaching hospitals in the USA acquires an iatrogenic, or doctor-caused, disease that usually requires treatment and leads to death in one in thirty cases. All too often, the rest of the Western world inexorably follows the example of the United States, sometimes years later, so there is no justification for smugness outside America. Half of these cases of iatrogenic disease result from complications of "correctly" prescribed drug therapy; and most alarmingly, one in ten is the result of what are considered to be appropriate diagnostic procedures. In other words, doctors make their patients sick while they are trying to find out what is wrong with them.

2 Clinical Ecology — The Safe Alternative

WHY ARE WE SO ILL? █

In the general practitioner's surgery, when the viruses, broken limbs, pregnancies and other diagnostically straightforward cases have been excluded, 80 per cent of the remaining patients by some estimates cannot be given any worthwhile treatment. That may mean that on some days half of all the patients who come looking for help from their family doctor cannot be helped. That is a terrible failure rate for any self-respecting professional to have to live with. Imagine how long an engineer designing aeroplanes or dams would survive if he was wrong half the time. And if it is unsatisfactory for the patient, rest assured that it is just as disturbing for the doctor.

It was inevitable that a few doctors, perhaps more adventurous or more persistent than the majority of their colleagues (innovation has never been welcomed by the medical profession), should search for some explanation, some common thread, to account for this enormous number of sick people, in every developed country in the Western world, who seemingly have no hope of getting useful treatment from orthodox medicine.

These doctors are arguing that it is no longer good enough for the medical profession to close ranks and proclaim that it, and it alone, is the sole repository of all health knowledge, when it fails so often. They reason that there has to be some common factor, something shared by millions of people in many nations, of many different ethnic and socioeconomic backgrounds, of all ages and both sexes, something that is creating in them sicknesses that are usually rare or unknown in the undeveloped world, or that resist all conventional attempts to treat them.

"Healthy people", Ivan Illich wrote, "are those who live in healthy homes, on a healthy diet; in an environment equally fit for birth, growth, work, healing and dying". And if we accept that, in the right environment (barring accident or congenital illness), we all have the capacity to function at optimum efficiency, then it is surely reasonable to assume that anything polluting that environment has the potential to make us function at less than optimum efficiency.

Only two things seemed to be shared by all these disparate people: they all had to eat and drink, and they all had to breathe. Could it be then that the very food and water we consume and the air we breathe, are in some way responsible for all these seemingly unrelated diseases, as well as for all those less clearly defined disorders like headaches, depression, tiredness, fatigue, apathy and the numerous aches and pains that seem to plague so many people that they are taken for granted? Could there, in short, be some environmental cause, previously quite unsuspected, for all these apparently untreatable illnesses? Could they be untreatable simply because we are still ignorant of what causes them?

CLINICAL ECOLOGY — THE MISSING LINK ■

It was to deal with this new notion — that many of the common diseases in Western society are caused by the environment — that a totally new approach to medicine came into being in the United States about forty years ago. It was called clinical ecology — "clinical" because that means diagnosing and treating real people's diseases and illnesses, as opposed to conducting contrived, artificial experiments in the laboratory; and "ecology" because that is the branch of biology that deals with the relationships between organisms (in this case, people) and their environment.

So clinical ecologists are concerned, by definition, with treating patients when something has gone awry in their relationship with their environment, usually because of something they have eaten, drunk, inhaled or touched. To many people this means something to which they are allergic, although what we are talking about has very little to do with allergy as it is generally understood.

If it is a clever name semantically, it has turned out to be a very unfortunate name in almost every other respect, because no-one, apart from those who are involved in it, has the faintest idea what it means. It bothered the Americans so much (and they coined the name!) that they changed it to environmental health. Other countries have not followed suit, either reasoning that the alternative sounds like the people who come round from the council to see why your drains are smelling, or that it is more productive to tell people what you do than to discard an otherwise excellent name. In Australia and New Zealand, the name clinical ecology still prevails, and it is used throughout this book.

A WORLD TO WHICH WE CANNOT ADAPT ■

In recent years there has been an enormous surge of interest in food and in diet generally, an acknowledgment at last that what we eat largely determines not only the quality of life, but the time and manner in which that life will end.

If it is correct, as many maintain, that the degenerative diseases of the West are the price we pay for our diet, and that primitive people escape those diseases because their diet has never changed, then we in the West must be the victims of incomplete or inadequate adaptation.

Whether to environment or food, adaptation is one of the most basic rules of life and humans down the millennia have proved themselves to be very adaptable. It is a principle of Darwin, from which few demur, that humans and all living species possess remarkable powers of adaptation to a changing environment. But adaptation in this context is geared to the gentle pace at which nature changes, not to the frenetic pace at which we have changed our environment and eating habits over a few generations. The parents of many people alive today were born well before the first steel roller began the disastrous process of mass-producing what has aptly been called "denatured" flour, which is at the hub of the refined carbohydrate diet that is taking such a terrible toll.

For almost the whole time that humans have inhabited the earth, they have eaten much the same kind of food, drunk the same water and breathed the same air. Only relatively recently, in evolutionary terms, has the course of their progression changed, when they ceased to be exclusively nomadic hunters and gatherers and began farming. For the first time, they altered their eating habits, even though not very substantially: they simply organised their old eating habits better.

THE DISASTROUS FOOD REVOLUTION ■

Then in little more than fifty years, a mere blink of the eye, a food revolution began that is still in progress and whose final consequences we can only imagine. It began with the excessive refining and processing of bread — white bread became fashionable, not because it was nutritious, but because it was white and therefore allegedly pure. The second stage was the introduction of chemicals into the food supply (more than 3500 of them at the last count). Now we are faced with the increasing use of substitute ingredients, sham foods that get much of their taste and appearance and nutrients not from nature, but from a chemical factory.

Today we can plainly see that primitive, undeveloped people on their unprocessed, unrefined, unadulterated, chemical-free diet are free of degenerative disease; and that civilised, technologically superior, "fortunate" Western society, living on a diet that is almost diametrically opposed to the primitive diet, is riddled with diseases that contribute to 60 per cent of deaths.

There is nothing new in the notion that some foods can make us ill. Hippocrates established this 2300 years ago, when he accurately pinpointed cow's milk as the cause of much illness in his patients. However, we are talking about something much worse than true food allergy. People in primitive societies don't die from cirrhosis of the liver, nor from most of the cancers that afflict Western populations. They don't get stroke or heart disease if they are living on their traditional diet (though they do as soon as they convert to a Western diet). Diabetes does not exist. Some might starve to death, but they don't suffer from the collective death wish of millions of affluent and not-so-affluent Westerners who gorge themselves on foods with which their systems cannot cope.

Bowel cancer is a classic Western disease, the result of too much food, too much fat, too little fibre and deficiencies in essential nutrients. Add to this the increased risk of large bowel cancer from heavy consumption of beer and you have a totally avoidable disease, caused almost exclusively by the food and drink that we voluntarily ingest.

THREE MILLION CHEMICALS
POLLUTING THE WORLD ■

At the same time as the first murmurings of concern over our food were being heard, fears were being expressed about what we were doing to our environment. Twenty-five years after the publication of Rachel Carson's devastating exposé of the dangers of pesticides, *Silent Spring*, it is hard to remember (if indeed we remember at all) the impact it had at the time. Today, the proliferation of new chemicals has got so out of control that it defies comprehension.

A new chemical compound is synthesised and added to the environment at the rate of one a minute in the United States alone. The American Chemical Society's computerised registry lists more than three million entries (about 63,000 of them in common use), almost all of which were unknown at the end of the Second World War. How can anybody keep track of what their potential might be for harming the environment? It would be difficult enough if every new chemical were properly tested, but that is impossible. As we shall see, even the tests on which governments rely before granting approval for a new chemical can be fraudulent.

Even "fresh" food like the modest apple may have been sprayed up to fourteen times by the time you get it home, and you ingest traces of those fourteen sprayings when you eat it. These chemicals often pass through the skin of the fruit, so that neither washing nor scrubbing, and least of all the perfunctory rubbing to put a shine on it that some people seem to think is the yardstick of a good apple, can remove them.

ADAPT OR PERISH ■

After barely two generations, it is clearly impossible for our bodies to have adapted to almost any of the chemicals that we encounter daily. If the price we pay for moving too fast is high at the individual level, it is even more serious when viewed across the whole human race. In the history of our planet, thousands of species have become extinct because of changes not nearly so profound as those which the human race has had to contend with, especially in modern times.

One of the world's great anthropologists, Richard Leakey, has warned,

> *People feel we are here by predestination and that because we are humans, we will be able to survive even if we make mistakes. In fact, there have been thousands of living organisms of which a very high percentage have become extinct, and there is nothing to suggest that we are not part of that same pattern.*

Most people are aware that many chemicals have the potential to cause serious, sometimes fatal, consequences. The disastrous dioxin leak at Seveso, the horror of Bhopal and the tragedies of thalidomide and Agent Orange, have conditioned most people to believe that where chemicals are concerned, almost anything is possible. These are poisons that anyone, expert or lay, can see to be deadly.

Seeking to identify and then eradicate all those substances that interfere with our ability to function as we were intended, clinical ecologists go a long step further. They believe that the myriad chemicals in our food and drink and in the atmosphere, as well as countless chemically treated products and the chemicals themselves which release their molecules ("outgas" is the jargon) in our homes and workplaces, are potentially harmful *even when toxicologists have declared them harmless to humans in any quantity, or when they are present in such microscopic amounts that they have never been considered a threat.* For most doctors this is an entirely novel concept. Clinical ecologists believe, too, that very ordinary foods, even without chemical contamination, are responsible for many of the symptoms and illnesses, both physical and mental, that afflict Western society. This too is a very novel idea for most doctors. We are not taught that bread or potatoes or oranges may be responsible for every symptom that every organ is capable of producing!

For those who have no previous knowledge of clinical ecology, it takes a very considerable credibility jump to accept this. It has been known for centuries that food can cause a true allergic reaction, but what clinical ecologists are talking about is something completely different. The foods that cause ecological illness produce none of the classic proofs of allergy. There are no elevated antibodies, no tests that reveal anything when subjected to the scrutiny of the pathologist. The only evidence so far is the clinical evidence, the thousands of patients whom we see and successfully treat using an ecological approach, patients who failed to get better when they were subjected to the methods of conventional, orthodox medicine. Their trouble stems not from bacteria or a virus, but from wheat and potatoes, sugar and coffee, eggs and beef, tomatoes and bread; from the formaldehyde in permanent press clothes and in the ironing aid Fabulon; from the aftershave a patient splashes on his face, the liquid wax on the school floor, the plastic chairs in front of the television set, or the Acrilon carpet.

Clinical ecologists know that nylon can trigger daily

migraine attacks and backache; that potatoes are responsible for such deep depression that other doctors, not understanding the problem, have prescribed electric shock treatment. Fumes from a gas heater left under a house, even after the gas has been disconnected at the street, can induce extreme irritability and uncontrollable crying bouts. Sponge rubber can bring on headaches so severe that a writer can hardly string two sentences together. The plastic in telephones can trigger headaches almost as severe in office workers. Pork can be responsible for a dizzying array of symptoms from impaired hearing, loss of equilibrium and migraine to asthma and arthritis.

People don't think of blaming food or chemicals when their children look pale or have dark shadows under their eyes. They don't blame the fluorescent lighting when they are tired and irritable halfway through the day. They don't think that something in the environment is responsible for their epilepsy or diabetes, their high blood pressure or insomnia. They don't suspect these things because in most cases there is no obvious association, no apparent cause and effect.

But these are the patients who are the failures of doctors practising only orthodox medicine. Even in a country with a small population such as Australia, there are millions of such patients. In Britain the numbers run to tens of millions; in the United States probably hundreds of millions. That is an awful lot of people who spend their lives functioning well below their optimum, suffering from a galaxy of disorders and illnesses, and being given no worthwhile help by their doctors.

3 Making Sense of Illness

CARING FOR THE WHOLE PATIENT ▌

Although clinical ecology is a relatively new approach to medicine, it is in many ways a return to the old-fashioned kind of general practice of fifty years ago, when doctors were just as concerned with *keeping* their patients healthy as with curing them of their illnesses, and when they looked at them both as whole people and as symptoms in need of investigation.

Clinical ecologists look at their patients' total relationship with their environment, and not only at what they eat and drink or what they are exposed to in the air they breathe. They are involved in improving the quality of their patients' lives in every way, through exercise, relaxation and coping with stress, as well as through diet. Their primary concern is to identify the causes of chronic illness when conventional diagnostic methods have found nothing organically wrong, and then to eliminate those causes. The usual treatment is deliciously simple: identify and then eliminate! If that isn't possible with chemicals, or if it would mean leaving a good job or moving house to comply, then neutralising drops — tasteless, odourless and completely free of any unwanted side effects — are placed under the tongue for a few seconds each day. It would be hard to find anything less threatening.

A BRILLIANT HERESY ▌

One of the earliest books on clinical ecology was written in 1905 by an Australian physician, Francis Hare. Hare and an American allergist, Albert Rowe, noticed the importance of eliminating certain foods from the diet as a way of speeding up recovery after a number of illnesses. These included ulcerative colitis, bronchial asthma, eczema, migraine and others for which dietary control had been thought irrelevant.

The real importance of the observations of Hare and Rowe was that they led to the realisation that the ability of a particular food to trigger an illness did not necessarily have anything to do with its nutritional content. Indeed, two foods could have identical carbohydrate, protein and fat contents, yet one would provoke symptoms in a patient, while the other had no ill effects at all. Even more confusingly, the same food divided into two would trigger symptoms in one member of a family yet produce none in another member. Some other quite unsuspected and unrelated factor had to be at work.

Not much research was done to take this intriguing notion further. The rebirth of clinical ecology came in 1951, when American allergist Dr Theron Randolph published a paper in which he maintained that people can react not only to apparently safe chemicals in the most minute doses, but to *any* common food; and that when this occurred, there was no evidence of any kind of allergic reaction in the conventional sense of the word. For many doctors, and particularly Randolph's fellow allergists, it was heresy!

More years passed and then in 1976 a British psychiatrist, Dr Richard Mackarness, who by good fortune had once been a journalist and knew how to write for lay readers as well as his peers, alerted millions to the existence of clinical ecology in a remarkable best-seller called *Not All in the Mind*. Mackarness, now retired and living in Australia, was one of the first doctors to establish that some of the troublesome symptoms in his most difficult patients had a physical cause, the result of foods and chemicals that they had ingested or inhaled, and not a psychological cause at all. This ran quite contrary to conventional thinking in psychiatry, even though Freud himself always maintained that one day a physiological cause would be found for most mental illness.

The irrefutable proof was that by identifying and removing "unsafe" foods and chemicals from the patients' diets and environment, using a technique that Theron Randolph had described, patients who had previously resisted all attempts to treat them effectively made what often looked like a miraculous recovery. It didn't matter whether the tests were carried out blind or even double-blind, when neither the patient nor the person administering the test are aware of the identity of the food being given.

When these patients reintroduced the "unsafe" foods or food chemicals into their diets, or chemicals into their personal environments, the symptoms and illnesses returned. They usually stayed well as long as they avoided the troublesome substances (which were frequently harmful only to them and not to anyone else in their families or workplace). The disorders from which they had suffered covered almost the whole spectrum of physical and mental illness. It was an extraordinary concept.

DISCOVERING CLINICAL ECOLOGY ■

As clinical ecology began in the field of allergy (although their paths quickly divided), it was logical that many of its new adherents should come from the ranks of the conventional allergists, but this was not necessarily the case, particularly outside the United States. A much broader cross-section of the medical community became involved, notably ear, nose and throat specialists, who found that clinical ecology was effortlessly providing answers to many of their most intractable cases. Specialist physicians and general practitioners then began to follow them into the fold.

Perhaps not surprisingly, a number of doctors embraced clinical ecology because they themselves overcame their own illnesses and symptoms by using an ecological approach when conventional medicine had failed. I came across it almost by chance. I had read about it (and there was precious little to read), but had never thought that it had very much to offer a consultant physician specialising in psychiatric and so-called psychosomatic illnesses.

Many of the patients who were referred to me for hypnotherapy, which I was using in my practice, were obese. To reduce their weight, I advised them to fast and to eliminate foods such as sugar from their diets. I found that often, with no other treatment, they were losing not only weight, but also their depressions, asthmas, skin rashes and many of the other symptoms that had been bothering them. Once they had lost weight, they were advised to stay on a restrictive diet and to "avoid any food that upsets you or causes symptoms". It was the crudest form of therapy, but almost miraculously it usually worked!

When I later met Richard Mackarness — who had himself been helped by Theron Randolph when he was on the point of giving up his practice because he was so sick and had received no help from normal medical therapy — I could see that I was missing something very important in my own work. It turned out to be one of the most exciting and challenging steps that I have ever taken in medicine, and certainly one of the most rewarding for my patients.

To see a seemingly endless procession of demoralised, drugged, sick, desperate people, with every imaginable illness, mental and physical, coming into my rooms, clutching enormous files, the testimony of all that they had been through; and then to send them on their way in due course, in most cases restored to health and usually helped to the point where they could lead normal lives, defied description.

They arrived at the end of their tethers, not infrequently having been told by their family doctors and a string of specialists that there was nothing that could be done. They departed, often without drugs of any kind, with new hope and wonder. The follow-up, often over many years, confirmed that this was no seven-day wonder, but a lasting answer that was available nowhere else in medicine.

WHO CAN BE HELPED? ■

How relevant, then, is clinical ecology? How many people can it help? We know that the breakdown of our ability to cope with the environment in which we live and work, and to adapt to the ever-increasing load of chemicals in the air that we breathe and the food we ingest, is already occurring on a massive scale. Hospitals and doctors' surgeries are cluttered up with patients manifesting illnesses that are not properly diagnosed, effectively treated or in many cases even minimally relieved.

We know that up to half of all general practitioners' patients cannot be helped except, for example, by drugs to suppress the symptoms, while the underlying cause continues and the disease expression relentlessly progresses. Dr Theron Randolph put that figure as high as 80 per cent in many practices and, after a quarter of a century as a doctor, I would not dispute it. At the same time, three of the best-researched American clinical ecologists have estimated that as many as half of the typical GP's patients suffer from one or more food intolerances which have a direct impact on their health and well-being.

My own experience, and that of most of my colleagues around the world who have adopted clinical ecology in their practices, is that the majority of chronic illnesses that do not respond to conventional therapy, and for which no satisfactory diagnosis has been made, are the result of food or chemical intolerance and the reactions that result from it. At the least, these are a significant component of the illness. The symptoms may be extreme or relatively mild, but they are never insignificant for the person who has to live with them.

NEVER TAKE BEING UNWELL FOR GRANTED ▮

Most of us have almost forgotten what it is like to function at optimum level. Headaches, fatigue, backaches, anxiety and insomnia have come to be taken as an almost inseparable part of modern life, something with which we are supposed to put up and shut up. They are nothing of the sort! In the majority of cases, they come about because our systems haven't adapted properly to some very ordinary food or chemical substance, which might be anything from the Gladwrap in the kitchen, to the formaldehyde in the can of Fabulon, to the preservative in a TV dinner.

Clinical ecologists are always doctors. They simply take ecological factors into account in the way they practise medicine. First, orthodox methods of diagnosis are used to establish whether or not there is any organic explanation for the illness or the symptoms. Only when a thorough examination finds no explanation for any of the symptoms, do we investigate whether some environmental factor, which may be food or chemicals or both, is implicated. In my experience these patients, many of whom the doctor genuinely believes have nothing wrong with them, are the victims of ecological illness. They will recover, either completely or to a substantial degree, if they are treated accordingly.

MEDICINE, THE MOST REACTIONARY PROFESSION ▮

Why, then, when doctors are offered a method of treating so many of their intractable patients, which has few, if any, side effects, which is highly cost effective, and which can be closely monitored by the patients themselves almost indefinitely, do they not seize it gratefully with both hands? Why is it like wringing blood from a stone to get many members of the medical profession even to acknowledge the existence of clinical ecology and all that it means, let alone allow their patients the opportunity of enjoying the benefits of it?

The reasons are complex and sometimes quite illogical, but it is important to understand them. Public pressure is the most formidable weapon to bring to bear on any reactionary body that resists change almost by divine right, and my own profession can sometimes be the most reactionary body of all. Probably the greatest disservice this attitude performs is that by the pressure it brings to bear on them, it effectively denies many relatively young doctors the opportunity to consider the chance of exploring clinical ecology for themselves — and they would be the most likely members of the medical profession to be willing to consider a new approach.

Doctors rarely feel comfortable when they are asked to venture into unknown waters. The claims by increasing numbers of doctors, who see in clinical ecology one of the most important developments in medicine this century, are very disturbing to many conservative doctors. They feel personally and professionally threatened by a method of treatment that runs contrary to many things they were taught and have practised throughout their careers. Their instinctive reaction when faced with something new and different is to ridicule and reject it.

When in 1798 Edward Jenner described a successful method of inoculating people to protect them against smallpox — then a major killer — his paper was rejected by the Royal Society because it had too many case histories of real patients, too little laboratory research. He had to publish his findings at his own expense. Pasteur was ridiculed for his strange reports that some diseases were caused by micro-organisms invading the body. When Semmelweis suggested that the incidence of child-bed fever, which claimed countless lives, could be greatly reduced if doctors would only take the trouble to wash their hands before delivering babies, especially when they came directly to the delivery room from dissecting corpses, many physicians were so offended that they refused to take any notice.

There are certainly sound reasons for caution with new treatments. Conservatism helps to protect patients from untried and potentially dangerous therapies, some of which would have had disastrous consequences if they had been blindly accepted. That is hardly the case with clinical ecology, which has now been practised by many very eminent doctors for half a century. Nor does caution guarantee infallibility: it does no harm to remember that it was doctors who endorsed thalidomide after it had been "fully" tested, without demanding the tests for teratogenicity, or birth defects, that are now mandatory.

HOW DOCTORS ARE TAUGHT ■

From a personal viewpoint, the responsibilities that confront doctors are so formidable that they are immeasurably reassured by being able to carry out their jobs in accordance with rigidly defined procedures that they know are approved by their peers. They obey what they have been taught with little, if any, critical analysis, clinging to the concepts and methods that they were taught as students. It takes great determination and courage to break out of this shackle.

As medical students we are trained to investigate until we make a diagnosis, and investigation means finding some abnormality in the pathology or X-rays or measurements, such as lung spirometry. Until we can find an abnormality, we haven't got a disease or diagnosis; and until we have a disease, we can't treat it.

Doctors still accept this view of illness and treatment, believing rigidly in what is called the law of parsimony. This means, quite simply, that a single problem must have a single cause. This single cause, single effect approach to medicine and science colours everything that the majority of doctors do in their practices. In consequence, a doctor who is faced with a problem that has no immediate, obvious cause, heads off in search of some injury or change in the functioning of an organ. Often the doctor finds nothing of the sort, because it does not exist, and ends up prescribing drugs to alleviate the symptoms.

It is still more confusing when doctors are faced with multiple symptoms affecting multiple systems in the body, but symptoms that seem to lack any common thread. There is nothing in their training to help them deal with this predicament. Their training requires them to find convenient and tidy pigeonholes, when in reality many patients have disorders that cannot be neatly pigeonholed.

Most people suffering from food- or chemical-caused disorders have an array of symptoms without clear-cut connection between them. The headache patient, for instance, may be prone to depression, and the hyperactive child may suffer from chronic eczema. What is more, there is no dividing line between physical and mental disorders, almost a heresy in medicine. And when people present with a headache, or arthritis, or depression, for example, those symptoms may be the principal, though rarely the only, complaints.

PINNING ON THE NEUROTIC LABEL ■

A doctor who cannot find a single cause to explain an array of symptoms often concludes that the problem must be psychological. It exists only in the mind of the patient, therefore the patient is neurotic, or schizophrenic, or a hypochondriac — there is no shortage of labels. Before telling the patient this, however, the doctor sends him off on a round robin of pathologists, radiologists, specialists and the rest. They either confirm that there is nothing wrong, or if there is, that nothing can be done about it.

(Food sensitivity and intolerance *can* involve organic problems so that tests like spirometry, which measures lung capacity, are abnormal. The same applies to some psychosomatic diseases such as asthma. Sniff a plastic rose and everything that follows is the fault of the plastic — but the spirometry is abnormal and can be detected immediately. Similarly in migraine, no matter what the cause, there is a change in the blood vessels in the final expression.)

All these experts will have acted correctly according to their lights and professional standards. Most will probably have prescribed a few more drugs along the way. By the time the patient gets back to the GP with this battery of tests behind him and a file half a metre thick, he is probably feeling much worse than before he started. He still has his original symptoms, plus the side effects of the drugs that have been prescribed, and he is now probably thoroughly depressed into the bargain. Indeed, often the doctor will recommend that he consult a psychiatrist as the final option, before the patient is written off as totally beyond help.

This is the condition of most patients when they arrive at the rooms or surgeries of doctors who take an environmental approach to sickness. What a tragic waste of time and money it is, and what pointless suffering!

NOT ALL IN THE MIND ■

Clinical ecology rejects the blinkered attitude with which medical schools have saddled the medical profession, that there is generally one cause for one disease. It rejects it because it is patently inadequate for so many of the patients who come to our surgeries seeking help.

Doctors who practise clinical ecology emphatically state that the great majority of these patients, whether in paediatrics, internal medicine, surgery or psychiatry, are suffering from potentially reversible disorders that are in no way imagined, or psychosomatic. These disorders are due to interactions with natural and synthetic substances in the environment (substances existing at levels that do not trouble the majority of people) or, in many cases, with ordinary food. Once we grasp the concept, it is exquisitely simple, even though we may not understand fully what is happening — and this has never been a criterion for rejection! If it were, the pharmaceutical manufacturing business would long since have gone out of business.

Even if the whole area of clinical ecology were nothing more than a fertile grazing field for hypochondriacs, as the most cynical imply (which is clearly nonsense), that would be no reason to discard it. Hypochondriasis itself is a miserable condition that almost always resists treatment by any conventional means. I long ago lost count of the number of patients, dismissed as "hypochondriacs" or whose symptoms are regarded as psychosomatic by their doctors, who have made a total and permanent recovery when their symptoms have been managed ecologically.

The most commonly voiced criticism of clinical ecology among those doctors who know enough about it to offer any criticism is that the clinical, empirical results (two of the most pejorative words in the medical vocabulary) are not supported by equivalent findings from the laboratory or by sufficient rigorously controlled double-blind testing. What they really mean, of course, is that clinical ecology is a threat to their claimed right to be the sole arbiters of how people ought to be treated. The arrogance of it, when you view it in this light, is stupendous. To claim to know how to treat sick people is excellent; to insist that nobody but you has any worthwhile answers until you concede that fact, when half of your patients are getting nothing from you but a bill and an assortment of prescriptions that are as likely to make them feel worse as better, is insulting to both the doctors who *are* finding new answers and to their patients.

Those who understand the role that environmental factors play are neither "fringe" doctors, witchdoctors, nor charlatans, as the establishment too often seems to imply. We are qualified medical doctors, many of us highly qualified. We not only want to help our patients with a modality that we know is successful, but we also wish to help our colleagues to achieve the same satisfaction.

Of course clinical ecology will benefit from more controlled, experimental studies. No responsible scientist, whether a medical doctor or not, would attempt to negate the importance of well-executed and well-documented research. In fact there have been many double-blind studies, something that is often conveniently ignored. However many of the doctors who apply clinical ecology have neither the time nor the money, nor indeed often the aptitude, for research. Like all my colleagues, my principal concern and obligation is to help my patients to get better. We are already embarrassed and worried enough by the excessive time they must wait before we can see them.

FAILING IN OUR OBLIGATIONS ■

Every time I stop treating people and spend time trying to replicate the same results in a laboratory, I am failing in that obligation to help people to get better. To dismiss the careful and honest observations of many doctors, who have now reported tens of thousands of cases over half a century, on the sole grounds that what they are doing has not been tested in the laboratory, shows an approach to medicine that I believe lies very uneasily on the shoulders of doctors who are obliged, both by law and, in many cases, by oath, to make their patients well as their primary responsibility.

Theron Randolph has helped more than 30,000 patients to recover using the clinical ecology approach, and he is still ridiculed by many of his colleagues. However, they would accept his work overnight if it could be replicated with white rats and endlessly repeated double-blind studies.

For myself, I am not a laboratory technician and, essential as research is, it is unreasonable to expect me to behave as though I were, at the expense of my patients. I will not allow animal researchers or anyone else to dismiss the clinical evidence of many thousands of patients as "only anecdotal evidence, not scientific", and therefore by implication as worthless. Like Dr Richard Mackarness, "until the men in white coats, working with white rats, come up with the answers that will satisfy everyone", I will rely on the proven effectiveness of the treatment, when effectiveness was dismally lacking before.

In all the criticism of clinical ecology, it has never seriously been suggested that there is anything wrong with either the diagnosis or the treatment, provided a thorough investigation has already established that there is nothing organically wrong with the patient. The criticism rests on one ground alone, that it departs from the conventional method of diagnosis and treatment of illness. That is a very flimsy foundation on which to base an argument that results in the denial of relief to countless thousands of patients.

I am not sure how to convince doubting doctors that this is a field that deserves their close attention. Clinical ecology does not replace anything in the practice of medicine, but rather reinforces existing methodology.

The simple solution is to include clinical ecology in the syllabus for medical undergraduates. In a modest way, each year the Australian Society of Environmental Medicine introduces about sixty previously sceptical doctors to environmental medicine through training courses and an annual scientific meeting. It is a small number out of the 25,000 doctors practising in Australia, but it is a vital step towards what should become a routine part of every medical student's training.

Research funds may be slow coming. There is unlikely to be much support from the pharmaceutical manufacturing industry (a traditional source of research funds), which uses the funds that it dispenses as a powerful and persuasive weapon to maintain its markets. The patients of clinical ecologists eventually spend very little on antihistamines or any other drugs. There is no profit from a therapy which consists primarily of omitting things rather than taking them. If clinical ecology were to be routinely introduced into the practice of every GP as a normal method of diagnosis and treatment, it would save the nation a fortune. It would also pose a significant threat to the pharmaceutical industry. Consequently, clinical ecologists have been cut off from one of the largest sources of research funding.

PATIENTS ARE PEOPLE! ■

I don't believe that I paint too harsh a picture of medicine as it has developed over the last few decades, or of the attitude of most doctors to anything that falls outside the scope of their training or experience.

What is the real purpose of medicine? To cure the sick, or to prevent them from getting ill in the first place? The answer surely must be both, but it is far more than a philosophical question. In the old days, doctors used to pay regular visits to their patients at home, offering advice on diet, hygiene and general health, answering many questions that no-one today would think of going to a GP's surgery to ask. Since the Second World War, GPs have withdrawn into their practices, doing fewer and fewer house calls, almost never giving medical guidance about our increasingly dangerous environment.

More and more, doctors specialise in one part of the body, with little concern for the whole person. It is a convenient, and of course a lucrative, way of dividing up the labours and the spoils of medicine. There is nothing intrinsically wrong with specialisation as such. What is so short-sighted is specialising to the point where anything beyond the subject of the specialty is given no more than token acknowledgment.

Even GPs, who are traditionally responsible for the overall health and welfare of their patients, often scorn a holistic approach to medicine (where the *whole* patient is treated, rather than an ache in the back, leg or stomach in isolation). In a busy practice it is convenient to find tidy pigeonholes for every symptom and disorder. Their attitude changes radically once they realise that, far from complicating their practices, clinical ecology allows them to treat successfully the many patients they could not help before, who repeatedly came back looking for a panacea their doctors could never give. Few, if any, of the doctors who are introduced to clinical ecology at the courses of the Australian Society of Environmental Medicine ever turn their back on it again. Rather, they embrace it gratefully.

SHARING OUR PATIENTS' JOY ■

Those of us who are not prepared to see patients denied the help that this approach can offer, who have seen the joy of patients and their families when they discover they can be made better, will not be daunted. An ecological examination for food and chemical intolerance should be a fundamental part of the GP's tools of trade. When this is adopted — and no-one is naïve enough to think that it will happen overnight — it will revolutionise diagnosis and treatment, as it has already done for increasing numbers of doctors.

Clinical ecology needs to be taught. Simple as it is in

theory, commonsense alone will never lead a doctor to the correct conclusions. That is the principal reason why it isn't used by every doctor in the country today. You have to know what to look for, then how to test for it and treat it. Everyone needs to be his or her own detective, for the wonder of clinical ecology is that each of us is involved, and must be involved, for it to succeed.

> *It seems to me to be necessary for every physician to be skilled in nature and to strive to know, if he wants to perform his duties, what man is in relation to the food and drink that he consumes and to all his other occupations, as well as their effect on everyone else. Because if he doesn't know what effect these things have on a man, he cannot know the consequences that result from them.*
>
> *If he doesn't pay attention to these things, or paying attention doesn't understand them, how can he understand the diseases that befall man? For man is affected by every one of these things and changed by them in numerous ways. The whole of his life is subjected to them, whether in health, convalescence or disease. Nothing else, therefore, can be more important than to know these things.*

These may sound like the words of a twentieth-century clinical ecologist, but they were written by Hippocrates more than 2000 years ago. They are as relevant today as they were then.

4 Understanding Ecological Illness

THE THINGS THAT MAKE US ILL ▮
The illnesses and symptoms that concern us in clinical ecology are mainly caused by chemicals (some of which are in our foods) and foods that our systems cannot tolerate. Unlike, say, acute poisoning, they do not affect everyone; and frequently those who are affected, are not all affected in the same way. In a typical family of four, two members may react to the same thing with different symptoms, while two may have no reaction at all.

Muddying the water even more, symptoms are usually also "masked", or hidden, by which we mean that there is no obvious association between the illness or the symptoms and the substance that causes them. And heaping confusion on confusion, the reactions are caused not only by consuming or inhaling harmful substances, but often by *not* consuming or inhaling them! It is no wonder that ecological illness is almost never suspected by chance.

The problems fall loosely into four categories, with a lot of overlap. There are the reactions caused by

1. food, frequently common foods that we eat every day;
2. chemicals in our homes and workplaces;
3. chemicals polluting the ambient environment;
4. (bridging food and general chemicals) the chemicals in our food.

Whether chemicals or foods are involved, they affect us broadly in the same way, interfering with the natural defences of our immune system.

THE COMPLEX WORLD OF IMMUNITY ▮
Immunity is very difficult to explain in lay language, but it is so important to an understanding of clinical ecology that we must

try. The immune system is our body's main line of defence. Its primary function is to protect us against infections and cancers by identifying and then destroying any foreign substance that enters our bodies and threatens our well-being. It is an organ of extraordinary complexity (see diagram on pages 34–5) but even a very general understanding will help to explain much about ecological or environmental illness that would otherwise remain a foggy mystery.

The *immune system* is an organ, but it is spread throughout the body, unlike the kidneys or the liver, which are single entities and which most people readily identify as organs. *Immunity* is the body's ability to resist harmful substances that get into it, such as disease-producing bacteria or viruses. Whenever one of these substances, or antigens as they are called, enters the body by any route, specialised cells react in order to get rid of it and so protect us. When we talk of the *immune response*, or the *immune reaction*, we mean the body's production of cells and antibodies in order to do this.

Besides bacteria and viruses, there are many other substances that provoke the same response. Poisons (which are chemicals) in the sting or bite of snakes, spiders and insects have this effect, as do many drugs and serums. The antivenene for snake bite, for instance, which is produced in horse serum, can occasionally result in a very dangerous reaction. Pollens and grasses also produce a reaction in some people, which results in the familiar allergies of hayfever and asthma.

The Role of the White Blood Cells   This highly efficient defence mechanism is largely the responsibility of several types of white blood cells in the blood. (The red cells, which contain haemoglobin and carry oxygen, are not involved.) The average healthy human has between 5000 and 10,000 *leucocytes*, or white blood cells, per cubic microlitre of blood. Each cell measures between seven and twelve microns in diameter (a micron is one thousandth part of a millimetre), and we have billions of them.

Three main types of leucocytes are involved in immunity, each with a particular role. The most numerous are called *neutrophils* and comprise about 60 per cent of all white blood cells. They are manufactured in the bone marrow and when infection is present, particularly bacteria (which are their main targets), there is a massive increase in their number. Each neutrophil contains a small granule of enzyme (enzymes promote chemical change). A mass of neutrophils moves through body tissue from the blood to the area of infection. Once there, they swallow up the bacteria and destroy them with their enzymes. Then the neutrophils break up. Pus is the accumulation of dead neutrophils, bacteria and dead tissue. Neutrophils are macrophages: "macro" means "big", and "-phage", means that they devour things.

The second type of leucocytes are the *lymphocytes*. These are small, round cells that circulate in both the blood and the lymph, and their role is to channel and filter fluids from the tissue back into the blood, ensuring that any impurities have first been removed. When impurities build up in the lymph nodes (or lymph glands, as they are also known), the lymph nodes become enlarged and painful. In tonsillitis, for example, the lymph nodes in the neck are swollen and sore. Poisons from the infected tonsils have got into the lymph and from there into the lymph nodes, which increase in size as huge additional quantities of lymphocytes are manufactured in them to combat the infection.

Lymphocytes account for nearly 40 per cent of all white cells and there are two types, known as *T-cells* and *B-cells*. Both come from stem cells in the bone marrow, but some go to the thymus, a gland in the chest, where they mature into T-cells (T for thymus). The B-cells mature in a different way, probably in the bone marrow. (The name B-cells does not come from "bone", but is a historical curiosity. In birds, lymphocytes that are independent of the thymus multiply and acquire their special properties in a unique organ called the bursa of Fabricius. Humans and other mammals do not have this bursa, but the name B-cells has persisted.)

B-cells respond to invading antigens in a very complicated way, by changing into plasma cells, which in turn produce proteins that are known as antibodies. These attack and destroy or neutralise the antigen. So it is not the cells themselves that attack the antigen, but these protein antibodies, which detach themselves from the cells in which they have grown.

How Antibodies Function   The antibody works either by dissolving the bacteria, by changing the surface of the antigens so that a lot of them clump together where they can easily be found by neutrophils, which digest them; or by attaching themselves to the surface of the invading viruses or poisons in such a way that they smother them and destroy their harmful effect.

Unlike the B-cells, which unload their antibodies, T-cells

ELEMENTS OF THE IMMUNE SYSTEM

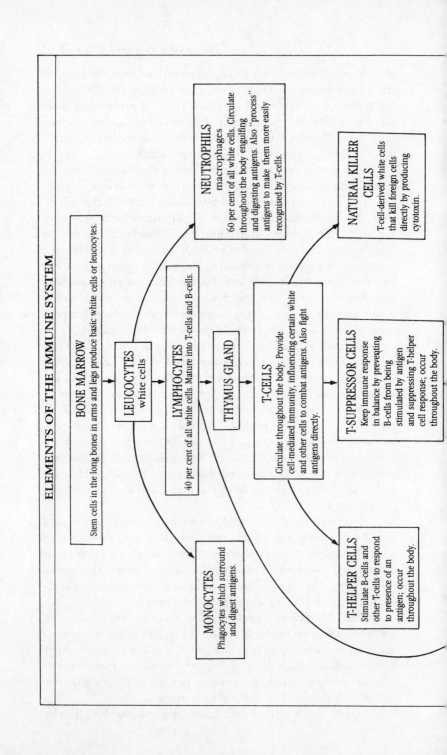

BONE MARROW
Stem cells in the long bones in arms and legs produce basic white cells or leucocytes.

LEUCOCYTES
white cells

LYMPHOCYTES
40 per cent of all white cells. Mature into T-cells and B-cells.

THYMUS GLAND

T-CELLS
Circulate throughout the body. Provide cell-mediated immunity, influencing certain white and other cells to combat antigens. Also fight antigens directly.

NEUTROPHILS
macrophages
60 per cent of all white cells. Circulate throughout the body engulfing and digesting antigens. Also "process" antigens to make them more easily recognised by T-cells.

NATURAL KILLER CELLS
T-cell-derived white cells that kill foreign cells directly by producing cytotoxin.

T-SUPPRESSOR CELLS
Keep immune response in balance by preventing B-cells from being stimulated by antigen and suppressing T-helper cell response; occur throughout the body.

MONOCYTES
Phagocytes which surround and digest antigens.

T-HELPER CELLS
Stimulate B-cells and other T-cells to respond to presence of an antigen; occur throughout the body.

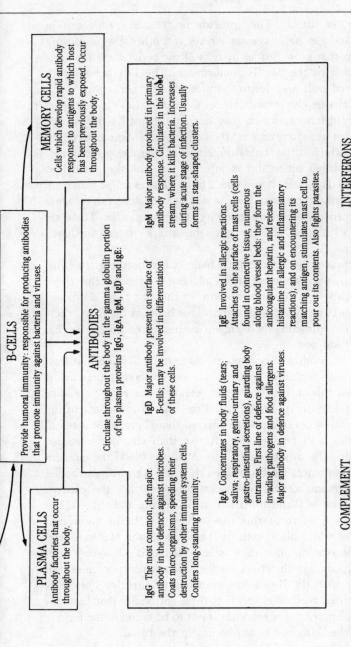

B-CELLS
Provide humoral immunity: responsible for producing antibodies that promote immunity against bacteria and viruses.

PLASMA CELLS
Antibody factories that occur throughout the body.

MEMORY CELLS
Cells which develop rapid antibody response to antigens to which host has been previously exposed. Occur throughout the body.

ANTIBODIES
Circulate throughout the body in the gamma globulin portion of the plasma proteins IgG, IgA, IgM, IgD and IgE:

IgG The most common, the major antibody in the defence against microbes. Coats micro-organisms, speeding their destruction by other immune system cells. Confers long-standing immunity.

IgA Concentrates in body fluids (tears; saliva; respiratory, genito-urinary and gastro-intestinal secretions), guarding body entrances. First line of defence against invading pathogens and food allergens. Major antibody in defence against viruses.

IgD Major antibody present on surface of B-cells; may be involved in differentiation of these cells.

IgM Major antibody produced in primary antibody response. Circulates in the blood stream, where it kills bacteria. Increases during acute stage of infection. Usually forms in star-shaped clusters.

IgE Involved in allergic reactions. Attaches to the surface of mast cells (cells found in connective tissue, numerous along blood vessel beds: they form the anticoagulant heparin, and release histamine in allergic and inflammatory reactions), and on encountering its matching antigen, stimulates mast cell to pour out its contents. Also fights parasites.

COMPLEMENT
A series of some 20 proteins with enzyme activity that occur throughout the body. They augment antigen/antibody reactions and are involved in inflammatory reactions and in combating micro-organisms.

INTERFERONS
Occurring in infected cells, they are the first line of defence against invading viruses. Proteins made by cells when under viral attack; serve to inhibit the multiplication of a broad range of viruses.

go in to the attack. They provide protection against certain bacteria and especially against viruses and other disease-causing organisms that grow inside the cells of the body where the antibodies made by the B-cells cannot reach. The T-cells can attack the infected cells and destroy viruses inside them.

T-cells are also responsible for some unusual delayed hypersensitivity reactions, which may not appear until a day or two after the antigens have entered the body. In the Mantoux test, for example, which is the standard method of diagnosing tuberculosis, the antigen tuberculin is injected into the skin, which is "read" two days later. If you take a biopsy and examine skin from the site during those two days, it will be seen to be full of white cells primed to defend the body against the invader. These are T-cells, which go directly into the attack in cell-mediated immunity.

Compare this, on the other hand, with the allergist's familiar scratch test, where again an allergen — though this time, say, a pollen — is put into the skin. In this case there is no need to wait for two days: within minutes, or hours at the most, there is a reaction, provided there are antibodies in the system for that particular antigen.

For antibodies to be present, there must have been at least one previous exposure. If there are no antibodies present, it means that this antigen has never been encountered before. The reaction takes a little longer while the system is manufacturing the new antibodies. If the same antigen should ever appear again, the reaction will be very fast. As we shall see, immunisation ensures that the antibodies are present in the blood the moment the infection enters the body: even the time lag while antibodies are being manufactured may be too long to save the patient. There will be local inflammation with swelling and redness, but if a biopsy is taken at this time, there will be no significant increase in white blood cells as there was in the Mantoux test. This is because the immunity is not cell-mediated, with T-cells going directly into the attack, as they did against tuberculin, but humoral, with the B-cells involved only indirectly. They have manufactured antibodies and it is these antibodies that fight the invasion. Therefore the evidence is not to be found in the form of cells on the skin, but as antibodies in the blood.

Phagocytes and Other Cannibals All the white cells involved in immunity work together in an immune response. B-cells produce far more antibodies if T-cells are present, just as T-cells attract macrophages, the big cells that gobble up clusters of antigens.

The third main group of white cells leading the fight against the invading enemies that threaten our bodies are the *monocytes*. Far fewer in number than either the neutrophils or the lymphocytes, they are produced in the bone marrow and also occur in lymph glands, the liver and the spleen. They act as phagocytes (from two Greek words meaning to eat cells), by surrounding the harmful invaders and digesting them.

With very rare exceptions, the leucocytes are very specific to a single antigen. There are, for example, many different flu viruses, each one antigen-specific, which means that each one provokes an antibody which is only effective against that particular virus, even though the virus itself is almost identical to other influenza viruses. The main reason why it has so far proved impossible to eradicate flu as one of our most common illnesses is that the flu virus is highly adaptable. It needs to change only infinitesimally to beat the existing antibodies in our systems.

It used to be thought that the exact composition of each antigen was "memorised" by messenger cells called mediators, which make the first contact with an invading antigen. It was believed that this "memory" served as a template from which the appropriate lymphocytes or other cells were synthesised. The mediators would come across an influenza virus, for example, and then armed with an exact description of it, would order up the appropriate neutrophil or antibody. We now know that the process is even more amazing. The genes that control the origin of the white cells already contain all the information needed to create antibodies, for example. In other words, we acquire specific antibodies genetically, even for antigens that were encountered by previous generations!

When the Immune System Fails The immune system is usually highly efficient. Otherwise, we would succumb to relatively trivial diseases, just as many Aboriginal and primitive people die when they are exposed to diseases like the common cold or measles, which are common in Western societies, but very rare in theirs. They have not experienced these diseases before and so have no appropriate antibodies to fight them off. This can also occur because of prolonged non-exposure, even among people who could be expected to have considerable resistance. It often happens in very isolated places, such as on an island or in a remote settlement, where the local inhabitants are rarely visited. When visitors do arrive, they may bring with them viruses such as flu or measles, which can again result in severe disease and even death because of the lack of immunity.

Occasionally, the immune system can react to the very thing that it exists to protect — its own body. An illness called auto-immune disease develops, sometimes with very serious consequences. In this disease, the immune system does not recognise as safe substances the naturally occurring proteins that make up our body, and it reacts to them as it does to any other foreign proteins, by attacking them.

Sometimes, on the other hand, the antibodies are not powerful enough, or they are swamped by the sheer weight of the antigens. When the immune system has a severe malfunction, as in diseases such as Acquired Immune Deficiency Syndrome (AIDS), rare and often swiftly fatal diseases slip past the normal defences of the immune system without encountering any resistance.

How Food Affects the Immune System   The immune system is not always correct in its perception of a threat. Allergy, as we have said, is an inappropriate reaction to any substance that the immune system wrongly reads as being potentially dangerous. All food and chemical intolerance (as opposed to food and chemical poisoning, which is quite different) is the result of the immune system wrongly interpreting those foods or chemicals as threats to the body.

For example, in a normally functioning digestive system, the protein in food is broken down by digestive enzymes such as protease ("-ase" identifies an enzyme, just as "-ose" identifies a carbohydrate), as it works its way through the seven metres of intestine. Because we cannot absorb the proteins in the form that we eat them, they have to be digested, or broken down into their component parts, first to polypeptides (which are not absorbed in a healthy person), then to peptides (of which only some of the smaller ones can be absorbed), and finally to amino acids (which are readily absorbed).

There are twenty-four amino acids in all, of which fifteen can be synthesised, or manufactured, by the body. The remaining nine, the essential amino acids, cannot be manufactured by the body and so have to be ingested in the diet. All twenty-four amino acids join together in different sequences to produce the different proteins that the body needs to make muscle and tissue, for example, or are burned up to provide the energy we need.

The precise significance of protein levels in the diet is still debated. A 400-patient study in Adelaide, conducted by the CSIRO's Division of Human Nutrition, reported in 1986 that a high-protein diet may significantly increase the risk of contracting bowel cancer. One implication of this is that the human digestive system just cannot cope with the business of converting too much foreign protein into amino acids, and the undigested proteins left behind in the gastrointestinal tract irritate the lining of the bowel so that cancer develops.

There is now very good evidence that foreign protein of many foods is able to pass through the gut and directly into the bloodstream, where it travels to any of the organs or tissues in the body. These proteins are recognised correctly by the immune system as foreign and are treated in precisely the same way as any other invader, such as a virus or bacteria. Which organ is affected appears to be entirely a matter of chance. This explains why an egg, for instance, can evoke a swollen face in one person, migraine in another and asthma or arthritis in others.

More About Antibodies There is still very much about the immune system that is not understood, but among the components that can be measured accurately are the antibodies, or immunoglobulins, as they are also known. Five immunoglobulins (abbreviation: Ig) have now been identified, each performing a specific role. The immunoglobulin IgA, for example, protects the mucous membranes; IgM protects the bloodstream; IgG, or gamma globulin, gives protection against certain bacterial and viral infections and contains most of the antibodies in the system; and IgD appears to be involved only in certain bone marrow cancers.

The immunoglobulin of greatest interest to us is IgE, the most recently discovered (in 1966), and the antibody activated in the presence of all the substances like pollens, dusts and danders that cause, for example, the classic allergies of asthma, hayfever and eczema, as well as in the presence of foods that produce the familiar allergic reactions.

THE NARROW WORLD OF THE ALLERGIST ■
There should be a simple definition for allergy, such as an inappropriate reaction of the immune system. In fact, defining it

has posed a challenge to allergists for at least eighty years. Just how much at variance many of these authoritative attempts have been can be seen in the assortment of definitions suggested. The specialty of allergy, as it is practised today, developed with the increasing knowledge of the quite closely related specialty of immunology, which takes advantage of various phenomena of the immune system to give artificial immunity, or protection, against many diseases.

Immunisation makes use of the paradox that exposing a person to a disease gives protection against further attacks of that disease. By giving that first exposure deliberately, in a safe form, the patient has a far greater level of protection in the future. Immunisation primes the immune system to produce antibodies, and this is essential because there *is* no immediate immunity until after the first exposure. At the first encounter with the allergen, it takes time for the immune system to identify it and then produce the appropriate antibodies. If the invading allergen happens to be a deadly and swiftly acting disease such as smallpox or diphtheria, the patient is likely to die while the immune system is still working out what to do.

After the first exposure and reaction, however, there is a very high level of protection, because the antibodies are now in place, travelling constantly around the blood system and the tissue with all the other antibodies, just waiting for the same allergen to strike again. After a time, the level of the antibodies can fall away, but with re-exposure to the allergen (whether an artificial one or the disease itself), there is a very rapid rise in the available antibodies to combat it, unlike the first slow response.

(The best known of the true allergies are the so-called "atopic triad", the unwelcome trilogy of hayfever, asthma and eczema, and the reason why hayfever and asthma sufferers in particular often have to consult their allergists every year is that their sensitivity switches from one pollen to another very frequently. A search must be carried out annually to identify the new pollen so that fresh protection can be given.)

We can see, then, that there are two ways of conferring immunity. Either a person contracts the actual disease and survives it, or the same microbe (whether bacteria or virus) is deliberately introduced into the body, which is immunisation.

What Happens When We Immunise Immunisation can

take three forms, all of which have the one aim of getting the allergen safely into the body without actually causing the disease. There is no point in carefully injecting a disease into a patient and leaving him with such a virulent form of it that the patient never recovers. But it is because the immune system is fighting even this safe exposure that we often experience unpleasant, feverish side effects as the antibody–antigen reaction, or struggle, occurs.

In the first type of immunisation, a live but weakened form of the infection is swallowed or injected, which provokes a response without inducing any dangerous symptoms. An example of this is the Salk vaccine against polio. In the second method, dead germs or bacilli of the actual disease are injected, as in the immunisation against typhoid. The dead germs cannot multiply, but they do provoke a response and prime the antibodies to be ready for a future genuine invasion by typhoid.

In the third method, immunisation is given in a similar but non-virulent live form of the disease that tricks the immune system. Normally, as we have seen, immunity is very specific, but there are a few exceptions. Smallpox vaccination is the best known example of this third method; it uses not smallpox but live cowpox germs, which produce a very similar but much less dangerous disease. Edward Jenner, who discovered the smallpox vaccine, noticed that girls working with cows never seemed to contract smallpox. He deduced correctly that the cowpox allergens must be so similar that exposure to cowpox gave immunity against smallpox as well. (The word vaccine itself comes from the Latin *vacca*, meaning a cow.)

A Valuable Side Effect   During early work in immunology, a chance discovery became the principal tool of allergists. The researchers working on obtaining an immune response by injecting allergens in the form of dead germs found that, as an unexpected side effect, local hypersensitivity reactions occurred upon re-immunization of their patients, when, of course, the antibodies were present and elevated.

Allergists still rely on this phenomenon, although in a more refined manner, to establish whether antibodies are present to a specific allergen. The antigen can be injected superficially into the skin, or by scratching or pricking the skin and applying a drop of it. By a series of different dilutions, it can also be used to determine the *degree* of sensitivity rather than just a positive or negative reaction. Serial Dilution Endpoint Titration, as this procedure is known, is used extensively in clinical ecology to determine a patient's degree of sensitivity. In clinical ecology the diluted allergen may also be administered as a drop placed under the tongue.

If there is a red weal after a scratch test, or at some dilution in the Serial Dilution Endpoint Titration when it is given by injection, then the allergist knows that the antibodies to the pollen or dander being tested are present. In this way the substance that is causing the allergic reaction can be identified, because each individual antigen provokes its own antibodies.

Once the identification has been made, more allergens of the same substance are injected under the skin, taking advantage of yet another curious phenomenon of the immune system. Initially allergens are given in a very small dose, which is worked out accurately when the Serial Dilution Endpoint Titration method is used, or by guesswork when the scratch test is used.

As increasingly larger doses are given, the patient eventually reaches a point where he or she can tolerate quite large exposures and so can cope with exposure to the same substance when it is encountered in the real environment. The correct name for this procedure is hyposensitisation, or lowering of the degree of sensitivity, rather than desensitisation, because it is never possible to totally desensitise anyone.

True Allergy Lasts for Ever Because antibody levels never disappear, it does not matter in the case of true allergic reaction whether months or years go by between exposures. If you react now with hives, for instance, when you eat prawns, then you will always get hives when you eat prawns, no matter whether six weeks, six months or six years have passed since you last ate them. So important are these elevated IgE levels considered to be by allergists, that they are thought to be the sine qua non of allergy. Without them, they say, there is by definition no allergy.

The great flaw in this argument when applied to foods is that in only about 10 per cent of cases of hypersensitivity or intolerance is there any elevation of the IgE antibodies, or can specific antibodies even be detected! In the other 90 per cent, there are no antibodies present, no measurable evidence that there has been any change in the blood or in any part of the immune system. By definition therefore, say the allergists, there is no allergy, regardless of the fact that these 90 per cent have illnesses and symptoms which subjectively and objectively are indistinguishable from what the allergists choose to call an allergy.

Semantic Pedantry It is largely semantic pedantry, of course, with allergists claiming unto themselves exclusive rights to the word "allergy". On the other hand, if you develop a fierce migraine every time you eat a potato; if you fall asleep wherever you are, at any time of the day, every time you eat Chinese food containing monosodium glutamate; or if your normally docile children turn into uncontrollable hoodlums every time they drink cow's milk, or eat any foods that are coloured red; then by any rational understanding of the word, you and they are having an allergic reaction to potatoes, MSG, milk or red food dye. If commonsense were the only criterion, to say otherwise would be nonsense.

The problem would never have arisen at all if the leaders in the allergy field had reacted differently when the revelations of the early workers in clinical ecology — all doctors — were becoming known. Indeed, the irony is that before it acquired its present very narrow meaning (that there is no allergy without elevated IgE), the word allergy did indeed embrace everything that the clinical ecologists are concerned with today. It was not until the discovery of the skin scratch tests at the beginning of the twentieth century, which the allergists immediately monopolised, that they themselves changed the definition of the word to suit their own purposes.

Much worse, they decided to belittle the significance (and the scientific evidence) of this new and exciting concept that offered hope to the 90 per cent of food-intolerant victims to whom neither they themselves, nor conventional medicine, had anything to offer. This attitude unquestionably held back acceptance of clinical ecology — and still does — by years, particularly in the United States, where most of the pioneering work originated.

In the United States, a bitter and most unprofessional struggle is still raging as the conventional allergists fight to preserve their incomes and their monopoly, and to deny the very existence of "allergy" or intolerance that doesn't fall within their blinkered definition. And the real victims are not those dedicated doctors who want to put clinical ecology to use, but the millions of ordinary people around the world who are denied all that it has to offer them.

The Search for a Compromise   The solution that the early doctors practising environmental medicine adopted was nothing if not pragmatic. If allergists refused to concede that without elevated IgE antibodies, there was no allergy, then there would have to be two kinds of allergy. This would at least acknowledge that both involved a breakdown in the normal functioning of the immune system, even though in different ways.

The allergies of the traditional allergists, who demanded demonstrable evidence such as elevated antibodies or skin reaction, would be known as "fixed" allergies — fixed because, regardless of the time between exposures, or the size of the dose, the reaction was always essentially the same. You ate the forbidden prawns, for example, and you developed hives. The other allergies, which took account of the 90 per cent of apparent food allergies disowned by allergists because nothing could be demonstrated by any known laboratory procedures, were called "cyclic" allergies, because they tend to come and go in cycles. These are the intolerances with which clinical ecologists are most concerned.

Criticising the intransigence of conventional allergists in not even conceding that there may be more to intolerance than raised levels of immunoglobulin, is not to belittle the importance of their work. Millions are plagued by true allergies and some, such as asthma, are potentially dangerous. The allergist who by training is expert at identifying specific allergens out of the thousands that might be responsible, and then at providing immunity against them, is far better qualified than any other medical specialist to carry out this work. It is painstaking and time-consuming and requires the special talents of a physician, a detective and a chemist all rolled into one. It is a special irony that of all the branches of medicine which one might expect to be opposing the burgeoning of clinical ecology, about the last is allergy.

If the word "allergy" is ruled out to describe whatever is happening in environmental illness, the English language is not much more helpful than it is in finding an alternative to clinical ecology. Hypersensitivity, intolerance and maladaptation have all been suggested, and some doctors, in spite of allergists' protests, persist in using "allergy". My own preference is for intolerance, which comes close to describing what we are talking about, and that is the word that we have used throughout this book.

5 Stress, Addiction and Food Intolerance

THE PERSONAL FACTOR ▮

One of the most perplexing aspects of intolerance and allergy is why some people react to certain substances and others do not. We are all exposed to an immense number of foods and chemicals that are known to be capable of causing intolerance, but not all of us react in the same way to them, or even react at all. Probably 20 per cent of people will never be troubled by anything they eat, drink or breathe as long, of course, as they are not being exposed to them in such excessive quantities that they are actually being poisoned.

Some people live long lives surrounded by the worst kind of pollutants, smoking heavily, eating the unhealthiest foods, drinking like fish and yet miraculously remaining disease- and symptom-free until they die. Others become intolerant of a food or chemical which they are exposed to in only minute doses, even though they have a healthy diet that is nutritionally correct in every way, never smoke and never drink, and live in the purest of environments far from any city or chemical pollutants. These victims rightly grumble that it is manifestly unfair.

The explanation lies in two simple but critical words: individual susceptibility. It is a phrase that crops up repeatedly in clinical ecology because it is fundamental to understanding what happens in food and chemical intolerance. There must be individual susceptibility. We must, for whatever reason, have the ability to react in a particular way, and it is because not all of us have that ability that not all of us suffer in the same way, or even at all, from chemicals, various foods, cigarettes, alcohol, even heroin and infectious diseases.

The existence of individual susceptibility explains why some people can use heroin and never become addicted to it, or require a dozen exposures as opposed to just one before they develop an addiction. It is why not everyone succumbs in an epidemic of a disease that is potentially fatal. We can see individual susceptibility at work in such everyday situations as people's reaction to the sun. Brown-eyed, dark-haired, bronze-skinned people get browner but blue-eyed, red-haired, freckled, fair-skinned people just burn. In between these two extremes is a spectrum of others who don't have such clear-cut reactions.

Individual susceptibility is still poorly understood. Only occasionally can we can see an explanation for it, as in the case of orientals being able to consume large amounts of rice. If you put a Caucasian on the same diet, he would quickly be in trouble. We know that this is because orientals have greater reserves of certain enzymes than Caucasians, and this gives them better metabolism and the ability to digest large amounts of rice. The reason why the Japanese have one of the lowest rates of alcoholism in the developed world (despite the much higher than average level of stress in their lives) is because half of them cannot metabolise alcohol properly. They get drunk very quickly and not wanting to be seen drunk, they don't drink.

THE ROLE OF HEREDITY ■

There is no doubt that heredity and genetics play a large part. Thirty per cent of people in Western populations are born with an innate tendency to be intolerant and allergic. If both parents suffer from an allergy of any kind, their children have a 70 per cent likelihood of being allergic as well, though not necessarily to the same substances as their parents. What we inherit from them is not so much the intolerance itself (though migrainous children tend to have migrainous parents, and similarly with asthma), as the propensity to become allergic or intolerant.

A history of true allergy (that is, allergy that allergists accept as allergy) also predisposes people to have the kind of cyclic intolerance that is part of food and chemical intolerance. The severity of the symptoms and the part of the body affected depend on the individual and can rarely be forecast any more accurately than the particular substances that may cause a reaction.

THE UNBORN BABY ■

Age, sex, damage to the immune system and general health are all probably significant as well in determining individual susceptibility. I believe that even the developing environment of the unborn baby plays an important part in deciding intolerances in childhood and later life. There is ample evidence that the critical time in the development of food intolerance is the first months of life. Not only is the immune system very immature at this time, but a baby's intestines are very permeable and allow some of the large protein molecules in food to pass into the baby's body. They cross into the baby's blood stream where they become screening agents for any future foreign proteins that get into the system.

This is why breastfed babies have a higher level of immunity than other babies, not only against foods to which they would be sensitive, but against many infectious diseases, viruses and bacteria. They are acquiring their mother's immunity and it is one of the most important reasons for encouraging breast-feeding.

The other side of the coin, however, is that as well as immunoglobulins, other foreign proteins may also slip through the baby's intestinal lining. The chances of this happening to the breastfed baby whose mother is not food sensitive are small. But it is quite possible for a baby to inherit food sensitivity in the womb. That sensitivity may be to cow's milk for example, because the mother-to-be is consuming cow's milk. If the baby goes straight on to either cow's milk or a formula containing cow's milk, there is a much greater chance of the baby becoming food sensitive for the rest of its life. The problem can be avoided if the mother, whether pregnant or breastfeeding, avoids foods to which she is allergic or intolerant (this is one of many reasons why these mothers should never smoke). In particular she should avoid drinking excessive amounts of cow's milk if the baby is to be quickly put on to a diet of cow's milk. The problems caused by cow's milk (see Chapter 11) are legendary and fill many books.

Not until a baby is six or seven months old has its digestive tract matured enough to handle the majority of foreign proteins. This is one of the most important reasons for encouraging breast-feeding until at least this age, without introducing any other foods, unless of course this is not indicated for any medical or nutritional reasons. Eggs, dairy products and wheat cause more trouble in children than any other foods, and they should be the last to be introduced — particularly cow's milk. Unfortunately, they are also almost invariably the foods that are introduced first.

ILLNESS AND THE CANARY FACTOR ■

Illness also contributes to susceptibility. You often find, for example, that an asthmatic becomes that way after having an attack of infective bronchitis which, as it were, weakens the lungs and allows them to become the organ where the symptoms of the intolerance will appear.

It is possible that some people simply have more critical measuring equipment than the rest of us and are better detectors of substances that have the potential to cause trouble and intolerance. Their bodies may be sensing something that could have a cumulatively harmful effect on a lot of other people as well. One writer described these people as acting like an early warning system for the rest of us, like the canaries that miners used to take down the pit with them to detect methane. (It isn't altogether a happy analogy: the canaries were supposed to keel over at the slightest whiff of methane, but there were many cases of miners being gassed while the bird went on chirping.)

In 1979, the medical journal *The Lancet* suggested that food fads in childhood (when children won't eat a particular food) may be a subconscious protective mechanism against potentially harmful allergens and other substances. Forcing unwilling eaters to finish up their food never had anything to commend it apart from satisfying the frugal instincts of the parents: maybe it is sometimes positively harmful as well.

One recurring factor in a serious ecological approach to illness is that a patient must be seen as a complete entity and not simply as a sore throat or a headache or whatever. If it makes the doctor's job more demanding, as it certainly does, it also makes it much more interesting and satisfying. Treating a person and not an organ has much to commend it.

We have seen that individual susceptibility is one of the vital ingredients in any environmental or ecological illness. It will come as no surprise to know that any injury to the immune system can also drastically affect our ability to cope properly with substances that ought not to present any problems. The system is extremely susceptible to injury to or disruption of the highly complex and finely tuned molecular traffic that is constantly moving around it. Viral infection, a serious accident and the trauma that follows it, drug therapy (including even normally prescribed antibiotics), sudden weight loss and thyroid disease are just some of the situations that can damage the immune system and result in an inappropriate reaction to some food or chemical.

STRESS: THE CURSE OF MODERN LIFE ■

The life-situation that is one of the most potentially harmful of all to the immune system is stress. Stress, as we shall see, can come to plague us in many guises. It can disrupt the immune system so that food and chemical intolerance take hold; but food and chemical intolerance are also among the most powerful factors that *cause* stress in the first place.

In 1936 Hans Selye, who was professor of experimental medicine and surgery at the University of Montreal, in Canada, carried out research on experimental animals using various stress-inducing agents, including heat, cold and poisons. He proved that chronic stress leads to chronic illness, and the reverberations that followed this discovery have never subsided.

Stress became a trendy word, part of the jargon of living in the twentieth century and in a frequently frenetic society. It also came to be equated, quite wrongly, with nothing more significant than the occasional pressure of a difficult job, or a row at home. In truth, it is much more and much more serious.

Each one of us reacts differently to stress. Each one of us has a personal stress capacity, a threshold that we go past at our peril, and this capacity can be filled in an almost infinite number of ways.

Imagine that our ability to tolerate stress is a bucket. Into that bucket go all the stresses in our lives — illness, being unfit, losing a job, financial problems, bereavement, excessive drinking and all the problems and miseries that go with it, examination nerves, family disharmony, tension in the office, too many medications, chemical pollutants in the atmosphere, at work or at home, even extremes of heat and cold. The list can be endless.

It is well known that the weather can trigger violent extremes in behaviour, perhaps the most literal example of environmental illness. In various parts of the world, hot, dry winds have a notoriously enervating effect on those in their path. In Los Angeles, for example, the Santa Ana wind has such an effect on people that mystery writer Raymond Chandler wrote, "Meek little wives feel the edge of the carving knife and study their husbands' necks." The Los Angeles police know from bitter experience that when the Santa Ana wind blows, the rate of violence, murder, child-beating and molestation, road accidents and suicides soars.

In Los Angeles, the winds are caused when air rushing down from the high inland plateaus is heated by compression as much as 3°C for every 300 metres of descent, but that bare statistic conceals a host of unanswered questions. What is known is that this highly antisocial phenomenon is the result of an absence of negative ions in the atmosphere and we shall see in Chapter 24 how disruptive this can be even in a household situation.

In Jerusalem the Sharav wind has the same effect as the Santa Ana, sending humidity plummeting by up to 40 per cent in as many minutes. Research has been going on for twenty-five years into brain biochemistry, neurotransmitters and oxygenation in the lungs and brain tissue to try to establish the precise effect of the Sharav. While the researchers still have far to go, they have found that many people experienced dramatic changes that left them feeling, in the words of one Los Angeles policeman, "that things are going crazy". It is little wonder that such phenomena can have an effect on the vulnerable, highly sensitive immune system.

FINDING THE COUNTERBALANCE ■

Just as important as this negative input is the counterbalance: the steps that we take to offset stress, such as learning to relax, counselling, talking over problems, proper diet, keeping fit, adequate sleep and so on. Hans Selye insisted that stress is only harmful when we constantly encounter frustration and failure, and our struggles are unsuccessful. The stress involved in successful activity leaves virtually no scars, but only a feeling of exhilaration and youthful strength, even at a very advanced age. This is why some people can insist on their hundredth birthday — truthfully — that they feel only half their age or less.

As long as the sum of negative stressors, less the balancing effect of the positive factors, does not take us past our personal threshold, or cause our bucket to overflow, homeostasis, or a general state of being well, is likely to be maintained. But let the total negative stressors go past that threshold, and beware the price that must be paid!

It is the cumulative effect that is all-important. It is the cumulative effect that explains why even an apparently minute exposure to some substance, or an event in our lives that on the face of it doesn't appear to be too traumatic, can tip the balance, allowing the bucket to overflow and in the process sending the immune and nervous systems haywire. Understanding this critical fact, that it is the *total* stress load that is of paramount importance, makes much that seems illogical about ecological illness fall into place. It is why doctors practising clinical ecology strive so hard to ensure that their patients back away as far as possible from their stress threshold.

ADAPTATION: THE WAY WE PROTECT OURSELVES ■

Selye found that all living organisms, from mice to men, respond in three stages to stress, and he called this the general adaptation syndrome. In the first stage, animals showed alarm and went into something very like surgical shock. Then, in the second stage, if he continued to apply the stressor (extremes of temperature or poison), the animals recovered and moved into a stage of resistance, or adaptation, as they tried to restore homeostasis in spite of the stressor: they tried to find a way of adapting to it. Finally, usually much later, they moved on again, this time into an exhausted stage from which there was no recovery because the pituitary and adrenal glands, the very resources that permitted adaptation in the first place, were now exhausted.

Selye called these three stages the *alarm reaction*, the *stage of resistance* and the *stage of exhaustion*: all three would come to have special significance in clinical ecology.

The general adaptation syndrome can be seen at work in a soldier sent to the front line for the first time. As he endures his baptism of fire, there is an immediate and very acute reaction — terror! His fear prepares him for fight or flight, or "paralyses" him so that he is completely immobile and so less likely to be seen by the enemy. The fight-or-flight mechanism is one of the most primitive and basic mechanisms in every living creature, an instinctive reaction that has its origins, in the case of humans, in their very earliest days as hunters and the hunted. In war, soldiers are not allowed the option of flight, or there would certainly be a mass exodus at great speed from the battlefield. The greater fear of the retribution that will certainly follow such an action keeps the soldier in his trench.

THE THREE STAGES OF ADAPTATION ▮

The initial *alarm reaction* lasts for only a limited time, however, and as men on the battlefield find to their surprise, they adapt and move into the *stage of resistance*. They find that they are no longer terrified by the battle raging around them, or even unduly bothered, as they were a short time before, by the sight of their dead comrades. If anything, many of them find themselves elated and excited, convinced that they can take on the entire enemy force single-handed.

Later still, there is yet another change, but this time with no accompanying elation. The soldier begins to degenerate into the third stage, the *stage of exhaustion*, which is marked, as the name says, by breakdown and exhaustion. His system can no longer go on with the pretence that there is nothing to be afraid of. Now the fear is as real as it was when the soldier first came up to the front line and he is shell-shocked and not infrequently deranged, quite unable to muster any more courage. Once he is in this state, neither the passage of time nor rest will make any difference: he will never return to the stage of adaptation.

In the First World War, before the complexities of stress and war neurosis were understood, men were given the Victoria Cross in stage two, then shot for cowardice in stage three.

In later research, Selye and others noted that individual rats reacted to stress in quite different ways. Some became aggressive in the face of the stressor, some withdrew into themselves (they had nowhere to escape to physically), while others just froze and cowered. It suggested that specific adaptation, or individual susceptibility, played a major role within the overall framework of the general adaptation syndrome. In later experiments, Selye was also able to prove that one of the most prolonged and intense stressors to which humans are subjected is allergy. He was referring, of course, to fixed or true allergy, because at that time allergy in the sense of intolerance was still largely unknown; but we know now that it is equally relevant when we are discussing food and chemical intolerance.

WHAT PRICE ADDICTION? ▮

We can see, then, that stress is a double-edged weapon, provoking intolerance because of its destructive effect on the immune system, and being in turn provoked by this same intolerance. The next step in understanding what is going on in food intolerance, and to a lesser extent in chemical intolerance, requires a walk down a very unexpected pathway. We must venture into the most unlikely world of drug addiction, because it is here that we shall find the key to unlock the last of clinical ecology's secrets.

It was Dr Theron Randolph, the former allergist and the man who nearly half a century ago first described clinical ecology, who pointed out that food and chemical intolerance reactions were remarkably similar to the reactions of drug addiction. Although most people associate addiction with heroin and the other hard drugs, there are in fact many other substances to which we can become addicted, and the addiction in each case is very similar — in fact it differs only in the degree of severity. "Any man and any mammal will develop an addiction if certain substances are introduced into the body in sufficiently large doses for sufficient length of time", observed Nils Bejerot, an American authority on addiction.

Substances other than heroin might take longer to become addictants, and the symptoms they produce might be less severe (although even this is by no means inevitable), but in every other regard there is no difference. Eating or inhaling them leads to pleasure, abstinence to withdrawal symptoms. There is an immediate improvement of these withdrawal symptoms if the substance is taken again, and a delayed hangover when it is omitted or does not arrive on time. In the end, over a variable period of time, there are only unpleasant negative symptoms, no longer any stimulation.

At the root of all the illnesses and disorders that are caused by the food we eat is this concept that *any* substance taken, as Nils Bejerot put it, "in sufficiently large doses for sufficient length of time", can lead to addiction and all its attendant symptoms — which *are* the symptoms of food intolerance. There has recently been strong support for this food addiction hypothesis, with the discovery in laboratory experiments that some of the substances involved in the digestive process work in an opiate-like manner.

The Pyramid of Addiction   Randolph described the relative addictiveness of many substances as a pyramid (Fig. 1). At the apex of this pyramid are the naturally occurring opiates, heroin and opium (when Randolph drew his pyramid, the deadly synthetic drugs of addiction that now vie with heroin for the

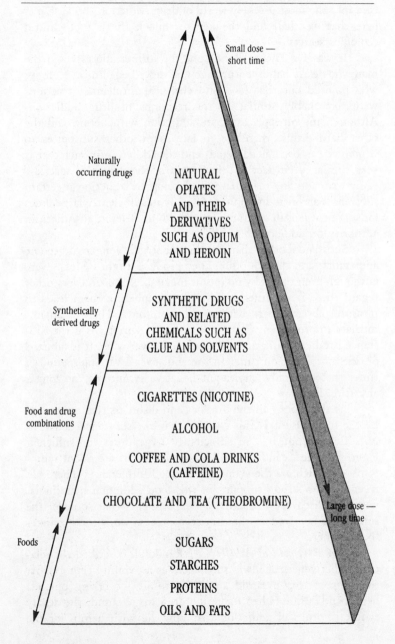

Figure 1.

THE PYRAMID OF ADDICTION

Small dose —
short time

Naturally
occurring drugs

NATURAL
OPIATES
AND THEIR
DERIVATIVES
SUCH AS OPIUM
AND HEROIN

Synthetically
derived drugs

SYNTHETIC DRUGS
AND RELATED
CHEMICALS SUCH AS
GLUE AND SOLVENTS

Food and drug
combinations

CIGARETTES (NICOTINE)

ALCOHOL

COFFEE AND COLA DRINKS
(CAFFEINE)

CHOCOLATE AND TEA (THEOBROMINE)

Large dose —
long time

Foods

SUGARS

STARCHES

PROTEINS

OILS AND FATS

claim to be the most addictive substances were unknown); and at the bottom are oils and fats. In between is the whole spectrum of more or less potent addictants with which we are likely to come in contact.

Next in potency after the natural opiates and their derivatives are the synthetic pain-relieving drugs, such as pethidine and Fortral (pentazocine), which *are* addictive and usually legally prescribed, even when they are abused. Ranking level with these are the chemically related substances that glue-sniffers abuse. (Glue-sniffing got its name because the fad started with people sniffing the glue in model aeroplane kits and finding that they could achieve a very quick "high". Now they sniff everything from petrol to aftershave, and it can sometimes be a deadly pursuit.)

Farther down the pyramid again, there is an even wider range of substances, which usually take still longer to bring about addiction, but which can still be highly addictive. They include cigarettes, alcohol and food–drug combinations, such as coffee and cola drinks (both have caffeine as well as their food content), which are more addictive than any foods themselves.

At the base of the pyramid, but still addictive, are the foods in decreasing order of involvement in addiction: sugars, starches, proteins and oils and fats.

How Ordinary Foods Become Addictive Randolph went a stage further to explain perhaps the most confusing part of clinical ecology, which is the mechanism that converts intolerance to a food into a seemingly quite unrelated symptom or illness. It is very easy to make the association between a food that doesn't agree with us and, say, indigestion or stomach-ache. It takes a much greater leap of the imagination to grasp that a food that we probably eat every day, which certainly has no obvious ill effects on us, can be responsible for every imaginable ill from migraine and insomnia, to arthritis and schizophrenia.

Nobody knows for sure exactly what is happening physiologically when a food to which we are intolerant — or more probably, a protein of that food — escapes from the gastrointestinal tract and forces it way through the gut wall into the bloodstream. From there it makes its way to any one of the organs or tissues in the body, and the place where it settles will be the source of all the symptoms and illnesses. If it settles in the stomach, the symptoms are likely to involve the gastrointestinal system; if it settles in the brain, then the manifestation will be in the form of migraine, headache, or any of the mental disorders, and so on.

Regular and Repeated Exposure an Essential Factor

We have seen that regular and repeated exposure is an important factor in any food-triggered ecological illness. We can put it even more strongly, and say that it is an *essential* factor. With most foods, this means they must be consumed at least twice a week, and the more frequently they are taken, the more likely they are to be incriminated. When a food is eaten this often, it is always present in the gastrointestinal tract, because it takes up to ninety-six hours for food in the average Western person, living on a typically Western diet, to make its way through the tract. A person will never be entirely free of it, or of its products of digestion, before another "dose" is put into the system. The majority of people have not been free of cow's milk, for example, since they were in nappies.

In time, it is postulated, this interminable consumption of one particular food wears down the digestive system's ability to cope with it efficiently. It may take months, it may take years, but sooner or later in a number of people an undigested part, or an incompletely broken down protein or complex carbohydrate or fat, will wear down enough of the gut wall to force its way through.

We have already seen how the protein, for example, in the food that we are eating is progressively broken down by digestive enzymes in a normally functioning digestive system, as the food works its way through the intestine, a journey that can take anything from twenty-four hours to four days.

In a carbohydrate food, such as sugar, there is no protein, but the same procedure is occurring. In complex carbohydrates there is a long branching chain of simple sugars (instead of amino acids, peptides and polypeptides) and these should ideally be digested by enzymes and broken down to individual sugars, such as fructose, sucrose or maltose before being absorbed. When absorption takes place before the complex carbohydrate has been properly broken down, the reaction is the same as with improperly digested protein. In time it forces a way through the gut wall. The same thing happens with complex fats and the enzyme lipase which, in a correctly functioning system, breaks the fats down into fatty acids before absorption. After the gut wall has been penetrated in this way, it will always be a "weak spot" for that particular foreign protein, for instance, unless it has time to heal. The description may be unscientific, but the picture, I think, is clear.

Very much the same thing happens with chemicals, when they are ingested in food or drink. Eventually, instead of passing harmlessly through the digestive process, a few molecules of the chemical manage to get through the gut wall and again, in sensitive people, the stage is set for the illness or disorder to manifest itself. The main difference is that chemicals are more readily absorbed than foods and do not need to be broken down by digestion for absorption to occur.

FOOD ADDICTION ■

Theron Randolph overlaid the concept of addiction onto Hans Selye's studies of stress, and his findings so correlated with all that he had seen in his own clinical work that many of the pieces of the jigsaw slipped into place for him. Randolph renamed Selye's three stages of stress so that they fitted more closely the experiences of victims of food and chemical intolerance. Selye's first stage, the alarm reaction, he called the *preadaptive stage*; stage two, the stage of resistance, become the *adaptive stage* (which he further subdivided into *adaptation* and *maladaptation* to represent the ups and downs of addiction); and stage three, which Selye called exhaustion, was referred to by Randolph as the *postadaptive stage*.

The physical and emotional symptoms that are produced by any form of addiction, whether to hard drugs, wheat or potatoes, usually follow a pattern that consists of two phases: one "high" or stimulatory, the other "low" or depressive. That is the reason why drug addicts fluctuate, sometimes wildly, between extremes of mood, sometimes hyperactively elated, often almost suicidally depressed. The lows (Randolph's *maladaptation*) are the withdrawal symptoms.

Victims of ecological or environmental illness, whether they are suffering the effects of food or chemicals, characteristically swing from one side of the spectrum to the other. Randolph plotted the "ups and downs of addiction", as he called them, on a scale of +1 to +4 on the stimulatory side, and −1 to −4 on the depressive side. Again, these −1 to −4 stages represent the withdrawal symptoms. This is misleading in one sense because it tends to imply that the different stages on both sides of the spec-

Figure 2.

THE PENDULUM OF ADDICTION

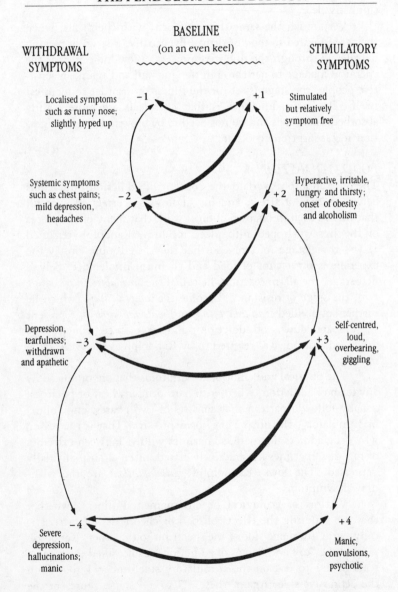

BASELINE
(on an even keel)

WITHDRAWAL
SYMPTOMS

STIMULATORY
SYMPTOMS

Localised symptoms
such as runny nose;
slightly hyped up

−1   +1

Stimulated
but relatively
symptom free

Systemic symptoms
such as chest pains;
mild depression,
headaches

−2   +2

Hyperactive, irritable,
hungry and thirsty;
onset of obesity
and alcoholism

Depression,
tearfulness;
withdrawn
and apathetic

−3   +3

Self-centred,
loud,
overbearing,
giggling

Severe
depression,
hallucinations;
manic

−4   +4

Manic,
convulsions,
psychotic

trum are clear-cut. In reality, they nearly always overlap and there is merging and blurring as patients' moods and symptoms fluctuate.

Let's assume that a patient is at that critical point in her life when she is on the verge of developing intolerance to some substance, say wheat, which she has been consuming in one form or another, particularly bread, for the last twenty years or so. To follow the progress in Figure 2 of what happens to her, we always start at the base line, even though this is a state with which few of us, certainly as we reach adolescence and adulthood, are likely to be familiar. Randolph nicely called it "The kind of normal behaviour which children usually expect from their parents and teachers, and parents expect from their children. We all expect it from our co-workers, business associates and friends — and rarely get it!"

The First Acute Reaction If this improbably placid person begins to develop an intolerance (by which we mean, of course, an addiction) to some food or chemical, an unpleasant, acute reaction is likely to be experienced soon after ingesting or inhaling it. In the case of our patient, she feels clammy and weak shortly after eating the three slices of brown wheatmeal toast that she has had for breakfast every morning for as long as she can remember.

On the chart, this patient is still at the base line, for there has been no move towards adaptation. The acute reaction may last for days, weeks, or even months if the exposure is very frequent. Each time the brown toast enthusiast has breakfast, she feels clammy and weak.

Almost imperceptibly, however, the victim begins to adapt. The body rarely allows a regularly experienced symptom of this kind to continue without attempting to adapt to it, so that it no longer causes distress. Gradually, she moves into phase +1 and has taken the first step, albeit unknowingly, into the risky waters of addiction and intolerance. It is often very difficult to detect that the patient is anything other than normal in this phase, because she is likely to be all the things that people take for granted in the well-adjusted individual — lively, ambitious, enthusiastic, amusing and considerate. The unpleasant acute reaction, the clamminess, has disappeared now and indeed our victim sounds like the paradigm of the ideal woman.

Though no-one, least of all the patient herself, recognises

it, this is not her true character and simply maintaining it is stressful, with all the attendant problems that we have seen come in the wake of stress. The symptoms may have gone, but neither the intolerance itself, nor the stressor have disappeared. They have merely gone underground and the unpleasant symptoms have been replaced by a rather forced jollity that can be compared to the effect of the first couple of drinks at a party.

Masked Intolerance   We say now that the intolerance is "masked", or hidden, because there are no longer any unpleasant symptoms to associate with the food. There is no obvious cause and effect and when symptoms do occasionally occur, they are most likely to be associated with a withdrawal symptom because the food *has not* been eaten. It is very difficult, unless you are looking for it, to make any association between clamminess and something that has not happened!

Masking is one of the most confusing aspects of environmental illness and more than any other, it is the factor that has left this course of sickness unrecognised for so long. How it was discovered for the first time is itself a story of luck — luck that it happened to one of the very few people in the United States who knew what to make of it (see box).

Through his experience with eggs Herbert Rinkel had learned one of the most important lessons in clinical ecology, that symptoms caused by food and chemical intolerance actually improve when more of the same food is taken. They improve because they are the product of addiction and as every drug addict knows, shooting up instantly takes away the unpleasant withdrawal symptoms from the previous hit whose effects are wearing off.

Because of this, when a staple food, for instance, is the cause of the intolerance and is eaten several times a day, the withdrawal symptoms can be kept at bay for years, even indefinitely. It is only when the food is for some reason not available, or paradoxically when it is consumed in unusually large amounts so that the total stress load goes over that person's threshold, that the unpleasant symptoms of intolerance begin to emerge. Until then, everything is masked, not only from the outside world, but even from the victims themselves.

The mother who says proudly that cow's milk used to make her son vomit soon after she first introduced it into his diet, but that she persisted and now he can not only tolerate it, but even

HOW MASKING WAS DISCOVERED

Herbert Rinkel was a doctor with a passion for making cause-and-effect observations in his patients, an outstanding clinical investigator in the field of allergy. He was already married when he entered medical school in the 1920s and because they were hard up, he and his family subsisted mainly on eggs as their principal source of protein. His father, who was a farmer, sent Herb and his wife 144 eggs a week! With what we know now about the hazards of eating any food regularly and frequently, the Rinkels were clearly heading for an egg-induced environmental illness, though of course at the time, they knew nothing of this.

At about this time, Herb Rinkel developed a severe nasal allergy and profuse nasal rhinorrhoea, or runny nose. He went to various physicians, but none could find the cause or give him any treatment that had any effect. To say that the Rinkels knew nothing of the possible ill effects of food is not quite true, because there had been work done on food allergy and he was aware of this, at least enough to wonder whether he might have such an allergy. He suspected eggs, but when he drank six raw eggs mixed in a blender, there was no

reaction. He could not know that he had already passed into the stage of adaptation and that his symptoms were withdrawal symptoms, the result of not eating eggs at the appropriate time, not of eating them.

Several years later, however, he was still suffering from his runny nose and still trying to find an explanation. He had never lost his suspicion that a food allergy was at the root of it and he was working now on the possibility that it might be a combination of foods that were responsible. He decided to avoid them to see if he improved, and one of these foods was eggs.

Now, as we shall see, one of the characteristics of food intolerance is that if you avoid the offending substance for about five days, or long enough to get it completely out of the system, and then reintroduce it, the effect is usually very abrupt and sometimes very severe. There is a swift and acute reaction. This characteristic is put to use in diagnosing the precise food that is responsible for the intolerance.

Herb Rinkel avoided eggs for five days and then went to a birthday party and had a piece of angel cake, whose ingredients included eggs. Within minutes he had collapsed. There were other doctors at the party, but none of them could explain it. His pulse, blood pressure, respiratory rate and other vital functions were all normal and the only symptom was that he was lying on the floor unconscious. When he recovered a few minutes later, no-one was more astonished by what had happened than Rinkel himself.

It was a stroke of fortune, at least for all those who would benefit from Rinkel's later work and research, that it was he who experienced this reaction, because it started him thinking on a different tack. Could it be that he was indeed allergic to eggs, as he had first suspected, but that as long as he went on eating them every day, the symptoms did not appear, at least until the effect of them began to wear off?

He took himself off eggs again for five days, and then repeated what he had done before and ate them on the fifth day. Once more he collapsed unconscious. After that he began experimenting with his own patients who had resisted all conventional therapies, working on the assumption that they were the victims of masked allergy, as he called it, with symptoms that were caused by eating foods that they were not even aware were harmful to them because the link between food and symptom was hidden. His success astonished him.

seems to like it, is talking about masked food intolerance. Her son is at phase +1 on our chart. She is doing him no favours by continuing to make him drink milk, even though the symptoms are now masked, because sooner or later, the adverse reactions will begin to set in. There is also ample evidence that ignored intolerances frequently develop into more serious intolerances to a much wider range of substances.

Many city dwellers also experience masking of chemical pollutants in the atmosphere, although they are usually not aware of it. People who live their lives in an atmosphere that is frequently polluted and smoggy often become adapted to it and tolerate, for example, the ozone, an air pollutant that occurs both indoors and outdoors. If they notice anything at all, it is likely to be that they are less troubled by the pollution, and seem to suffer fewer acute respiratory illnesses, than visitors from the country. The reality is that city dwellers do not have any greater protection against ozone and other environmental pollutants than country dwellers. It is simply that the symptoms they would normally expect to experience have been masked. The chemicals are continuing to do their damage, however, and eventually chronic symptoms will emerge.

"I Feel Great — What's Wrong with Me?" While the patient experiences the +1 phase of adaptation, he will not seek help. And indeed, viewed subjectively, why should he? Who goes to the doctor when they feel well? If he were to suspect that something was wrong and did go to a doctor who was aware of the problem of food intolerance, it could quickly be identified and nipped in the bud, but this rarely happens. Most doctors would look sideways at a patient who told them, "Doctor, I used to have headaches, but now I feel terrific — better than I've felt in years. What's the matter with me?"

But for every adaptive, or stimulatory plus stage in the table of ups and downs, there is a corresponding maladaptive, or depressive minus stage. Usually — though not invariably — once a patient has progressed to the simulatory level +1, he will sooner or later swing to −1 on the maladaptive scale, before slowly returning to the base line. Or, like a pendulum, he may swing backwards and forwards between the two sides before returning briefly to normal and starting the whole cycle again.

The symptoms at the maladaptive phase −1 are more definite than the rather woolly +1. They are the localised responses that most people associate with the expression "allergic responses" — runny nose, asthma, wheezing and various eye and ear problems. Herb Rinkel was at the −1 phase when he was suffering his egg-induced runny noses. Commonly, the victim is also slightly hyped up for a while, and then develops a low-grade headache before finally returning to normal.

Loud, Self-Centred and Unpleasant: the +2 Level If the time that the victim of food and chemical intolerance spends in +1 is likely to be unexceptional to his friends and associates, the same cannot be said at +2, to which he will certainly graduate if he continues to eat or inhale the substances to which he is intolerant. Months, or even years, may pass before this happens, and when it does, it is generally subtle and not immediately obvious. Gradually, however, the patient's personality is no longer the thoughtful, energetic wit of +1.

Now the alertness and activity have degenerated into a tense, jittery state. He is likely to be argumentative, loud, self-centred and generally a pain to have around. He often has sudden fits of sweating or flushing, followed by chilling, and he is frequently hungry or thirsty. At this stage any of three major health problems may also appear: hyperactivity in children, obesity and alcoholism.

Those who are addicted to food invariably crave the food to which they are addicted, even though they have no idea what they are doing. They do not know they are addicted, or even food intolerant, and they have little control over their actions. Whether they are children or adults, they are likely to describe the food that is harming them as their favourite food and it is the food that they are always raiding the fridge to find.

Because it is often refined carbohydrates to which they are addicted and which are causing their intolerance reactions, they often stuff themselves with bread, sugar, or sugar-containing foods without consciously understanding their craving. But their unconscious mind makes sure that they know which food is their addictant. Then, just like the junkie resisting any attempt to take away his supply, and so resisting most treatment, the food addict rejects any idea of staying away from bread, or whatever, or of changing his diet. As a result, excessive kilojoules are consumed and those which are not burnt up as energy are stored in the body as adipose tissue, or fat. The weight goes up and we have the condition that is known as obesity.

The third serious health risk that is encountered at +2 is closely related to the problem of obesity, and that is alcoholism. This is the time when alcoholism develops and typical +2 symptoms are all too familiar to those who have to live and work with people who have a serious drinking problem.

Alcoholism is often a heightened form of food intolerance. In this case, the alcoholic is reacting to the foods from which the drink was made, rather than to the drug-like effects of the alcohol ethanol itself. (See also Chapter 27.)

None of the symptoms combine to make the +2 personality an ideal husband — or wife, for just as many women as men graduate to this level. Nor are they much use to any employer. Their grating manner and self-righteousness will probably have turned most of their clients away. Unless the +2 victims are careful, they run the risk of losing both their families and their jobs, yet they probably have no idea what is wrong, or where to turn for help. Any conventional medical check-up almost invariably finds nothing wrong. "Try and take it easy and have a holiday", is likely to be about the only constructive advice such patients get, plus, of course, a prescription for a tranquilliser.

Many doctors, unaware of what is happening, shrug their shoulders and dismiss the patient as an inadequate personality. Yet telling him to pull himself together is likely to be no more effective than telling an alcoholic that he should stop drinking because it is ruining his life.

Problems Doctors Despair of: the −2 Level Because people tend to swing to and fro between the corresponding positions on the plus and minus scales, the +2 patient usually reaches the −2 level before long. If the −1 reactions can be categorised as local intolerance manifestations, those at −2 can accurately be described as systemic responses, because they affect the body's system as a whole, rather than individual parts of it.

At the −2 level we find many of the problems here that doctors despair of being able to help, and many that are dismissed as psychosomatic, including chest pains, mild depression, tiredness and general fatigue, headache, backache and neckache. Fatigue, or lack of energy and drive — a very important symptom — is remarkably common at every level of food and chemical intolerance. It is one of the most frequent non-specific symptoms and is invariably associated with illnesses and other symptoms where the pathology reveals nothing wrong.

If the cause of the trouble is food or chemical intolerance, the +2 and −2 phases are usually the limit of most people's journey up the stimulatory ladder, although they can swing wildly from one to the other, returning occasionally to the base line or more usually only to +1 and −1. This is because the withdrawal symptoms take over before they progress any further. Many of those addicted to substances higher up the pyramid of addiction do, of course, go on to +3 and −3, and the extremes of +4 and −4, and a few food and chemical addicts share the journey with them. Many more have fleeting and alarming visits to these higher levels.

Something Definitely Wrong: the Final Phases By +3, there is something very clearly wrong. Victims are loud and overbearing, and seem as though they are drunk, even when they have not had a drink at all. Sometimes they giggle stupidly, and give the general impression that they are decidedly odd. They are totally self-centred, impossible to live with and disastrous leaders, in spite of the fact that superficially they sometimes seem very dynamic. They are incapable of making sound judgments. Most of us know one or two +3s: hopefully we don't have to work for them or live with them.

The down-side to +3 is −3. Here again the symptoms are just as disturbing to the patient as those in the +3 adaptive stage. This is the point where depression can take over, with much tearfulness, sadness and sullenness. It is an emotionally unstable phase, with victims unable to concentrate or think clearly, withdrawn and apathetic. It often leads to physical illness, and at its most severe, it slips almost imperceptibly into −4.

At −4, there is severe depression, with suicidal tendencies, hallucinations and delusions. This patient very obviously needs to be hospitalised and closely supervised. At +4 they are also very sick, clearly in need of hospitalisation if the symptoms are more than transient. These patients include the classic cases of psychosis and in lay language, they are quite mad. Their limbs are likely to flail, they may even have convulsions and their behaviour and thought patterns are bizarre.

When we, as doctors, see patients in this condition returning to normal, simply by excluding something from their diet — patients who believed that they were mad, but whose only disability, when their symptoms are stripped away is gross intolerance and whose "madness" is entirely organic — that is one of the most moving experiences in medicine, for both physician and patient.

Blind Adaptation There is one other possible course of events that complicates the picture even further and makes it still more unlikely that the intolerance will be unmasked. We have seen that there is normally a warning that intolerance symptoms are about to develop, an acute reaction to the potentially harmful food or chemical. But if there has been a long and regular exposure to the food responsible for the intolerance reaction, say to cow's milk which has been drunk since infancy, there may be no acute reaction at the first, preadaptive stage. Instead, victims go immediately into the +1 adaptation phase, where the symptoms are masked and all that they experience is pleasant and mildly euphoric.

This is known as blind adaptation, because there is no warning. Because the symptoms at +1 usually feel normal, these patients are likely to drift into the much more unpleasant symptoms at −2 before anyone is aware what is happening. Even when doctors are constantly looking for environmental causes for illnesses and unexplained symptoms, they may miss the blind adaptation unless they are on their guard for it. If few sufferers from food intolerance can be of much help to their doctors, the victims who moved straight into a state of blind adaptation are even less likely to be able to give them any clues.

The inability to give the doctor any clues or even suspicions as to what is causing the symptoms, complicates diagnosis in ecological disorders. Even when the patient knows that he is unable to tolerate, say, cow's milk or wheat, he can be trapped by ingesting them unwittingly. Even with new labelling requirements, it may not always be obvious that a processed food contains milk or a milk by-product: if it was included in one of the ingredients supplied to the final manufacturer, as opposed to being put there by him, it does not need to be shown on the label. And there is no way of knowing whether milk is a part of a recipe in a restaurant or at a friend's dinner party.

Similarly with corn, it is relatively easy to avoid eating corn or any other product where corn is obviously an ingredient. But what of the person who cannot eat corn safely who unknowingly suffers a reaction every time she licks a postage stamp because the glue on the stamp contains corn?

THE RELENTLESS CYCLE OF ADDICTION ■

All addicts, whether on drugs or chocolate, establish a routine that revolves around the length of their particular cycle of addiction, or the time between "fixes" during which they can maintain their high and stave off withdrawal symptoms. Intolerance, or addiction, to foods and chemicals is no different to any other addiction: when the addictant, whether it is heroin, tomatoes or coffee, begins to wear off, the withdrawal symptoms, which are frequently the symptoms that we look on as illness, begin to take over.

Unless we have been taught to be suspicious, we would never think of blaming something that we *haven't* taken, rather than something that we have, for those symptoms.

It is much simpler to maintain the high if you are addicted to a dollar bar of chocolate than to heroin, costing $150 or more for half a gram, but the need to set a routine so that the addictant is always available before the withdrawal takes place, is exactly the same for food and chemical addiction as for heroin if the addict wants to stay free of withdrawal symptoms.

Usually, the higher the addictive substance on the pyramid of addiction, the shorter the cycle is likely to be. Some heroin addicts may have their fix only once a day, but most of them are experiencing withdrawal symptoms for most of the twenty-four hours until the next fix. It is only the cost and the difficulty of getting heroin that delays the time of that fix. With food and chemical combinations particularly, such as coffee, the cycle may also be very short, even as short as twenty minutes, so that to maintain the high the addict must have an almost constant intake of coffee while he or she is awake. It is not uncommon to have patients drinking thirty and more cups of coffee a day.

At the other end of the spectrum is, say, broccoli, with a cycle of perhaps twenty hours, which can cause problems of its own. If withdrawal begins twenty hours after broccoli has been consumed, to stay free of unpleasant symptoms, the addicted person must eat broccoli at least every twenty hours. Broccoli for lunch may have considerable appeal, but broccoli for breakfast and at four o'clock in the morning seldom has much to commend it!

Another common example is our patient addicted to wheat. If she has a ten-hour cycle of addiction, eating bread containing wheat at breakfast (7 a.m.), lunch (midday) and dinner (7 p.m.), together with the biscuits and scones that she will invariably nibble in between, will ensure that there are no withdrawal symptoms until 5 a.m. the following morning (that is, ten hours after dinner and the last exposure to wheat). At 5 a.m., however, she will probably wake with a symptom such as a headache that she can't explain and which will last until breakfast, when for some reason that she cannot explain either, the headache disappears. All that has happened, of course, is that she has fed her addiction — taken her fix — with the morning toast and marmalade. How common it is to admit that we just don't function normally in the morning until we have our coffee and toast!

If the cycle of addiction to wheat is only six hours, however, the pattern will be different if meals are still taken at the same times. Now withdrawal symptoms can be expected at 1 a.m. and at any time of the night before breakfast, as well as one hour before the 7 p.m. dinner — if afternoon tea doesn't have wheat in it.

What will probably happen in this case is that for some months the sufferer will wake at 1 a.m., perhaps with an annoying headache, then fall asleep and wake again before dawn, not properly rested and still with the headache. Sooner or later, this person will almost certainly eat bread just before going to sleep, without consciously being aware that this has anything to do with an addiction or even with the symptoms, and this will carry her through until four or five the next morning. Before much longer, she will probably get up at this time because her morning headache is worse when she lies in bed thinking about it. She will gravitate to the bread bin, her headache will go and she will have established the pattern that for the time being — and it may be for years — will keep her free from the maladaptive symptoms.

It is remarkably common to wake at about 2 a.m. and visit the refrigerator or bread bin, perhaps have a bowl of corn flakes or some other cereal, and then return to bed and sleep, just as it is no coincidence that the asthmatic whose illness is due to some ecological factor often wakes with an attack at about 2 a.m., needing relief from his inhaled medication.

Already, in all these cases, addiction or intolerance to simple foods has begun to dominate its victims' lives. It is inevitable that it flows over into their work and relationships with their families, if they are never getting a proper night's sleep.

Spacing Meals Because food addicts quickly learn (often subconsciously) that avoiding a meal makes them sick, they can be very short-tempered if their meals come late or do not contain the food that they crave, which may be as basic as potatoes. As the reason for their behaviour is rarely understood until it has been explained, they just seem to be getting increasingly bad-tempered.

Food addicts become expert at arranging their eating schedule (again usually subconsciously) so that it always includes the particular food to which they are addicted and intolerant. A cow's milk addict, for instance, who is usually also addicted to the whole spectrum of dairy products, may always have a bowl of cereal just before he goes to bed. He doesn't realise that it is the milk on the cereal, not the cereal itself, that he is craving, even if he understands that he is craving anything.

A woman who is a sweet or chocolate addict (I call her a carboholic) will ensure that there is always a supply in the house, and probably by the bed and near the television. If she inadver-

EGGS, COFFEE AND COKE — DISASTER!

Eggs are a frequent source of intolerance reaction. Some egg addicts, to maintain their high, must have eggs for breakfast, in their mid-morning sandwiches, at lunch, during the afternoon and for dinner, and even then they will always wake up with some withdrawal symptom.

For business people, with this and many other food addictions, the special danger time is lunch, particularly if they are not aware of their intolerance. If they have lunch without eggs, for instance, or skip lunch altogether, they may find themselves unable to stay awake, or as happened in one case, be quite incapable of giving intelligible dictation. Next morning, normal again after eggs for breakfast, they get angry with their secretary for not taking accurate shorthand!

Coffee is one of the commonest addictants and causes endless problems to the coffee sensitive. Some coffees contain 2.5 per cent caffeine, which even in modest amounts (say two or three cups a day) can affect the heart rhythm, the diameter of the blood vessels, coronary circulation, blood pressure, urination and many other bodily functions. (Coca-Cola and the other cola drinks, which contain caffeine as well as their food content, are almost worse than coffee, because they include, in the case of Coca-Cola, a worrying 10 per cent and more of sugar, as well as many other chemicals.)

Typically, after a lifetime of drinking coffee without any unpleasant side effects, a person suddenly cannot tolerate it and begins to suffer headaches and sweating, for example, whenever he drinks it. He is usually unwilling to accept what commonsense tells him, that the coffee is causing the headaches and bouts of sweating. He will reason that coffee has never been a problem before, therefore there must be some other explanation.

If he continues to drink coffee, say at a rate of ten cups a day or less, the acute symptoms of the preadaptive stage will quite soon abate and the intolerance will become masked. There will be no more unpleasant symptoms, as long as the coffee is there at regular intervals, but our victim has now moved to +1 in the ups and downs table, and the coffee has become a significant stressor. Only if there is a sudden increase in the level of stress (if, for example, he is taken ill with a virus, or has severe financial worries, or drinks two or three times the normal dose of coffee); or if he is deprived of coffee, will the unpleasant symptoms temporarily return.

Coffee is one of the main reasons why many people have headaches at the weekend, or when they are on holiday. What has happened is that on every other day of the week, they drink their coffee fairly early in the morning before they leave for the office. Though they don't understand it, this also happens to be the time they need to take their first fix of the day in order to ward off the withdrawal symptoms as the stimulatory effect of the last coffee from the night before begins to wear off. At the weekend, or during holidays, on

the other hand, they are likely to sleep in, say for an extra hour, which means that they have not had their fix on time. They immediately begin to suffer withdrawal symptoms and the headache and other symptoms return.

The usual cure is to have a cup of coffee and if this does the trick and takes away the headache, most people will be unlikely to associate the unpleasant pain or the sweating with the coffee. Indeed, to the contrary, they will see only that coffee must be good for them because it takes away their headache!

Every alcoholic knows this trick and can space his or her drinks to avoid the withdrawal symptoms, or hangover.

tently runs out, there will be the same panic that the smoker experiences when he finds that he has no more cigarettes in the house. I have a patient who has driven more than 10 kilometres in the middle of the night to buy chocolates when she has run out.

People with short addiction cycles, who need to eat at least once during the night, often maintain that they are night owls, and even become night workers, when before nothing would have kept them from their eight hours' sleep each night. They begin to stay up very late, and the reason, of course, is that in this way they are able to get the food that they need to postpone the withdrawal symptoms that they would otherwise suffer in the early hours of the morning.

Many addicts, including food addicts, become expert at manipulating the exact amount of a substance that they need to stay high, or relatively normal, for as long as possible. Not too little, or the withdrawal symptoms will start to appear; and not too much, or the unexpected stress will again bring on an acute attack. Coffee can be measured accurately, and the daily dose can be varied according to the need, from half a cup a day, to more than forty cups. Alcoholics are expert at controlling their dose, usually by learning not to eat and drink at the same time. Because all alcoholic drinks, except for neat alcohol, are a food–drug combination and because the food fractions are often as troublesome as the alcohol ethanol, eating makes it difficult to control with any precision the amount of food that is being ingested. This is why the alcoholic must control his dose, because if he underdoses, he is likely to pass straight to the severe symptoms of the −3 level; and if he overdoses, he may well find himself in the equally unpleasant adaptation stage of +3.

Coming Down from a Permanent High As the permanent high begins to wear off, as in time it nearly always does, and simple foods lose their ability to keep a person in a constant state of stimulation, more serious problems begin to arise. The first indicator is likely to be an increase in the frequency of intake and the amount of the triggering food. The dose gets larger as the cycle of addiction gets shorter and the withdrawal symptoms become more unpleasant. Next, there will be a gradual progression up the pyramid of addiction, to take advantage of more rapidly absorbed substances, such as sugars and alcohols. Rye in whisky is absorbed faster than rye in bread!

How long it takes for this stage to be reached varies from person to person and depends on the same factors that led to the initial intolerance — individual susceptibility, the extent of other intolerances and the total stress load being experienced. The higher up the pyramid of addiction the substance involved, the sooner this dominating maladaptive stage is likely to arrive, and if the initial intolerance was triggered by an event such as a viral infection or an emotional upset, these same factors will frequently play a part.

As victims move into the last stage of stress — Hans Selye's stage of exhaustion, and Theron Randolph's postadaptive stage — most food and chemically intolerant patients will at last belatedly take their troubles to their doctors. They will invariably say (and believe) that the onset of the dominant withdrawal symptom marked the onset of their present illness and most doctors will concentrate exclusively on this symptom. A few sufferers do suspect that food is the cause of their problems, though without knowing which food, and they choose a form of therapy which is fraught with danger. They simply stop eating, and even if anorexia nervosa does not follow, there are likely to be serious difficulties caused by the abrupt loss of weight and dangerous undernutrition, both of which can trigger the beginning of yet more intolerance reactions, and the whole cycle starts again.

It becomes increasingly difficult to maintain the stimulatory adaptive stage and a progressive decline begins as the maladaptive reactions set in with increasing frequency and severity. Unless remedial action is taken, it will lead inexorably into Hans Selye's final stage of exhaustion. Just as in the first stage of addiction, when intolerance resulted in an immediate and unpleasant acute reaction as soon as an unsafe substance was ingested or inhaled, now again there is no protection against the stressor, no masking, and the reaction is swift and disagreeable. The cycle of addiction has finally turned full circle.

The clinical ecologist would be immensely helped if there were illnesses, even symptoms, that could be pointed to and labelled with conviction as environmental disorders. But there is nothing so simple! Because every organ and tissue in the body can be affected by food and chemical intolerance, we find every disorder and symptom that these organs and tissues are capable of manifesting.

If the target organ is the skin, the blood vessels and cells are likely to swell and break down, often oozing their contents. The result is a rash. Eczema with its itching redness and oozing, weeping skin is one of the most familiar examples. It is so unpredictable that it may involve almost the total surface of the body, or it may be localised to a small area like the back of the hand or the foot. Why this localisation occurs in the way that it does is not known.

If on the other hand the blood vessels and tissues of the brain are affected, the symptoms are likely to be headaches, migraine, tiredness and depression. If the mucous membrane lining the nose, the sinuses or the bronchial tree are affected, the glands produce surplus mucus, which we try to get rid of by excessive sneezing, nose-blowing or coughing. In the lungs, asthma can result. It is all a question of chance, of individual susceptibility or perhaps of some organ or tissue weakened by previous illness or injury.

SYSTEMIC WITHDRAWAL SYMPTOMS ▮

Although the number of symptoms that can be experienced is high, there are some systemic withdrawal symptoms (which affect one or other of the body's entire systems, as opposed to being localised like a rash on the back of the hand) that are even more commonly encountered. When one or more of these symptoms appear, after the possible organic explanations have been eliminated, there is all the more reason for suspecting an ecological cause.

Headache The headache and migraine that so often accompany ecological illness can affect any part of the head. They are often accompanied by nausea, vomiting, dizziness and blurring of vision and they most commonly result from exposure to specific foods and/or environmental chemicals.

Fatigue We have already mentioned that fatigue (which can be described as excessive or abnormal tiredness that is not relieved by reasonable rest) is probably the most common single symptom in ecological illness. It is frequently at its worst in the morning, gradually improving as the day wears on. It is often associated with headache, muscle pain, oedema (swelling of the tissues), irritability, depression and "brain fag", or mental exhaustion.

Muscle Pain (Myalgia) Myalgia often accompanies both fatigue and headache, especially when it involves the nape of the neck and when it is a symptom of what is known as tension/ fatigue syndrome. Myalgia, though, can involve any of the muscles in the body and not infrequently it appears with tinnitus (ringing in the ears), dizziness and loss of equilibrium.

Joint Pains and Arthritis Joint pains and restriction in the movement of the joints are common symptoms in ecological illness, and any form of arthritis, rheumatism or gout can be triggered by, and certainly worsened by, specific foods and simple chemicals. Many apparent cases of rheumatism and arthritis are only look-alike symptoms of environmental disorders — but they look so much alike that they can deceive even doctors specialising in the field.

Cardiovascular Among the many cardiovascular symptoms that are directly related to ecological illness are arrhythmic heartbeat (irregular rhythm, missed beats or extra beats), tachycardia (increased heart rate), palpitations, high blood pressure, shivering and flushing, and oedema. Arrhythmia in particular is encountered at any of the adaptive or maladaptive phases in the table of ups and downs (Fig. 2, Chapter 5).

Brain Fag, Impaired Thinking These include mental confusion, forgetfulness, indecisiveness, impaired comprehension in reading, shortened attention span, moodiness, sullenness and dysphasia (loss of coherent speech).

Depression Depression, accompanied by impaired responsiveness, disorientation, sleep disturbance, poor judgment and sometimes amnesia, is characteristic of the more extreme forms of ecological illness that may often be relieved simply by eliminating certain items from the diet, or avoiding exposure to certain chemicals.

Other Symptoms Hyperactivity, irritability, nervousness, jitteriness, excessive hunger and thirst, ulcerative colitis, diarrhoea, constipation, insomnia, restlessness are all often encountered. Sometimes debilitating and usually distressing symptoms can affect the upper respiratory tract, the nose, sinuses and throat, producing the lower respiratory complaints of coughing in bronchitis, and wheezing and shortness of breath in bronchial asthma, with all its complications.

Obesity and alcoholism, one the result of addicting foods in their edible form, the other in their drinkable form, are frequently associated with ecological illness, as we have seen.

As a very general rule, if only mild symptoms, such as nasal catarrh, are present, there are likely to be only a few intolerances (occasionally only one) involved. While at the other extreme, where the symptoms can be so disabling that it is difficult or even impossible for the victim to continue functioning normally, there are usually multiple substances implicated, needing only very low levels of exposure to trigger the reactions.

Sometimes we encounter people who seem to be intolerant of just about everything. There are few patients more disturbing and frustrating for a doctor than the victims of exquisite or extreme intolerance. Conventional therapy is useless and it is distressing to know that one is helpless to do anything to relieve their very real fear and suffering, particularly when such patients are frequently children (see box).

THE CRUEL MIMIC ■

Many of the symptoms of ecological illness mimic other diseases and disorders, sometimes with disastrous results for their victims. Patients with the very common tension/fatigue syndrome that results from food and chemical intolerance — many of them children — also complain of abdominal pain so severe that they are sometimes hospitalised and have extensive investigations and X-rays. Some have even been operated on because of the persistent pain, and of course at surgery no physical abnormality can be identified.

THE TRAGEDY OF THE TOTAL ALLERGY SYNDROME

Sixteen-year-old Jackie* was a tragic case when she came to me. Gasping for breath, racked by pain, she spent much of her life on her bed, a victim of the mercifully rare total allergy syndrome and a miserable example of the ultimate price that some must pay for being born into our polluted world. Not only was she unable to tolerate almost any food, but she was exquisitely sensitive to numerous chemicals: simply to survive, Jackie was compelled to withdraw from all contact with the outside world.

When I first saw her, it was at my home in the country, for there was no way that she could have come into the city. Her parents had already uprooted the family and moved into a specially prepared house away from the polluted city to try to ease her suffering. She arrived with her father and with a full-size oxygen cylinder on the back seat of their car, from which she was breathing through a mask. Even with this, she was cyanosed, her skin bluish, short of breath and quite severely distressed.

She got out of the car with difficulty and we sat in the garden because I knew that in the house there would be things that would affect her, even though it is ecologically a good deal safer than most homes. She had taken only a few steps when she collapsed on to a rug, where she lay, now deeply distressed. Even the effort of making this visit to me left many of her joints swollen and extremely painful for three months.

The treatment that was eventually prescribed required a multiple approach by a number of doctors, including a conventional allergist, because she had many classic allergies as well as her numerous food and chemical hypersensitivities, or intolerance reactions.

Many of her chemical sensitivities were such that she had to avoid the chemicals entirely because the usual hyposensitising drops achieved nothing; and the yeast Candida albicans turned out to be a major problem, as it often does in severe intolerance (see Chapter 30). This aspect did improve significantly after a course of nystatin, the antibiotic that is specific for candida.

After numerous unsafe foods had been identified, strict dietary control helped and our combined efforts, coupled with inspiring persistence by Jackie

*True names of patients have been changed throughout the book.

and her parents, saw her able to control her more debilitating symptoms and to live a reasonably normal life, restricted though it necessarily still was.

Why one person should be singled out for reactions of this

severity must be largely a question of individual susceptibility. In Jackie's case, interestingly, her mother was also severely intolerant. Probably everything just came together in the worst possible way.

Others are so nervous and irritable that they are put on a continuous regimen of debilitating tranquillisers. They may complain of leg pain and be diagnosed as having rheumatism or arthritis. For the majority, the only treatment they really need is an exclusion diet that leaves out a few foods or food ingredients.

One of the most disturbing of these mimicking disorders, which has long been thought to be psychosomatic, is ulcerative colitis, an inflammatory disease of the colon that is disabling and occasionally fatal. It is marked by agonising abdominal pains and intermittent bloody diarrhoea. The truth is that many of the diagnoses of ulcerative colitis are tragically wrong. In many instances, it is not psychosomatic at all, with the mind influencing the body to produce the disease, but more accurately it is somatopsychic, where the disordered function of the body influences the mind and the behaviour.

A common method of treating ulcerative colitis that is still widely used involves the surgical removal of the colon, or part of the colon, which necessitates either a colostomy or ileotomy. Both are operations that can be psychologically devastating to the patient.

Surgery may well be necessary if symptoms persist, even with a clinical ecology approach, in order to prevent complications such as cancer developing. But in many cases of ulcerative colitis, this major surgery is completely unnecessary. The solution may require nothing more traumatic than taking a patient off cow's milk, or some other food to which intolerance has developed.

A change in diet, or the surgical creation of an artificial anus in the wall of the stomach? What has to be done before the medical profession at least tries this frequently successful therapeutic approach before it resorts to the disfiguring and psychologically appalling treatment with the scalpel? Even if it only works for a handful of patients, it would surely be worth trying. The reality is that it *is* successful in many more cases than just a small percentage.

THE PUZZLE OF NEURASTHENIA ■

A less traumatic, but more common ecological disorder, involves a cluster of symptoms including fatigue, muscle and joint aches, drowsiness, difficulty in concentration, nervousness and depression, as well as irritability, pain in the chest, headache, insomnia and gastrointestinal problems. Individually, they are all common enough in ecological illness; but what marks them out in this case is that they are all found at the same time. For some reason, women outnumber men with this problem by 2.5 to 1.

What makes this particularly interesting is that the syndrome is almost identical to a common functional disorder known as neurasthenia, or psychasthenia, whose cause has always been controversial, although the disorder is generally thought to be psychological in origin. It was once thought to be the result of "exhaustion" of the nerve centres. Enlightened physicians have now shown that it often responds to an ecological approach, where before it was usually considered to be untreatable. By either removing some substance from the diet, or removing the patient from exposure to an "unsafe" chemical, the "neurasthenia" disappears.

In one study, male workers exposed to diesel jet fuel (a common source of ecological illness because of its fumes) were diagnosed as suffering from neurasthenia with significantly greater frequency than a control group who were not exposed to the fuel. But when they were moved from that work and away from the diesel-polluted environment, they recovered spontaneously. Their only illness was intolerance of diesel fumes.

Other studies have shown painters (another high-risk profession for ecological disorders), after long exposure to organic solvents, suffering significant cognitive impairment, meaning that their ability to think and reason was diminished. They had difficulty in concentrating, poor short-term memory, emotional instability and irrational motor coordination. Once again, however, removing them from contact with the solvents was all that was required to reverse the symptoms.

That this happens should be no surprise, for ecological illness affects the brain and the central nervous system with the same facility as it affects any of the joints and muscles of the body, or the linings of the respiratory and gastrointestinal tracts.

A quite closely related problem may be involved. Autonomic dyspraxia means that the autonomic nervous system (that part of the nervous system that controls the functions over which we usually have no control, such as heartbeat and peristalsis) is not working correctly and this in turn can also result in the symptoms of ecological illness.

SYMPTOMS MAY CHANGE ■

Masking can be responsible for symptoms appearing to lessen, as well as often removing them altogether. Symptoms are certainly less directly related to the true cause of the intolerance as the years pass. I have patients who, after suffering from hayfever for decades, found to their delight that the hayfever gradually lessened — only to have that delight turn to dismay as they realised that the hayfever had been replaced by increasingly severe asthma or eczema.

One patient, a woman who had suffered from asthma for forty years, found that it was suddenly replaced by a distressing intolerance to polyester. There was not even the gradual transition which usually occurs. When she first came to see me, just wearing polyester clothing caused a new spectrum of symptoms, although she didn't know it at the time. If all her clothes happened to be made from polyester, which they sometimes were before we pinpointed the trouble, she experienced tongue swelling that was sometimes so bad that it almost choked her, as well as swelling of the face and lips and a serious itch all over her body.

With children it is common for the nature of the reaction to change with time. Many cases where allergy and intolerance appear to have been outgrown are in fact only a change in the symptoms. Cow's milk, for example, may produce colic in an infant, then wheezy bronchitis as the baby grows into a young child, and nasal catarrh and migraine when the child reaches adulthood. Stopping bed-wetting is a common milestone along the road from young childhood intolerance to, say, cow's milk, to chronic hayfever or urticaria.

Only very occasionally, as with true allergy, do patients spontaneously lose their intolerance and their symptoms. Far

THE PROBLEM WITH AMANDA

A typical case history from my files will illustrate the problems that patients have to face when they are overtaken by intolerance. Amanda was in her early forties when I first saw her, a housewife with an active interest in the family business, a sports complex. Extreme as some of her symptoms might seem to be, none of them were exceptional for someone suffering from several food and chemical intolerances simultaneously, as is often the case. Amanda's problems were manifold — weepiness, depression, fatigue and an odd inability to sit up straight at times, compounded by headaches, nausea and "strange feelings in my head".

Fasting followed by challenge testing to identify the offending foods (see Part Two) soon pinpointed the cause of her problems. She had already suspected that the bread she bought in the supermarket was affecting her adversely, though she could not tell precisely why, and when we tested for wheat, it was clear how right she was. Within half an hour of eating it, she developed feelings of heat all over her body, then nausea and vomiting and the strange feelings in her head which particularly

bothered her, with a marked pulse rate of almost 120 per minute.

Disconcertingly, the feeling in her head began to spread all over her body in a way that she found extremely unpleasant, but was unable to define. The vomiting was repeated and then a headache developed. She had taken the test meal of wheat bread in the evening and the symptoms persisted until she went to bed.

She slept for a couple of hours and woke at 1 a.m. with what she called her typically severe headache above the left eye, a headache that almost invariably led to a migraine so severe that on occasions she had to receive pain-killing injections to relieve it. Eventually, she got off to sleep and woke still with the headache. All these symptoms, we were able to establish, were the consequence of eating wheat. They were not the result of some organic malfunction, as an array of doctors had tried to prove before she was referred to me at the eleventh hour, nor were they the result of some incipient madness, as her GP had begun to imply when nothing else could be found.

Wheat was not Amanda's only problem area. Strawberries

also provoked a full-blown migraine and, perhaps as the result of the increasing headache (although she herself felt that it was independent of this), she lost her ability to concentrate. At the same time, she felt inexplicably very weak as though everything was an overburdening effort; and she had a sensation of coldness.

Avocados (like strawberries, in plentiful supply in her native Queensland) were another source of trouble, we found. Masking had ensured that with the exception of bread, she had made no association between any of these troublesome foods and her intolerance reactions.

Tested with avocados, she began to experience bad reactions almost immediately and she wrote them down for me at the time. "I suddenly felt nauseated and dizzy, and came over hot and sweaty", she wrote. "It became much worse, and I found that my legs had gone weak until I quickly reached the point where I could hardly walk. Became very nauseated indeed, but did not vomit. Went to bed, but couldn't sleep. A feeling of coldness and became very shivery and had to warm up with a hot water bottle."

This was in the middle of the day and by mid-afternoon, she was fast asleep. When she

awoke, she had a strong taste of avocado in her mouth and once again felt nauseous. For the rest of the day, she was anorexic (she had no appetite) and had nothing more to eat. Next morning, she still had a strong taste of avocado in her mouth.

Dates turned out to be yet another source of intolerance. (I test only for foods that are frequently and regularly consumed, because this is a prerequisite before addiction can develop. In the questionnaire I had asked Amanda to fill out, she had mentioned dates as a food that she nibbled constantly when she was on duty at the sports complex.)

She ate eight dates for me and commented that just one would have been enough. Within ten minutes, after being cheerful and normal, she had what she described as a grade 2 depression (out of a maximum of 3). After twenty minutes, this had worsened to a very severe grade 3 depression. This took the next four hours to drop gradually back to what she perceived as grade 1.

At the half-hour point, when the depression was still at grade 3 in her estimation, she became extremely angry and irritable with everyone around her and this too took two and a half hours to subside. Her con-

centration deteriorated and after the first hour she was quite unable to concentrate on anything.

Also at twenty minutes, she developed a severe headache (which probably had something to do with the crankiness that at one point she said was so bad that she was ready to murder anyone who came along).

Amanda did not even need to eat certain cheeses to develop symptoms. If she just smelled a strong cheese (which meant that molecules of it were entering her system by way of her nose), she developed a headache, nausea and, as always, a feeling of general unwellness and fatigue.

Chemicals were also contributing to Amanda's intolerance reactions. To petrochemical derivatives, formaldehyde and particularly tobacco, she reacted

with weepiness, lethargy, depression, tiredness and an odd inability to sit up straight.

With sensitising drops, we were able to neutralise all the chemical problems (Chapter 26). Once the danger foods had been identified, it was simply a matter of ensuring that they were kept out of her diet for at least six months and then reintroduced very gradually, and never more often than once every four days. In this way, she ensured that her gastrointestinal system was entirely free of these foods before they were eaten again, so that the addiction did not creep back. Sometimes an offending food has to be avoided forever, just as foods that cause a true allergic reaction can never be eaten again, even after fifty years, without the risk of a reaction.

more often, the problem only worsens with time if it is ignored or not recognised. In classic allergy (that is, IgE-mediated allergy), the original symptom usually persists. Once hives have developed as the allergic reaction to eating prawns, they are likely always to be the symptom when prawns are eaten. In food and chemical intolerance, the symptoms not only worsen in severity as a rule but, with continued exposure or ingestion, spread to include symptoms in other organs and tissue.

POTENT DATES ∎

Amanda's experience with the dates was very similar to another test for date intolerance that I carried out on a girl in front of television cameras for the program "Sixty Minutes". She ate two dates and I warned the crew that the reaction would begin to occur between ten and thirty minutes later. I had underestimated the potency of those dates! Within minutes she began to react and the crew had to scramble for their cameras as she collapsed heavily into a chair. One of her symptoms was that she could hardly talk coherently, and after chattering away animatedly before she ate the dates, she was now stammering so badly that the words wouldn't come out. It was an impressive demonstration.

Another patient, Marie, a very unhappy young woman when she arrived at my rooms, was referred to me by her very caring family doctor who was at the end of his tether trying to fathom out how he could help her. Marie suffered equally debilitating symptoms to those of Amanda and about the only difference was that her particular intolerance was to sultanas, which she was addicted to and consumed in copious amounts every day. A battery of tests, numerous prescription drugs and referrals to four specialists had done nothing to relieve an array of symptoms, which included a feeling of hotness all over her body, migraine, acute depression, lethargy and fatigue. Her depression hung over her like a black cloud, and I was the last stop before she went into hospital for electric shock therapy.

When I questioned her, it was clear that not one of all the learned doctors she had spoken to had asked her a single question about the sultanas. Yet treatment could hardly have been easier. It consisted of eliminating sultanas and other related foods such as grapes and currants, from her diet. Nothing else was required and five years later, as I write, she is still symptom-free.

THE VALUE OF SIMPLICITY ■

One of the greatest attributes of doctors of past generations was the ability to see things in a simple, uncomplicated light. I like the example of the patient who arrives at the surgery with a red, sore, swollen finger, complaining that he can't sleep properly and that he has lost his ability to concentrate at work. The doctor examines him and the patient comes away with something to relieve the pain, a sleeping pill, an antibiotic for the infected finger, perhaps another antibiotic to control the effect of the first one on the yeast in the body, a laxative because the pain-killer may cause constipation and a tranquilliser to help him be more relaxed at work. How much easier it would have been if the doctor had just removed the thorn from his finger!

In clinical ecology, the thorn may be milk, wheat, or a

chemical, or whatever is causing the intolerance; yet trying to persuade doctors whose whole training encourages them to take the most tortuous route to effecting a diagnosis, that the simplest answer really is very often the correct one is a task of Sisyphean proportions.

I like the story — a true one — that beautifully illustrates what I mean. For years doctors have been intrigued by the fact that women who do a lot of running are amenorrhoeic, meaning that they have no monthly periods. Researchers have puzzled over this and come up with a variety of complex explanations and learned papers (some of which can only have come from scientists locked up in their laboratories whose knowledge of women athletes was minimal), like the thesis that women who run are much less feminine anyway.

The truth was almost laughably simple and it did not need any of these erudite scientists to reveal it. All that is happening is that women's breasts bounce up and down when they run. This causes breast stimulation, which in turn increases prolactin levels. The effect is exactly the same as when a woman is breast-feeding, when she is also usually amenorrhoeic. The tightest bra will not prevent this irritation, or stimulation, which the brain interprets as a baby being nursed.

At a recent conference, the panel of which I was a member was asked to give its views on the best way of monitoring immuno-suppressive therapy. In other words, how do we know when a patient being given hyposensitising treatment to neutralise intolerances is getting better?

The others on the panel gave correct but complicated answers, talking about the response to the level of the immuno-globulin IgE, and so on. When it was my turn to answer, I said simply, "When the patient says he feels better." It wasn't a particularly profound answer, but I was given almost a standing ovation by the audience of largely non-medical health-care experts. We get so far away from the patient, that we forget that in the final analysis, all that matters is the patient getting better and feeling better.

7 The Trouble with Food

EATING OURSELVES TO DEATH ▌

Once upon a time we ate because we were hungry. Now we eat because convention says that it is time to eat, whether we are hungry or not. As a result, about a third of all the people in the Western world — the "advanced" nations — are overweight and their children are fast heading in that direction, or are already fat. It is a cruel legacy to leave them with.

For once, the statistics tell the story with deadly accuracy. The National Health and Medical Research Council, the Australian body that recommends desirable levels of nutrients, has suggested that the average adult male needs a daily intake of 8900 kilojoules (2126 calories). The Australian Bureau of Statistics records that the average Australian male is actually consuming 4660 kilojoules (1113 calories) *more* than his energy needs.

When you recall that it takes a one-hour brisk walk to burn off the energy obtained from eating two thin slices of bread and butter, it is clearly wishful thinking that anyone is going to stay healthy and maintain the correct weight in any other way than by eating properly.

Many people in our society are literally eating themselves to death: about 60 per cent of all deaths are now attributed to diet-related diseases. Coronary heart disease, high blood pressure, stroke and diabetes are just four of these entirely avoidable diseases that claim so many lives prematurely and often painfully. Several of the most destructive of the seventy-five or so cancers are also diet related. (Lung cancer is the main cancer killer, but that's just wilful suicide.)

In primitive societies there is certainly a tremendous loss of life in the first years of life because of malnutrition and infection, but once they reach maturity these people are free of almost all these degenerative diseases. Obesity was almost unknown in such societies until recently, when they were introduced to Western food. Adults reached their maximum weight by their mid-twenties and then weight declined. You can probably count on one hand the number of men you know past their mid-twenties who actually grow slimmer. Even the gradual rise in blood pressure, which we take for granted in the West as we get older, is not seen in primitive societies. It is wrong to assume that this is a natural and unavoidable accompaniment to the process of ageing.

Not only do we eat too much, but we suffer from a diet that is poor in balance, lacking in fibre, far too high in fat and milk, and top-heavy with refined carbohydrates. Add to this the chemicals that contaminate our environment and which we can never wholly escape — chemicals that have no nutritional value whatsoever and many of which are toxic — and it is little wonder that we are grossly maladapted to our environment.

Every other species that has ever lived on earth has perished and become extinct if it became even a fraction as maladapted as Western man has. Only our unique ability to keep alive those who by natural selection would probably have died out — who may yet die out — has kept that fate at bay. But it is just bizarre to be proud of the fact that the talents of countless brilliant people are used, at a cost of billions that could have been so much better spent, simply to cure a handful of the horrendous diseases that existed in the first place only because of our stupidity and short-sightedness.

Many people find it very difficult, sometimes impossible, to accept that we are biological creatures like any other animal; that we *are* animals. To understand and accept this does not require an acceptance of Darwin's theory of evolution, or a rejection of the Biblical version of the Creation. Zoologically, we are just another species sharing this planet. Like every other creature on earth, we thrive on certain foods and not on others. Horses don't eat meat and lions cannot survive on grass. The food that we choose to include in our typical, conventional Western diet simply is not, for the most part, the food on which our particular species of animal, *Homo sapiens*, thrives.

Some get by perfectly well on the typical Western diet, because of individual susceptibility or for the other reasons that we have discussed, but many don't. The ecologically oriented doctor, the clinical ecologist, is concerned with those who don't thrive on this diet, and that means about 80 per cent of the population. Even if their symptoms never progress beyond mild and low-grade headaches, it must surely be better not to have a headache at all. Yet the attitude seems to prevail, even among doctors, that such symptoms are nothing more than an annoying and unavoidable part of modern living, to be tolerated without grumbling. What nonsense that is!

VEGETARIANISM — THE RIGHT APPROACH? ■

There is a continuing controversy about whether vegetarianism is in itself a healthier way of eating. Australia has a long tradition of eating meat, with a hardly veiled implication that non-meat eaters are in some way weak, which has been encouraged by the flagging beef industry in particular. It has much in common with the sugar industry, which also perceives itself as being under siege.

Nearly $9 million a year is currently being pumped into extolling the virtues of sugar and red meat in Australia, and almost without exception, those who are concerned with keeping people healthy condemn both products in all but the most modest amounts. "Feed the man meat!" was a jingle that the meat industry used (unsuccessfully, it now concedes) and it was quickly adapted by meat's opponents to "Feed the man a heart attack!" For whatever reason, red meat consumption has fallen by 20 kilograms a year in the last twenty years, but the average man, woman and child in Australia still manages to eat 82 kilograms each year. Australia is also ranked sixth in the world in the incidence of heart disease and the correlation between fat and heart disease is beyond dispute.

But is vegetarianism the answer? Its critics point out that as far as we know, there has never in the history of humankind been a culture that has thrived on an exclusively vegetarian diet to the extent that they refuse to eat any living creature, even a grub. Others respond that it is the *quality* of the vegetarian diet that counts and that we know enough today to ensure that the quality is high.

A number of studies have established that vegetarians have a significantly lower risk of dying from coronary heart disease than omnivores, those who eat everything. One study of over 10,000 Seventh Day Adventist vegetarians in California showed that their risk of dying from coronary heart disease was between a quarter and half that of the average age-matched Californian omnivore. Significantly, because it could be argued that Seventh Day Adventists have a lifestyle which tends to make them healthier people anyway, the vegetarians' risk of dying from coronary disease was also three times lower than for non-vegetarian Seventh Day Adventists, whose lifestyle was presumably similar in every other respect except their consumption of meat.

Vegetarians also appear to have lower mean blood pressure than non-vegetarians, which is desirable. The exact mechanism that produces these effects is not clear. It may be nothing more than the consistently reported observation that vegetarians weigh less than omnivores and have a lower incidence of problems with obesity, which we know increases the risk of many illnesses. There is evidence, however, that a vegetarian diet in itself has some protective effect, at least as far as heart disease is concerned; and if it consistently lowers the risk of obesity, it ought to be encouraged for that alone.

There are, of course, many different degrees of vegetarianism, from the vegans who will eat no animal products at all, including milk and eggs (some find the killing of animals so abhorrent that they won't even wear animal products or leather shoes); to those who will not eat the flesh of any creature, including fish, but do not exclude eggs, milk and other dairy products; to those many people who simply abstain from eating red meat.

Apart from eating no meat, vegetarians usually consume far more whole grain cereals, legumes and other vegetables than average. While on the plus side this may result in a significantly higher intake of fibre, potassium, vitamin C and vitamin E, with lower cholesterol, iron and vitamin B_{12}, it is also a fact that those who depend heavily on grains and legumes find it more difficult to achieve optimal balanced nutrition. The main risk they face is that their food base is too narrow. Inevitably, the more extreme the degree of vegetarianism practised, the narrower the food base; and the narrower the food base, the more difficult it is to achieve a balanced diet.

From the viewpoint of the clinical ecologist, one of the factors that is most likely to end in food intolerance is frequent and repeated exposure to the same food, and it makes no difference whether that food is eggs and meat, or wholegrain flour and soy. This need not be the case because there is a wide variety of fruits, vegetables and non-animal products available. It is just harder work and needs more time and imagination; in time, human nature being what it is, many people stop making the effort.

Vegetarians also tend to rely on wheat gluten in the cereal grains as their basic source of protein. There is nothing wrong with that except that gluten intolerance is a common cause of ecological disorders particularly coeliac disease, which is the outcome of wheat gluten sensitivity. In my experience, wheat is one of the highest maladaptive reacting substances, especially in evoking mental symptoms. I have produced full-blown psychosis with a test meal of gluten.

In brief, the vegetarian diet has much to commend it, but it is important that it remains a balanced diet, with as broad a food base as possible. The most extreme diets, such as fruitarianism, whose devotees eat a diet exclusively of fruit, rarely have much to commend them.

WHY SIMPLE FOODS AFFECT US BADLY ■

Once, not so very long ago, sitting down to a well-cooked meal was one of the simple pleasures of life. Today (assuming that the family even bothers to sit down to a meal together except possibly on Sundays), every meal can turn into a minefield for those 80 per cent of people who cannot be exposed to various foods, or chemicals in those foods, without reacting adversely to them.

Foods affect people badly for one of three reasons. Some people, a minority, have a conventional allergy, complete with elevated IgE antibodies, that produces a predictable reaction to the specific food-allergen (after it has been eaten once). Prawns and other crustaceans, fish and strawberries are among the foods that are commonly implicated.

A second group have what are called metabolic defects, which arise because of faulty metabolisation of a particular food, as with diabetics who cannot metabolise sugar properly. Metabolism involves both the breakdown of our food, which provides energy (called catabolism), and the manufacture of the complex molecules needed for growth and repair (anabolism).

It is the third group, however, which is by far the most common and includes all those foods that create problems of addiction and intolerance. It is this group that concerns the clinical ecologist. Medicine has never taken very seriously the notion that food or the ingredients in food may be one of the principal causes of illness. Those who have espoused the idea publicly have either been ridiculed and damned by their colleagues if they were doctors, or dismissed as ignorant and unscientific if they weren't. Even now, when there has never been a greater public awareness of the importance of diet, or a more profitable market for those offering new diets, orthodox medicine still views it as very peripheral in the overall business of making people well.

Yet the fact that we are largely the product of what we eat has been shown in countless studies. One of the forerunners of these was a famous demonstration of the relationship between diet, health and disease that was carried out in India in the early part of the century by Sir Robert McCarrison using rats. He placed the rats on the diet that was typical of the diet of the seven different districts of India, whose people he was studying. The health and physical characteristics of the people of each of these districts were quite distinctive, as were their diets. McCarrison a physician, ran his experiment for two years, which was the equivalent of fifty years in the life of a human. At the end of this time the rats, originally indistinguishable, revealed physical as well as health changes that mirrored those of the humans living on the same diets.

THE EFFECTS OF THE WESTERN DIET ■

It is well known that identical twins living in Japan, on a Japanese diet, have almost zero chance of getting cancer of the colon, which is almost exclusively a disease of Western societies. If one of those twins moves to Hawaii, however, and has a partially Japanese and partially American diet, the incidence of colon cancer rises. If that same twin moves on to the United States, and lives on an exclusively Western diet, the chances of contracting cancer of the colon become as great as for any native American. This same tendency has been found in Chinese who have moved to Americanised Taiwan, and Indians who have migrated to South Africa.

In East Africa a number of studies revealed that the diseases of civilisation were extremely rare in the indigenous population — or at least until the introduction of Western eating habits. Then obesity, hypertension and the whole gloomy litany of degenerative diseases began to appear. In one of these studies, conducted in both Kenya and Uganda, a reason was sought for the almost complete absence of high blood pressure in the native population, and for the fact that the blood pressure of the elderly was even lower than that of young adults, a complete reversal of the situation in the West. It was discovered that they rarely had access to salt and that their total daily intake ranged from only 1 to 4 grams, compared with up to 18 grams consumed by the average Westerner today. As consumption of salt goes up, so does the incidence of hypertension, or high blood pressure. The Africans who were studied, incidentally, used a salt substitute, which they obtained by burning plants that contained more potassium than sodium; even though they lived in the tropics and perspired freely, they never suffered from heat exhaustion.

Nearer to Australia, among the Polynesians, who inhabit the islands from Hawaii down to New Zealand and include the Tongans and Fijians, the development of obesity has reached alarming proportions on some of the islands which have adopted Western eating habits, and is often accompanied by adult-onset diabetes and hypertension. The Polynesians, and some other islanders, tend to become very obese and to develop a much higher incidence of diabetes than even Westerners on the same diet. The incidence ranges from almost three in every hundred among Samoan males to an astonishing 42 per cent in the tiny phosphate-rich republic of Nauru, on the equator. The Nauruans have mixed racial characteristics, but are dominantly Polynesian. Although they have the highest per capita income in the world (double that of Australia) or perhaps *because* of it (they can and do afford unhealthy and junk food), the life expectancy of their obese, diabetes-ridden males is worse than any on earth except that of the drought-ravaged Ethiopians.

In New Zealand, Polynesian Maori women, who have grown obese from Western eating habits (and compounded by their heavy smoking) have the highest coronary rate in the world, twice that encountered in European women. As well as the smoking, the main predisposing factor appears to be hypertension.

HOW OUR DIET CHANGED ▌

The main dietary changes that were introduced in Western societies, which paved the way for the development of all the degenerative diseases that plague us today, were a switch from complex carbohydrate, mainly vegetables, to refined carbohydrate; an increase in the cholesterol and animal fat content in the food that we eat; a fall in the dietary fibre; and a great increase in salt intake.

Overconsumption of fats, sugar, cholesterol, salt and alcohol, says the CSIRO's Division of Human Nutrition, is directly related to six out of every ten deaths in Australia.

Starting in the United States, like so many of the Western world's bad eating habits, the predilection for eating deep-fried foods compounded the problem. (Anyone concerned with the health of their families should put down this book at this very moment, head for the kitchen and consign the deep fat frier to the depths of the garbage bin: it is probably the most health-injurious piece of equipment in most modern homes.)

Recognising the dangers is one thing, but what is the ideal diet for humans? The short answer is the natural diet, as it is for any species on earth. But it is surprisingly difficult to know what our natural diet is.

If you want to find out what the natural diet of a wild animal is, you go to its habitat and observe what it eats. However, it is no longer possible, except perhaps for a few remote tribes in South America or New Guinea, to find any group of people on earth who have not been affected by civilisation and, inevitably, civilisation's dietary habits. Even such remote tribes are likely to have been touched by the fallout of pesticides and herbicides carried up to thousands of kilometres from the site of their spraying. So you have to make an educated guess at what such a diet would have been, and that guess would certainly be that it contained no refined food and, in particular, no refined carbohydrate.

THE MANY-SIDED CURSE OF REFINED CARBOHYDRATES ▌

By refined foods, we mean any food that we consume in a form that is different from its natural state, and this includes the entirely artificial foods that are not found in nature at all. Margarine, for example, is a totally contrived product, notwithstanding the fact that almost all margarines contain some milk (a trap for the milk sensitive who think that they are avoiding milk by eating margarine). It is a manufactured food, made by a complex chemical process from various vegetable fats and oils — normally liquid — to turn them into semi-solids.

It is the refined carbohydrates, sugar and flour, however, that have attracted the greatest opprobrium. In the past, from prehistoric times until little more than a century ago, the carbohydrate that people consumed was in the form of complex starch molecules. If sugar was used in a free form at all (as opposed to the sugar occurring naturally in fruits and other foods), it was a mixture of sucrose, glucose, lactose and fructose and other simple molecules. When flour (now the major source of starch in the Western diet) was eaten, it came complete with the bran and germ.

It was only for the sake of convenience, probably about 3000 BC, that people began to alter the form of these carbohydrates, grinding the grain into flour. Initially there was no harm in this, for the flour retained all its natural ingredients, including the fibre, so that it was just as beneficial as the raw grain. At about the same time, sugar began to be extracted commercially from sugar cane, and it was white. The notion arose that whiteness and fineness indicated not only improvement in the product as a source of nutrition, but status. Those whose flour was white and refined to the point where every ingredient was removed that did not enhance the appearance of the flour, had a certain social edge. (The ancient Egyptians prized white bread for the same reason, but at least theirs kept the germ.) It also, it must be admitted, kept better. Weevils have more sense than to try and live in white flour if there is any alternative.

Inevitably, the commercial appeal of these new products increased and so began the progressive destruction of all that was good in complex carbohydrate. It was probably, as one commentator has put it, the most significant, dangerous debasement ever to occur to our food supply.

In the course of manufacturing white sugar, all the fibre, minerals and vitamins are removed from the molasses, and finish up being fed to farm animals whose dieticians often show a great deal more sense than their colleagues in the field of human dietetics. The pigs grow healthy on it, while poor humans are left with nothing but the energy-rich, but otherwise nutritionally useless white sugar; and not only is it almost worthless from any dietary point of view, but it is an insidious and frequent trigger of disease and intolerance.

The price we pay for our concentrated white sugar and emasculated flour is obesity, high cholesterol, high acidity and a string of life-shortening, pain-inducing degenerative diseases. For the clinical ecologist, it is the cause of one of the most prevalent and harmful ecological disorders, hypoglycaemia, which ruins the lives of countless thousands of people and can be effectively treated only by the methods of clinical ecology (see Chapter 33).

FOOD PROCESSING — THE NECESSARY EVIL ▮

The ideal diet, in general terms, is one that is essentially un-processed, unrefined, free from artificial additives (which means colouring, preservatives, anti-oxidants, flavouring and so on), and which at the same time is as near to living as is possible and practical.

If you take a carrot, for example, and pull it out of the ground, it is progressively "less alive" from that moment. Once it has been taken out of the ground, you cannot put it back and make it keep on living. So the ideal time, nutritionally and nearly always as far as taste goes, to eat that carrot, or any other fruit or vegetable, is the moment it comes out of the ground or off the tree, provided, of course, it is ripe. At the other end of this spectrum, and about as far removed from the living state as you could imagine, is when the carrot turns up as hydrolised vegetable matter, an increasingly common component of pro-cessed foods, which is a process that has as its starting point the chemical decomposition of the vegetable.

For most of us, however, truly fresh foods are something we rarely encounter and eating them all the time is just not an option that we have. If we live in towns or cities, the most that we can hope for is a limited variety of fresh foods grown in our own or market gardens for a short period each year when they come in season. They have to be grown close enough to where we live to reach us before they begin to go off. If we relied exclusively on fresh food, we would be denied many tasty and nutritious fruits and vegetables. Those people living in the southern states of Aus-tralia would never have any of the marvellous tropical and sub-tropical fruits of Queensland. Melbourne folk would never see a banana except in pictures, and avocados would be as rare as truf-fles and certainly as expensive. Not only would our diets be very boring, but for most of us they would also be nutritionally de-ficient if we had to rely exclusively on foods grown sufficiently close to us to eat fresh. It is a myth that those people who have to eat a very narrow-based diet, such as the Eskimos whose natural diet is by necessity very high in oily fish, adapt and live healthily enough. In reality, the Eskimos suffer frequently from nutritional deficiency.

Our skill at processing foods allows them to remain viable and edible until they reach the table, and that may be weeks or even months after they have reached their peak of freshness. Freezing, drying and canning all allow this to happen. Processing makes food safe by destroying disease-causing micro-organisms like salmonella and clostridia, two common bacteria, which are potentially deadly. (The toxins produced by *Clostridium botulinum*, which causes botulism, are the most potent known poisons; and *Clostridium tetani* causes tetanus.) Processing also destroys fungi and natural toxins. As soon as foods have been harvested or slaughtered, they deteriorate rapidly because of what is known as autolytic decay as the tissue breaks down. It is autolytic decay that makes meat rot so quickly once an animal is dead, and the micro-organisms that multiply during this decaying process quickly render the food dangerous.

Processing also provides convenience. It is not so many years since conscientious wives spent hours each day slaving away in the kitchen to bring some variety to their diet. Modern processed convenience foods have freed them from many of those chores. Preservation also plays another important role in the household diet: it reduces wastage and therefore costs and it allows many foodstuffs to be grown in large quantities in ideal growing conditions, even if those are far removed from the consumer.

Milk is a good example. As late as the end of the last century, cows had to be kept in towns because there was no way of preventing the milk from souring unless it was delivered almost immediately to the customer. Today it would be all but impossible to find sufficient space in our major cities to keep the number of cows necessary to supply them with sufficient milk. Modern processing methods of pasteurisation and homogenisation, as well as the ability to preserve the cattle feed so that this in turn can be grown far from the cows, mean that dairy herds can be kept at almost any distance from the consumer and the food supply.

CHANGING THE APPEARANCE OF FOOD ▌

Processing does much more than keep food fresh for longer. By means of an array of chemicals, it can change the appearance, taste, shelf life and even the texture of foods. Improving — the industry's word, not mine — the appearance of food is commercially very important. We have clear expectations of how we expect food to look and if it doesn't match up to these expectations, we will not buy it. As in many cases the processing itself causes discolouration, it is frequently necessary to add synthetic colouring even to foods, such as peas, which one might reasonably think were the right colour to start with.

The extent to which we are influenced by the look of our food seems to be associated in part with the colour of natural foods that we are familiar with. That is why we hardly ever see blue food. Indeed many people are repelled by the idea of eating anything blue and even in children's sweets it is used very sparingly. Most of us who have been in hospital at any time will have experienced the depressing sight of white fish, white sauce, white potatoes and white ice-cream, all served up on white plates with a glass of milk in a white plastic cup. However well cooked it is, it is going to taste boring because it looks boring!

THE HIGH PRICE OF FOOD PROCESSING ■
Food processing may well be the lynchpin of modern eating habits, but it comes at a price. Because modern processing methods are almost inseparable from the use of synthetic chemical additives (more than 3500 of them are in use today worldwide), that price can be very high. Toxicologically, the great majority of these chemicals are harmless, and so far as intolerance is involved, most people are not affected by most of them. But most people *are* affected adversely by some of them and the challenge of clinical ecology is to identify which ones affect which people.

For the unsuspecting, food processing puts some strange things into simple foods. When you buy a packet of potato chips, you are getting a great deal more than a few cents' worth of potato solids. Even ignoring the fat in which they are deep-fried (and you would do well not to ignore it), there are residues of the antioxidants that prevented the cooking oil from turning rancid; the sulphur that stopped the potatoes turning brown after they were peeled; the copious quantities of salt that seem to be obligatory in chips; the synthetic flavourings that either reinforce a minute trace of natural flavouring (so that the words "natural flavouring" can be used prominently on the packet), or create the complete illusion that what you are eating is genuinely beef, bacon, prawn or cheese and vinegar. It is much cheaper to put in a chemical that smells like a prawn than to use real prawns. It is the chemicals in food processing that turn the family hotpot that grandmother used to make into the chemicalised brew, masquerading under the same name, that consists of stabilisers, emulsifiers, antifoaming agents, flavour enhancers, synthetic colours and who knows what else.

There is nothing inherently sinister about food processing as such. Processing is, after all, what we do to food in our own kitchens on a much smaller scale; and the standards of hygiene in the food factory are likely to be much higher than in most homes. It is equally nonsense to claim that all home cooking tastes better and is nutritionally better than all processed foods. Some people are terrible cooks and can almost boil the nutrients out of a boiled egg.

There are certainly losses of nutrients during food processing, wherever it takes place. Vitamin C and folic acid are unstable when they are heated in any circumstances, and all water-soluble vitamins (which include the B group and C) dissolve into the cooking water, with up to 70 per cent of vitamin C being lost. In the factory, these lost vitamins and nutrients can easily be replaced, in the home they rarely are.

The main problem areas with processed foods are that many of them contain excessive amounts of sugar, salt and fat; that consumers are duped by advertising into believing that foods are nutritious when they are manifestly not; and, most important from an ecological point of view, that many of the additives have become so commonplace in food that we are now eating them with the frequency and regularity that cause serious problems of intolerance.

CONVENIENCE FOODS — THE BILLION-DOLLAR INDUSTRY ■

Australians still have some way to go before they match the American experience, where the average family eats out or buys takeaway food for almost two meals out of three. The social consequences alone of never sitting down as a family to eat a meal (important because in most families, it is about the only occasion when the family comes together), are serious enough without the added problems of a diet that is increasingly composed of fat-fried, chemically tainted foods.

A convenience food, by definition, is any food that comes to the consumer in a more convenient form than if he were to buy the raw ingredients and make it himself. Even frozen peas are a convenience food in that it saves the customer having to pick and shell the peas, sort out the bad peas, and usually add mint to them. Convenience foods have to be prepared in such a way, whether they are single food items, or multi-product frozen dinners, that they look and smell just like (or better than) the natural product. Consumers would baulk if they opened a can of soup and found that all the ingredients had separated so that it looked like an unpleasant laboratory experiment, so antioxidants, emulsifiers and stabilisers have to be added to prevent this happening.

Colour, we have seen, is vitally important for consumer acceptance. That is why the very suspect chemical, alas, is sprayed on to apples to improve their colour, and why prawns are sprayed to make them pinker. It is why butchers and greengrocers put warm-coloured electric bulbs over their display areas and why vegetables often look much less appealing when you get them home than they did in the shop.

A whole new industry is developing that specialises in making foods taste and look like what they are not. The food processing industry has always been adept at taking cheap and plentiful foods and, by adding even cheaper natural and synthetic ingredients and chemicals, transforming them into "value added" products that are more profitable. But what is happening today goes far beyond that. Sometimes a simple chemical application is all that is needed, like the many "smoked" foods that have never been anywhere near smoke. They get their appearance (and usually their taste and smell) by being sprayed with chemicals.

One of the areas that is causing great concern is the increasing use of what are known as replacer ingredients. Whatever the finished product, many of them have a very small number of basic ingredients in common (soy is the miracle product of the age for the processors) and rely heavily on saturated fats. Our food base is growing ever smaller and that is nutritionally very undesirable.

We have imitation cheese made out of saturated and probably hydrogenated fat, while artificial colours and flavours give it something like the appearance of real cheese. Its low cost makes it appealing to fast food outlets like pizza bars. There are imitation tomatoes with absolutely no nutritional value apart from the calories in the sugar that makes up most of the product; and chemical tomato flavour-enhancers are a cheap alternative to the real thing. They allow manufacturers, as with potato chips, to get away with including a microscopic amount of real tomato because the chemicals provide the actual taste, while still being able to state legally that the product is "flavoured with real tomatoes".

Non-dairy creamers, which have none of the nutritional benefits of real milk and cream (for those who can tolerate cow's milk), have been introduced not only on airlines and in hotels and motels, but even in hospitals. They are relatively cheap and they last almost indefinitely, but they are not even a wholly safe alternative for people who cannot tolerate cow's milk: most of them contain a milk derivative to give them their white colour.

There is instant mashed potato that has nothing to do with potatoes and (mercifully still apparently only in the USA) even restructured baked potatoes. Inside is pretend mashed potato, reconstituted and with a great many additives and flavourings; while the skin is actually a waste product of peelings from potato canneries and from firms that peel potatoes for bulk sale to restaurants and hotels. These pieces of skin are then also reconstituted, stuck together with modified food starch, shaped until they are identical in size and weight, and sold to food outlets, which welcome them as an ingenious aid to portion control.

Fish sticks and crab sticks are reconstituted by being ground down to a fine mince and then extruded into their familiar shape after being flavoured, flavour-enhanced with monosodium glutamate, starched, salted, sugared and coloured. In this way, unsellable fish can be turned into a marketable and profitable product.

The Americans, ever ingenious, have turned out a 200 millimetre long reconstituted egg with a square end, again for restaurant and processing use. But even this is as nothing to the experiments being carried out in the United States by geneticists working in conjunction with the Kentucky Fried Chicken company. Because more people apparently want drumsticks than the company has drumsticks to sell, and fewer wings, the geneticists are working to produce a four-legged chicken. From past efforts, the chickens can take hope. Scientists earlier came to the conclusion that much of a chicken's energy goes into producing the protein needed to grow its feathers, so they developed a featherless chicken. This was easier than designing one with four legs, and it might have worked, except that the chickens became so nervous and neurotic, and developed so many pulmonary problems, that they began to shiver. And they shivered so much that they wasted more protein than they used growing feathers.

HIDING THE SLUDGE ■

Mechanically deboning meat has concerned health authorities since it first became technically feasible, mainly because it involves substantial amounts of bone being ground up and included with the meat. This is now widely practised, however, and at the end of the complex process, the meat comes out looking like an unpleasant slurry that is quite unacceptable as any kind of human food (or pet food for that matter, because dog and cat meats must look, smell and, for the fastidious owner, taste exactly like a similar product for humans).

By adding a protein to this sludge, however, the manufacturers can give it back much of the texture of normal meat. It has to be cooked quickly because of the risk of dangerous microorganisms in the finely ground bone and meat mixture; and then, when it has been "shaped", it is re-cooked and can be frozen and cooked yet again in safety by the consumer. This is a product that is particularly useful in convenience foods where the meat is partially camouflaged by sauces and gravy. The real concern is not the fact that very low quality meat can be passed off as an expensive cut, offensive as this may be to the few who discover what is going on. What is most worrying is the usually unacknowledged presence of all the chemicals that are needed to bring about this sleight of hand. (The only ingredients that need to be listed by law on the package are those included by the final processor: none of the chemicals need appear at all if they were put in by a company that *supplied* the final processor. Of course, because many of these foods are supplied to the fast-food industry and to restaurants, the consumer never knows anyway.)

PRODUCTS THAT MASQUERADE AS FOOD ■

The protein commonly used by processors absorbs and holds water and there is now a refinement to this, another synthetic substance called micro-crystalline cellulose (MCC), which, as well as absorbing and holding water, gives a pulpy texture. MCC is used as a filling in various bakery products that are normally filled with fruit or fruit jelly. They may have no fruit or jelly in them at all, but instead are made with the far cheaper MCC and are artificially fruit-flavoured and coloured. Consumers apparently rarely notice the difference.

No less worrying to those who cannot tolerate the chemicals

involved is a new material being put into certain so-called high-fibre breads, which consists of cellulose made from wood. It is just a refined form of wood pulp: loaves can now be made with cellulose replacing much of the far more expensive wheat. This fibre can also be used as a thickening agent in commercial soups, as a binder in sausages and an emulsifier in drinks as well as in many bakery products. It is a profitable by-product not of the food industry, but of paper manufacturing.

What is of concern with this product, as with so many phony foods, is that we have no idea whether the human body can handle fibre from cellulose in the way that it handles fibre from traditional sources such as fruit, vegetables and cereals. It may turn out to be harmless, but it may not: the trouble is that nobody knows and nobody knew when it was first put into food.

An even more unlikely source of a common food ingredient is the oil industry, which has now marketed a food yeast made on a substrate of petroleum by-products. Again the most profitable potential market is baking, although Amoco, the yeast manufacturers, expect to find many other outlets. As well as being exposed to petroleum in the environment, we are going to be eating it, as well; and because there is nothing to prevent it being legally labelled as a natural yeast, we will never know that it is there. Petroleum derivatives are already one of the most common causes of ecological illness.

Rich sauces are usually extremely high in sodium, or salt, just as many breakfast cereals could more accurately be described as sweets than nutritious foods. Many tinned products are high in sodium and have lost some of their potassium, two minerals which ought to be in ratio. There is a slight excess of potassium over sodium in the natural state, which processed foods should emulate. With some varieties of canned beans, for example, there is a loss of between 47 and 66 per cent of the potassium compared with the natural product, and an extraordinary 45,000 per cent increase in the sodium content!

Calcium and phosphorus are two other minerals that ought to be in balance in our systems but frequently are not, either because of processing, or because we have consumed too much Coca-Cola or other cola drinks (indeed many soft drinks) that are very high in phosphoric acid.

Now food scientists are experimenting with grinding chicken feathers to replace some of the flour in products like biscuits and cakes where they will not be noticed. It may not be what Shakespeare had in mind when he wrote of the slave who "gets him to rest, cramm'd with distressful bread", but he came very close to the mark if we are going to be fed bread containing petrol, wood cellulose and chicken feathers.

8 Doubtful Labels and Deceptive Advertising

The labelling and advertising of food is a constant source of frustration to anyone trying to avoid particular foods or food chemicals and to any doctor trying to treat food intolerance. Nobody can be expected to manage their food intake properly unless they are given all the information they need to make an informed decision, yet it is often very difficult to know what is in many of the things that we eat.

LABELLING REQUIREMENTS — THE CONSUMER'S RIGHT

Long overdue regulations, enforcing the listing of food additives (though not all of them, as we shall see) and requiring all ingredients to be shown on the label in descending order by volume, are a significant improvement on the former total absence of any information other than what was being used as a sales aid.

For years, manufacturers resisted giving any information on the specious and patronising grounds that consumers would not understand it. They argued this to the last, when they were being forced to show most of the chemicals in processed foods, insisting that giving the full chemical name (presumably implying that most consumers are incapable of reading and finding out the significance of words of more than two syllables), or simply the code number, would not help the consumer. The consumer, they argued, doesn't need to know that a product contains, say, butylated hydroxyanisole (code 320) because he or she won't know what it is or why it is there. But that isn't the point.

Apart from the fact that it ought to be the right of everyone of us to be able to identify, if we choose, all the ingredients in the food that we eat, we may know that specific chemicals cause intolerance or other problems. In the case of BHA, as butylated hydroxyanisole is known, which is used to delay rancidity and loss of flavour, we have a chemical food additive that is not tolerated by many people and that causes severe intolerance reactions in those who are susceptible to it. What is more, it should never be given to babies or young children, and it raises the cholesterol level of the blood.

If people know that they cannot tolerate it, or that they don't want their children to eat it, they have every right to know if they are unwittingly consuming it. As with nearly all additives, there is no way that any of the senses can detect its presence, at least until the symptoms begin. If it is listed by name or code number, those who want to avoid it *do* have the opportunity to do so in the food they consume in their own homes.

Food addiction and intolerance to food chemicals are so prevalent that there is no reason why the task of the consumers and their doctors should be made any more difficult than it already is. Manufacturers have for too long taken advantage of the public's naïve and misplaced trust in believing that because a substance is included in food, it must be entirely harmless or it wouldn't be there. If that were the case, we would never see a patient with food-chemical intolerance.

The requirement to list additives on labels does not cover all chemicals that go into food. It is still not necessary to list flavours, for example, a concession that was made after the manufacturers had successfully argued that their flavours were trade secrets. Protecting manufacturers from their competitors thus apparently became more important than protecting consumers from hidden ingredients: we know that many flavours are capable of causing severe intolerance reactions.

In Australia, ingredients need be listed only in decreasing order according to their volume in a processed food — the more of an ingredient there is, by weight, the higher up the list it must be shown. In the United States, the actual weight must also be shown on most foods, so that it is possible to know precisely how much of a substance is being consumed, as well as its presence in the first place. Listing the exact weight of a substance contained in a food has been bitterly resisted by Australian manufacturers (usually relying on the same argument that the information is misleading for the consumer).

Labelling requirements in Australia are such that only the final manufacturer must list the ingredients that it has added. If, for example, a manufacturer of baby foods buys ham from a supplier, and that ham arrives already treated with sodium nitrite, the presence of the sodium nitrite does not need to be shown on the label. For the mother trying to avoid giving her baby any chemicals or specifically sodium nitrite, her task is almost impossible.

Any additive that is even suspected of being harmful should be avoided. Appendix VIII shows the food additives that scientists suspect to be potentially harmful, usually on the basis of experiments with animals. Carry a list of them with their code numbers (often only this code is shown on the label) whenever you go shopping and make a point of refusing to buy any product that contains them.

No manufacturer has the right to put a chemical into a product if that chemical has been found to injure so much as one mouse in laboratory experiments. The common practice of waiting to see if the chemical has the same effect on humans, before withdrawing it, is outlandish. The food industry, however, mounts a very powerful lobby. Food processing constitutes the largest single sector of Australian manufacturing industry, accounting for nearly one in five of all manufacturing employees. Eight of the ten top-spending advertisers are corporations with food interests. Coca-Cola is so sure of its position in the marketplace that it has threatened to withdraw its product from an entire country rather than obey a government directive to reveal its secret formula. Coca-Cola's 12 per cent sugar content and its caffeine already make it a disastrous drink for most people. In addition, there is no way of knowing what else it contains that may lead to ecological illness.

FINDING OUT BY TRIAL AND ERROR ■
Reliable testing and unmasking can be very difficult when product ingredients change overnight, as they still can without any indication on the label. It is impossible to detect the difference by taste or appearance. This can happen, for example, with the listed ingredient "solid white vegetable shortening" in many processed foods. This shortening is a mixture of oils, but the oils vary, largely depending on their availability and price. It can happen that a patient intolerant of some vegetable oils, but able to eat others safely, finds a product that provokes no reaction. Then suddenly the patient begins reacting to the food. What may well have happened is that the manufacturer has introduced a new shortening, even though there is no change on the label.

If shortening is not labelled as being of vegetable origin, it usually comes from lard, which is rendered pork fat, but its source may also be beef or lamb fat. Many people are intolerant of one, but can safely consume the others. (In decreasing order of importance in food intolerance, pork is the worst offender, followed by beef, and then lamb.) Once again, the label is no help in steering such people towards products that contain their "safe" form of shortening. Almost all gelatin desserts, such as Gell-O, are also made from either pork or beef.

Vinegar on the label, when the source is not stated, means white grain vinegar. Those who are intolerant of wheat and yeast, as well as other grains and sugar may react to this. Malt vinegar, on the other hand, is made chiefly from barley with the addition of other grains such as corn and rice. Apple cider vinegar is free of both corn and wheat and is likely to affect only those who cannot tolerate apples. People with sensitivities to cereals ought to be able to identify from the label precisely which grain they are being invited to eat and not to have to find out by trial and error.

The non-dairy coffee whiteners are another example of confusion in labelling. To start with, as we have mentioned, it is usually a misnomer. Practically all coffee whiteners contain sodium caseinate to give them their whiteness, and sodium caseinate is a milk protein derivative. There is nothing on the label to indicate this to people who are trying to avoid milk products and who do not recognise casein for what it is. There should be no obligation on the manufacturer to spell out the significance of the ingredients listed, but there ought to be some restriction on using the description "non-dairy" on a product that includes a protein derived from cow's milk. Most manufacturers claim, or at least imply, that non-dairy whiteners are a dietary aid, when the truth is that most of them are 50 per cent sugar and 35 per cent fat, and weight for weight contain nearly twice as many kilojoules as cow's milk.

ADVERTISING'S MEANINGLESS WORDS ■

Most media advertising of foods, particularly on television, leaves a great deal to be desired. Try writing down the words of television food advertisements and then read them back, divorced from the pictures behind them. Most are worded at about the level of a slow-learning child of 10, and what little nutritional information given is worthless. Instead, there are meaningless words like healthy, natural, pure, nutritionally balanced and goodness. In the Newspeak of advertising, "natural" has even been used for cigarettes!

On children's television, the message is often even more offensive: most of the advertising is for nutritionally worthless junk foods, or foods that are heavy in fat like McDonalds products and potato chips, or laden with sugar like sweets. Parents have long complained that they are fighting a losing battle trying to inculcate some kind of food sense into their children, when they are simultaneously being exposed to television advertising that urges them to eat rubbish.

Attempts by the Sugar Board and the company that dominates the sugar industry in Australia, CSR, to sell the idea through its advertising that refined sugar is a natural, healthy product were correctly dismissed by the Australian Consumers Association as "a gross insult to the Australian community" (see Chapter 33).

DECEPTIVE PACKAGING ■

No amount of labelling can ever give the complete picture. What frozen dinner or packet of frozen vegetables mentions the pesticide and herbicide residues that are in virtually all commercial vegetables; or the hormones and broad-spectrum antibiotics in the beef dinners; or the tranquillisers and chemicals that speed up the rate of growth of chickens? All these will certainly be present in the packet along with the legitimate additives.

The pictures on labels can imply what the words are not allowed to say and fruit juices are a good example of this. A drink labelled "fruit juice" must not contain added water or more than 4 per cent sugar. "Fruit juice cordial", on the other hand, needs contain only 25 per cent fruit juice; while "fruit drink" has to have only 5 per cent fruit juice and the rest of the volume can be made up of water, sugar, artificial flavourings, preservatives and colours. All these must be included in the list of ingredients, but in all cases, the pictures on the labels may be identical, usually of the fruit itself.

The size of type can also give a false impression. One manufacturer produces an orange fruit juice cordial which is artificially coloured but carries a label depicting a fresh orange and, in large letters, the words "with vitamin C". It would hardly seem necessary to explain that one of the fruits that is richest in vitamin C actually contains it, but they are referring to the vitamin C that is added to replace all the vitamin C that has just been lost in the processing.

What is important about this product is that the hard-to-read small print states that the vitamin C level, at normal recommended dilution, is a minuscule 5 milligrams per 100 millilitres. An Australian Consumers Association test found only 2 milligrams per 100 millilitres, a quantity so small as to be almost irrelevant. In most cases this may not be of any consequence, but some parents who see the large lettering "with vitamin C" will certainly be induced to buy the product, believing that it will be nutritionally valuable to their children for that reason.

AVOIDING THE TRUTH ■

Rarely do labels stipulate whether sugar means cane sugar, beet sugar or corn sugar, yet it may be of vital importance to someone with certain sugar sensitivities to know which is present. Even with the purest sugar extract, there remains a very small amount of the parent substance, whether cane, beet or corn, but sufficient for the highly sensitive patient to react to it.

The word "unsweetened" on a label means only that no sweeteners have been added to the food during processing. The contents may already be high in natural sugars. And "no added sugar" is even more misleading because it refers only to sucrose. Any of the other sugars (and Americans claim to be able to describe sugar in seventy-one different ways for their labelling), such as fructose or glucose, may well have been added without needing to be listed on the label, or may be present naturally. The hypoglycaemic patient, in particular, needs to know what sugar is present, in any form, if he is on a strict low-sugar diet.

When several sugars are shown on the label, usually without the word "sugar" appearing at all, it is nearly always to hide the high sugar content. Shown only as "sugar", it might well mean that it has to appear at the top of the list of ingredients, which must be shown in decreasing order of volume. Broken down to sucrose, dextrose, fructose, lactose, maltose, corn syrup and many more, no one sugar is present in sufficient quantities to require it to be at, or even near, the top of the list. Consumers trying to shop for low-sugar foods can easily be confused.

The Beecham product, Ribena, a blackcurrant juice that is marketed as a healthy drink for children (in supermarkets it is often stacked with the baby foods, not the other fruit juices), is loaded with sugar, although marginally less than when the Australian Consumers Association reported that it contained more sugar than almost any other drink on the market. The potential harm that this excessively sweetened product is likely to cause to a child and its teeth must exceed any good that comes from the high vitamin C content (which isn't all that high anyway). Beechams no doubt argue that if mothers don't want to buy their children such a sweet drink, they have only to read the list of contents and they will see sugar listed as the first and therefore the most voluminous ingredient.

That alone certainly ought to make any caring mother put the Ribena straight back on the shelf, but it isn't quite as simple as Beechams imply. The first item listed is not "sugar" but "sucrose" and although this is strictly correct and although many people understand that sucrose is sugar, there are many others who certainly do not. Why cannot it just be listed as "sugar", which everybody understands? It is information that should not be denied consumers simply because their education does not allow them to understand that sucrose is synonymous with sugar.

PICTURES THAT DO NOT TELL THE WHOLE STORY ■

There are many people, of course, who hardly glance at the label and when they do, it is usually only to satisfy themselves that the picture on the front looks appetising. If they looked more carefully, they might be surprised that the modest-looking piece of fish in the photograph, for example, isn't all that they are buying. As a very typical example, there is a popular brand of frozen fish that comes with a white sauce, or as the blurb on the packet puts it, "tasty fish fillets with a delicious white sauce". Now anyone buying this might reasonably expect to get tasty fish fillets with a modest, but adequate, amount of the delicious white sauce to put over it.

In reality, a closer inspection of the fine print on the label reveals that the white sauce consists of 50 per cent by weight of the entire package, and that this innocuous sounding addition to the meal turns out to consist of skim milk powder, modified food starch, spices and colouring, salt, onion powder, bleached white flour, butter, natural flavour, monosodium glutamate (MSG), sugar, garlic powder, cooked lobster (a very modest amount of that), dextrin, dehydrated carrots, dehydrated onions, dehydrated tomatoes, yeast, dehydrated parsley, disodium inosinate (a flavour enhancer, specifically prohibited in or on foods made specially for babies and young children, though this fact is not mentioned on the label) and disodium guanylate (which is another flavour enhancer, also prohibited in or on food intended for babies and young children).

What a Pandora's box for anyone food or chemically hypersensitive! One can understand that a warning label on a packet of tasty fish fillets, to the effect that it contains chemicals that may be dangerous to babies and small children, would not exactly be the ideal sales aid; but the public ought to be informed that seemingly simple and safe foods may not be simple at all and decidedly harmful to anyone intolerant of them. Just reading the labels carefully, and owning a comprehensive additive code breaker that explains what the additives do and sets out any known adverse effects are probably the two most valuable steps that anyone regularly buying groceries can take.

9 The Chemicals in Our Food

SOME NATURAL HAZARDS AND UNEXPECTED CHEMICALS ▮

Dr John Knowles, the president of the Rockefeller Foundation in the United States, observed wisely that "over 99 per cent of us are born healthy and made sick as a result of personal misbehaviour and environmental conditions".

Personal misbehaviour is usually outside the responsibility of doctors and the best we can do is try to counsel those patients who are making themselves ill by the lifestyle they have chosen. Anyone who chooses to endanger himself and his family (and women are just as guilty as men), no matter whether by smoking, promiscuity, or in any other way, is usually well aware of the risks he or she is taking. Such people may argue passionately that they are in the grip of something too big or too addictive or even too enjoyable for them to control, but in the end, the solution lies in their own hands, not in a doctor's rooms.

But this is certainly not the case for the majority of the victims of intolerance caused by the hidden ingredients in food. More often than not, they are undetectable by any of the senses, and if you can't see them, touch them, hear them, smell them, or taste them, what possibility is there of avoiding them? Chemically, there is little difference between natural and artificial substances which perform the same role in food: in fact synthetic chemicals are probably purer. Both can cause adverse reactions in sensitive people if sufficient quantity is consumed.

The Troublesome Salicylates   Benzoates, amines and salicylates are all chemicals that are both manufactured and occur naturally. Benzoates and amines are closely related natural chemicals, with many medicinal and other uses; but it is salicylates that cause the most problems. As well as being a large family of benzene-related chemicals occurring naturally in most plants, they are also produced synthetically, and aspirin is probably the best known member of the family.

All salicylates, whether natural or synthetic, are a frequent cause of trouble for those who are intolerant of them, and there are very many who are. Ben Feingold's early treatment of hyperactivity in children, for instance, was designed specifically to exclude natural salicylates, as well as artificial flavourings and colours, and his concern was justified.

Most fruits, especially berries and dried druits, contain salicylates, with raisins and prunes containing the highest amounts, as demonstrated by a comprehensive survey conducted recently by the Human Nutrition Unit at the University of Sydney. As a rough but quite accurate guide, fruits with a less sharp flavour, such as pears, pawpaws and mangos, are often low in salicylates compared with, say, oranges, berries and pineapples. The one exception to this is that pears (like carrots) appear to have significant amounts of salicylate in the skin.

Salicylate content in vegetables varies widely, ranging from negligible amounts in celery, lettuce and cabbage, to top-scoring gherkins. Potatoes that have been peeled are free of salicylates, but the peel contains significant amounts, which probably explains why some patients can eat mashed potatoes without ill effects and then suffer after a meal that includes potatoes baked in their jackets. Fresh tomatoes (which, of course, are a fruit, not a vegetable) are low in salicylates, but most tomato products are high in them — whether as canned whole tomatoes, tomato sauce, tomato paste or tomato soup. This is probably because very ripe tomatoes are used, these are very concentrated foods, and particularly because many herbs and spices are added for flavouring.

Many herbs and spices contain extremely high levels of salicylates. Curry powder, for instance, has 218 milligrams per 100 grams (compared with say 4.4 milligrams per 100 grams for raspberries, which is itself considered to be high). Admittedly the amount of curry powder that is likely to be eaten is very small, but it is the total intake each day that matters.

Some coffees have very significant levels of salicylates. International Roast, Maxwell House Instant, Moccona Instant and Nescafe Instant in particular should be avoided by anyone sensitive to salicylates. (Andronicus Instant was found to be completely free of all salicylates.)

Salicylates are important in ecological illness, not only because so many people are sensitive to even the smallest traces of them and they are so ubiquitous, but because they appear in foods that are frequently thought of as "safe" when an exclusion diet is being worked out.

Other Natural Additives Other widely used natural additives include the food acids, such as citric, acetic and malic acids. They are used for flavouring and as aids in various manufacturing processes, such as setting jams and sometimes as a preservative. Foods are often fortified or "enriched" with nutrients, either as a sales aid, or to replace similar nutrients lost during processing. Margarine, for example, frequently includes added vitamins A and B, while flour, bread and some breakfast cereals receive a boost of various B vitamins.

Natural foods are often incorporated in processed foods, sometimes as a vehicle for other additives. Common among these are eggs, cow's milk, pork (including lard), beef (including shortening), yeast, corn, wheat, soy and peanuts. They may not appear on the list of ingredients if they were added at some stage before the final processing, or of course if the food is unwrapped, like some bread.

If the manufacturer purchases food colour in a milk powder base and doesn't actually add the milk, it is again under no obligation to list milk in the ingredients, yet for the milk intolerant person it makes not the slightest difference at what stage the milk enters the food. Such a person just needs to be told that the milk is present, especially when there is no visible means of detecting it.

Some processing involves foods being exposed to chemicals which are not strictly food additives. Rather it is their residues that cause the damage. Among these are the foods that are exposed to gas, usually ethylene gas, which is a petroleum derivative. Even minute traces of it will affect the many petroleum-sensitive people. Most bananas are artificially ripened in this way, particularly when they are sold far from the place where they are grown. They are picked green so that they can be transported before they rot, and are then artificially ripened by exposure to ethylene gas which destroys the green chlorophyll that identifies an unripe banana. This happens immediately before the bananas are distributed to the markets, so that if they are bought and eaten very soon after the gassing takes place, the ethylene content will be high and the fruit will be less tolerated by anyone susceptible.

This probably explains why some petroleum-sensitive people are sometimes able to eat bananas that have been gas-ripened, and sometimes not. They come to the wrong conclusion that gas-ripened fruit is therefore not the cause of any of their symptoms. Gas-ripened bananas can be detected quite easily. The naturally ripened fruit have black seeds and tend to have small, specked spots on the skin, in contrast to the gassed fruit which has immature white seeds and large blackened areas on the skin at places where they were bruised during handling or shipping.

To a lesser extent, tomatoes, apples, oranges and pears are all sometimes exposed to ethylene gas to speed up ripening. Coffee is also often gas roasted and the process of clarifying sugar involves gas liquid flame.

In his classic *Food for Naught*, Ross Hume Hall told an awful story of another way in which a chemical residue can be left behind in a food when it was not put there intentionally as an additive. The US Department of Agriculture was asked to help solve the problem of frozen chips that didn't taste or feel as good when they were baked in the oven (a commercially important method of cooking for a convenience food), as when they were deep-fried. The solution it came up with was at least novel. It found that by dipping the fresh-cut chips in a bath of freon 12 at about $-30°C$ ($-21°F$), then leaching them in warm water to remove as many of the sugars and soluble constituents as possible and finally frying them in oil, they could deliver them frozen to the retailer, looking and feeling like the ideal chip. The main weakness in the process is that freon 12 is almost identical chemically to a widely used dry-cleaning fluid and most health authorities stop short of recommending that food be prepared in dry-cleaning fluid, whatever the justification.

The two sure things about this bizarre adulteration of a widely bought frozen food is that neither leaching, frying nor freezing will totally remove the freon 12; and that no mention of its possible presence will ever be disclosed to the customer by the manufacturer.

FOOD PROCESSING ▮

Food processing dates back thousands of years. Butter is mentioned several times in the Bible (a processed food because it is not a natural product: cows don't make butter), and the Egyptians were brewing beer in 1500 BC and knew how to make raised bread. Even the use of chemicals in processing can be traced back to at least 1000 BC, when sodium nitrite was being used as a preservative.

But for all this early experience, it was not until as recently as the years immediately following the Second World War that processing as we know it, and particularly the widespread use of chemicals in food, came into its own. It is no coincidence that the prevalence of ecological disorders has soared in that time, nor that these disorders become increasingly more common as the chemicalisation of our food supply grows more pervasive and more complex.

Many food products would not exist at all without chemical additives: ham would be just salt pork without sodium nitrite, and most soft drinks would be nothing more than water without their chemical sweeteners, flavourings, colourings and preservatives. The further we get away from a natural product, the less likely we are to become adapted to it and the more likely it is to cause problems of intolerance. Sir Richard Doll, Regius Professor of Medicine at Oxford University, who was among the first to establish the link between cigarette smoking and cancer, has estimated that various components in our diet account for about 35 per cent of all deaths from cancer; and that food additives on their own are responsible for 1 per cent of all cancer deaths. And that is the very tip of the iceberg, taking no account of all the damage that is wrought through other diseases because of what we have chosen to do to our food and our environment.

ADDITIVES AND CONTAMINANTS ■

If chemicals are in food by design, they are called additives; if they get there "by accident", they are said to be contaminants. To call them an accident, however, is to go along with the Newspeak of the food processing industry, because they are very seldom there accidentally, if by that we mean by pure mischance. Almost invariably, what the industry and health authorities call contaminants are the residue of everything chemical that has come into contact with the food before it actually arrives at the factory of the final manufacturer, or in the shop if it is sold in its natural form, such as fruit and vegetables.

As an example, more than 21 per cent of sheep kidneys

tested in an Australia-wide residue survey in 1987 contained excessive levels of cadmium, a toxic heavy metal. Cadmium is a cumulative poison which replaces zinc, an essential body element. Its effects, when it is present in excess, can include interference in the development of the foetus, bone damage and certain forms of arthritis. Its half-life in the body is up to thirty years.

It is a very difficult impurity to avoid in Australia. It occurs in superphosphate fertilisers, particularly superphosphate manufactured from phosphate mined on the Pacific island of Nauru which supplies much of Australia's requirements. Probably the only safeguard that can be taken is to have much more stringent checking procedures to eliminate any meat which contains excessive levels of cadmium as well as other heavy metals and unacceptable herbicides or insecticides. That would be very expensive.

The most disturbing examples of contaminants are the numerous pesticide sprayings that most grown foods are subjected to. For the baker, the pesticide residues that come in the wheat he buys are "accidental" as far as he is concerned, and are therefore contaminants: the chemicals that he himself puts in to enhance the appearance, taste, shelf life and colour of his products are the additives. For the customer, it doesn't make the slightest difference how they get there.

Almost no pesticide can be removed from a food that has been treated with it, no matter whether by washing, rubbing, peeling and sometimes even boiling. Residues of every spraying remain and will be eaten by the consumer. Statistics say that the average Australian consumes as much as 2 kilograms of food additives a year, an enormous quantity if you picture it as a heap of chemicals piled up on a plate. The true figure is probably much higher: research in Britain has shown that the average additive consumption in that country is between 3 and 7 kilograms, with some people eating and drinking up to 15 kilograms annually!

Most of these food chemicals have been introduced without any real understanding of the effect that they will have on the human system. The director of the British Industrial Biological Research Association put it very succinctly when he observed that "food additive toxicology is not a science which seeks to understand the biological effects of chemicals upon humans, but merely a technology designed to produce animal test data sufficient to gain permission from governments for the use of the additives". In other words, if an additive is fed to white mice and rats and they don't die from cancer or give birth to deformed young, it moves quickly on to the market.

In fact, the situation is even worse than that. Just getting a single additive up to a standard acceptable to the European Economic Community authorities (the starting point for Australian Standards) can cost $750,000 and take three years, and unless manufacturers are looking for pan-European trade, they often don't bother. In the United States the position is just as bad. Most of the testing is done in commercial laboratories and, as we shall see when we are looking at the havoc wrought by environmental chemicals on our health, those results can be manipulated and falsified. One of the largest chemical testing laboratories in the world, Industrial Bio-Test Laboratories, was found guilty of giving its manufacturing clients (including some of the biggest multinationals) fraudulent figures to allow them to get products on to the market quickly.

Remember that Australia, like almost all relatively small nations without the highly sophisticated testing equipment and finance needed for this work, relies heavily on foreign research. Nobody knows how many chemicals are improperly and unsafely being sold and used in Australia on the strength of false Industrial Bio-Test data, for instance: the company suffered an unfortunate fire that destroyed its records on the night before the police moved in.

Exactly how these artificially synthesised molecules, which are put into our food and drink, come to be approved is a mystery to many experts, let alone to the layperson. If a new ethical drug (a prescription drug) is introduced on to the market, the toxicological studies have to be carried out over many years. The drug has to be given to animals and the animals have to be monitored for years and then killed to ensure that there is no disease state that has resulted from the drug. Then the drug must be tested on humans over a further period of years.

Even with these precautions, drugs with a horrendous list of unpleasant and even potentially fatal side effects can be allowed on to the market, as we have seen with amitriptyline (p. 8), so long as those side effects do not include cancer or deformed births. But at least the information is available to someone, somewhere. That certainly is not the case with the vast majority of the 3500 and more food chemicals that exist. And none of the regulations concern themselves with the possibility that a new

BUYING FROM HEALTH FOOD SHOPS

In general, the proliferation of health food shops in recent years (their number has increased by at least 500 per cent in ten years in Australia, and much more in other countries) must be a positive trend towards improved health. My advice is always to use organically grown foods whenever that is an affordable option. However, don't assume that because you buy something in a health food shop, it is untainted by chemicals. In particular don't assume that it will always be free from any risk of intolerance. As we have seen, it doesn't matter what the food is: if it is consumed sufficiently often, it can result in maladaptation reactions and intolerance.

Many "organic" farms still use herbicides, pesticides and fumigants on their products (and indeed may be ordered to do so by local or health authorities). Even if they escape having to use such chemicals themselves, their products may be affected if their property is within range of other places being sprayed for noxious weeds, for instance, particularly if the spraying is carried out from the air. They may also be using water that has been contaminated with chemicals.

Many herbs that are bought from health food stores, as well as most herbal remedies, also contain concentrated plant chemicals, which are as capable of producing side effects in anyone who is sensitive to them as any synthesised chemical. This does not mean that these herbs should be avoided, but that they shouldn't be dismissed as a potential cause of intolerance simply because they are herbal.

chemical substance might be responsible for any of the physical, mental and emotional disabilities and symptoms brought on by intolerance of them.

THE FALLACY OF "SAFE" CHEMICALS ■
Alarming as the quantity of chemicals is that we consume each year, it is rarely sufficient for any one of them to be considered by toxicologists as a threat to health. But then very few toxicologists are concerned with environmental diseases, or with the effect of even minute traces of chemicals on susceptible people.

Human epidemiological studies to establish the toxicity of

food additives prove nothing. (Epidemiologists specialise in establishing the incidence and likely cause of diseases in a community, such as a high rate of birth defects in regions that have been heavily sprayed with pesticides.) Tobacco smoking kills an appalling number of its lifetime users and maims even more, but it took about twenty-five years for epidemiologists to demonstrate this fact. The tobacco industry, however, can still produce its own epidemiological studies to show that everyone else in the world, except the tobacco industry, is wrong. But then it can even produce doctors willing to state publicly that smoking is good for you.

Even if only a small number of food chemicals are in use in a country (Australia has about 200 that have been approved and many more that do not have to be registered, notably the flavourings, which are considered to be trade secrets and so exempt from any control), the possible permutations when they are used in combination with other chemicals, as they usually are, and with foods are so numerous that the task of the epidemiologist is almost impossible. Sometimes there are more than thirty different additives in a single product. Potatoes alone have about 150 natural chemicals in them! All in all, the quantities of a specific chemical in a specific food are likely to be so minute, and the possible permutations so numerous, that no laboratory or mathematical experimentation is ever likely to prove anything conclusive.

Clinical ecologists know that individual chemicals are involved, because they test for them. They suspect them and then deliberately exclude them. If exclusion results in the illnesses or symptoms going away, and reintroduction brings them back, and if these results can be repeated over and over again (even when the patient has no idea what he is being tested for) then it is obvious that this particular substance is at least one cause of the symptoms.

Illness and symptoms can just as easily result from a small amount of many different foods and chemicals, or from a lot of only a few foods and chemicals; or even from a combination of a food or a chemical and another quite unrelated stressor, such as a virus, money worries or losing a job. We also know that any unnatural substance that we ingest or inhale is a stressor, prompting a reaction from the immune system.

Many patients do not react positively to individual chemical tests, but are still intensely chemically sensitive, simply because of the cumulative effect of a number of chemicals, or food-and-chemical combinations, to each of which they are *slightly* intolerant. I have a patient, for instance, who loves wine and drinks it with every evening meal. There is never any problem, except when he eats with a friend who has a dog, when he immediately begins to wheeze alarmingly. Normally animal dander has no effect on him either.

His trouble is that he is mildly intolerant of both wine and dander, and this intolerance is so mild that, except after fasting and testing, he is not aware of it. Only when he comes in contact with both the dander and the wine simultaneously is a quite serious reaction triggered. This synergistic effect is common, though often very difficult to identify. As every asthma sufferer knows, an emotional upset can set off an attack, even though the root cause of asthma remains organic.

SUSPECT TESTS ■

We tend to give misplaced credence to formal testing that is given a scientific imprimatur (and I don't mean the out-and-out fraud of companies like Industrial Bio-Test). Even when *in vitro* culture tests can identify something as serious as mutagenic effects, for example (meaning something that can cause mutation in an unborn child), this is far less significant than most people imagine. As the *New Scientist* pointed out in a recent timely warning, "They can at most detect a subset of a subset of cancer-causing chemicals and are irrelevant to all other toxic hazards".

In the toxicity tests on animals, on which food additive regulations are almost exclusively based (when they are carried out at all), the failure rate is very high. David Salsburg, of Pfizer Central Research in the United States, has suggested that animal tests are only 37 per cent successful in identifying the presence of carcinogens. Many of them are identified only after the substance has been allowed on to the market.

Thalidomide was subjected to numerous tests, although it was not specifically tested for its teratogenicity (its ability to cause birth defects), and none of them revealed its true danger. Only later, long after the product was being marketed around the world, was the full horror discovered of what it did to the children of many of the mothers who used it as a tranquilliser. Even then, as we now know, some manufacturers continued to market it long after this discovery, milking it of the last dollar before it was eventually banished from all European markets. It is still widely available today, without any warnings, in a number of Third World Asian nations that have not formally banned it, naïvely relying on the foreign companies that market it to safeguard the users.

If Salsburg's figures are correct — and his analysis seems to be very thorough — it means that results of animal tests are statistically wrong more often than they are right. In fact this is significantly worse than tossing a coin! The widest disagreement is in how to extrapolate from the results of tests on small laboratory animals in small groups to human beings in large groups who do not live in anything remotely approximating laboratory conditions. There are at least twelve accepted ways of going about this and the results of each may vary wildly.

I have long since come to the conclusion that from a clinical point of view — which means from the point of view of my patients — there is simply too much suffering in the community, too many illnesses and disabling symptoms that I can relieve by adopting an ecological approach to medicine, for me to worry about the purity of my science. I dream about the day when every doctor accepts the value of clinical ecology, just as every patient will understand the link between foods and chemicals, and their symptoms. If that day comes — as it will, though I am sure not in my lifetime — the indiscriminate use of chemicals in our food supply will be treated with a very healthy suspicion. At present that is almost non-existent because of the ignorance of most consumers about even the presence of chemicals in food, let alone their hazards.

AUSTRALIAN STANDARDS ■

Before looking at food additives in detail, let us look at the standards that apply in Australia. Unlike most other countries, all additives in Australia have to be approved before they can be used in food (except for a long list of exclusions, including the flavourings of which there are many hundreds). Elsewhere, the general rule is that an additive may be used, provided it does *not* appear on a banned list. The United States and the European Economic Community (EEC) countries are particularly reticent about banning additives that seem to be harmless only on the grounds of lack of long-term proof. The EEC even has a special category for additives that are permitted to be used pending further investigation!

Some countries are very strict in certain regards, slack in others. The French, for example, ban artificial colouring agents in all canned vegetables (which is why canned French petits pois are sometimes an anaemic pastel colour as a result of the canning process, though they taste good). On the other hand, the French are very lax about allowing almost any chemicalised foods into the country from outside.

The Australian system is an improvement on that of most other countries and its weakness is mainly in the level of enforcement that the government can bring to bear, particularly with imported foods. The legislation in Australia works on the premise that additives should be permitted only when their use is essential and when their safety in use has been established. It is an admirable goal, except that any manufacturer can put up a case for an additive being essential. In addition, the whole methodology for determining whether a substance is safe is suspect to start with.

THE ODD CASE OF THE BRITISH KIPPER ■

One example of how foreign foods can come into Australia unchecked, even when they contain chemical additives that are highly suspect, will make the point that enforcement falls far behind the letter and the spirit of the law. There was a time when the British kipper was made by leaving it for long hours in a smokehouse. Today, the filleted herrings are salted in less time than it takes to catch them and the smoky flavour, together with a good deal of the colour, comes from chemicals. In particular, most British kippers (almost all the kippers sold in Australia come from Britain) are coloured with the brown colouring agent, brown FK (code E154). This colouring agent is banned throughout Europe except in Britain, where its use in the highly profitable kipper business has allowed the kipper lobby to secure an apparently indefinite reprieve for it. In most cases, a ban in continental Europe would swiftly ensure that the British (or any other country flaunting common safety requirements) came into line; but the French and other Europeans look on kippers as one of the more unpleasant British eccentricities and since they import very few of them they don't trouble about it.

Unfortunately, the British do have a very lucrative export

market for kippers to all those countries where there is a strong showing of Anglo-Saxons and Gaels who can become quite emotional at the first whiff of a grilling kipper, and Australia is not left out. Again though, kippers slip through the net. Because nobody makes kippers in Australia and local smoked fish, such as tailor, are produced in very small quantities by the traditional smokehouse method, no application to use brown FK has ever been made to the National Health and Medical Research Council, which oversees the use of additives. Consequently, because of the Australian rule that an additive is banned until it has been specifically approved, brown FK is a forbidden product here. (The "E" prefix in the code number E154 signifies that it is on the EEC list, which was the basis of the Australian listing, but has not been approved in Australia.)

That should mean that not one kipper is allowed into Australia, but a quick glance at any supermarket shelf will confirm that the country is knee-deep in them. Why? Because, says the Federal Department of Health, kippers come in by the container load. This makes them the responsibility of the Customs Department, which insists that it has enough to cope with already, without becoming involved in the colour of kippers. What is more, the Commonwealth Health Department concedes that it would be physically impossible to check every single imported consignment.

The simple answer, to make anyone selling kippers responsible, seems to have occurred to nobody. And is it worth the effort? It most definitely is worth the effort. Research has proved that not one, but two of the constituent chemicals in kippers cause genetic mutation. It seems a high price to pay for the continued pleasure of having kippers for breakfast.

10 Tracking Down the Additives

Food additives are so important in ecological illness that we need to look at them in detail. Their purpose is varied but quite clear. They are chemicals that are introduced by manufacturers into food products either to make them more appealing to the consumer, and therefore more marketable; or to extend their shelf life; or to assist in the actual processing. Either singly, or much more often, combined with other chemicals, they are present in virtually all processed foods, which means anything in a tin, a packet or a bottle, in most dairy products and probably everything produced by bakeries or that is deep-frozen. For most people, on a conventional diet, this means that they can never get away from food and drink chemicals. Knowing that up to 80 per cent of the population cannot tolerate one or more of these substances without suffering an unpleasant reaction, we can see how every family in the land is likely to be adversely affected by them.

Additives can be conveniently grouped into five categories, depending on their purpose:

1. *Nutritional supplements*
2. *Preservatives* — including anti-oxidants, sequestrants and fumigants (irradiation is a preservative and is dealt with separately)
3. *Aesthetic agents* — the chemicals that are put there to make the product more appealing to the customer, including colours, flavours, sweeteners, enzymes, acidulants, alkalis and buffers
4. *Texturisers and stabilisers* — which generally keep the product looking palatable after processing and include emulsifiers, humectants, thickeners, surface-active agents, foaming agents and gums
5. *Processing agents* — including aerators, solvents, propellants, anti-caking agents, curing agents, leavening and drying agents, lubricants and dough strengtheners.

1. NUTRITIONAL SUPPLEMENTS ■

Many processed foods have added vitamins and minerals, often to replace those lost in the processing itself. Vitamins A, B_1, B_2, B_3, B_5, B_6 and B_{12}, as well as the minerals calcium, iron and phosphorus are the most commonly used. Some, for example the B group if they have been derived from yeast, can be troublesome to those who are intolerant of yeast.

2. PRESERVATIVES ■

Of all the food additives, preservatives can stake the most compelling justification for existing. We have already seen that in economic terms and as a means of ensuring that we have a much broader food base than would otherwise be possible, preservatives play a vital role in our diets. That they extend the life of most commercial foods and so have obvious consumer value is clear enough. They also appear to extend the shelf life of human corpses, which strongly suggests that we still have a great deal to learn about their persistence and the full long-term implications of their permanent presence in our bodies, quite apart from the ecological sickness that we know they cause.

Drying is an old and effective way of preserving food. Once, it was done in the sun or over a fire and by smoking, but today's modern methods, such as freeze-drying, remove all the water much more effectively and eliminate many of the dangers of bacteria. Freezing removes available water, without which bacteria cannot grow, and inhibits the autolytic enzymes that make a dead animal rot.

Nitrates and Nitrites   Nitrate has been used to preserve meat since at least Roman times. It changes rapidly to nitrite, which is the form that inhibits the growth of many bacteria, including *Clostridium botulinum*, the bacterium responsible for the lethal form of food poisoning known as botulism. With the introduction of canning technology in the nineteenth century, nitrate became indispensable because even today as many as one in twenty animals that are slaughtered carry *botulinus* spores, which then thrive in the ideal environment of the airless, sealed tin.

Since 1899, when it was found that nitrate's active constituent is actually nitrite, this is the form that has been extensively used, rather than the unrefined nitrate. By far its most important use is in protecting meat, but it is also widely used in curing hams and bacon. It is the nitrite that gives bacon and corned beef their characteristic pink colour.

Nobody suspected that nitrite might also have a black side in addition to its long-proven benefits. It was not until the 1950s that American researchers began looking much more closely at the substances that were being added to food, and one of the first chemicals they closed in on was nitrite. What they found was alarming: this unsuspected workhorse, which had been used for at least 1500 years, was capable of combining with amines — natural substances found in many foods and wine and produced in the human body — to form nitrosamines, which are a potent poison.

That was only the beginning. In the early 1960s, British researchers injected nitrosamines into rats and found that they had produced "one-shot carcinogens", capable of producing tumours after only a single exposure. From this came the long-remembered scare story that your morning bacon, eggs and coffee can give you stomach cancer. The theory (which was never substantiated by the research) was that the nitrite in the bacon might combine with the amines in the coffee, to produce the deadly nitrosamines. It is at least theoretically possible.

By 1969, even the American Meat Institute was warning that nitrites might form nitrosamines in cured meat. Later research showed that nitrites have been implicated in nausea and vomiting, dizziness and headaches, low blood pressure and collapse of the circulatory system. In sausages, they have been responsible for triggering asthma, and they are legally banned in Australia in foods that are specifically made for babies and young children. This ban does not, of course, prevent them from ingesting it in foods that are not specifically marketed for the very young. *The Lancet*, ever conservative, warned as far back as 1968 of "the gravest concern" about the presence of nitrites.

Yet nitrites are still being used and there is no indication that they will be outlawed, despite the increasing evidence that people who eat food containing a lot of nitrites may have a greater than even chance of developing cancer of the stomach or the oesophagus. The reason is very simple: nitrite may not be the only preservative that gives fool-proof protection against botulism, but it is certainly the cheapest. The food manufacturing industry argues very forcefully that the community is much better off avoiding certain death from botulism, rather than the still debated and certainly infrequent likelihood of death from nitrosamine-caused stomach cancer. The other illnesses associated with nitrites, they say, are not terminal and therefore of no significance compared with the danger of botulism. And that encapsulates much of the food additive debate.

Sulphur Dioxide and Sulphites Sulphur dioxide's history as a food preservative is as long as that of nitrite. The ancient Egyptians used the fumes of burning sulphur to sterilise their wine vessels and the Romans adopted the practice. It has been used ever since, right up to the present day, as an effective, cheap and convenient food preservative, with much wider application than nitrite. It has also been directly blamed for at least four deaths, acute mental and physical symptoms and a host of other very unpleasant disorders. What, then, is the truth about this substance that many would choose to see relegated to the one use of sodium sulphite that does not provoke bitter argument — that of fixing photographs?

Sulphites and metabisulphites are converted to sulphur dioxide, which is the active agent. It is permitted in a great variety of foods, in concentrations that range from 29 milligrams per kilogram in some beers, to 3000 milligrams per kilogram in some dried fruits. Since the dangers of sulphur dioxide became known, no safe level has been determined.

In spite of its age as a preservative, there is remarkably little known about sulphur dioxide, including the mechanism by which it works as a preservative. Free sulphite is believed to be the form that is responsible for the preservative action, even though total sulphite is specified in most food additive legislation.

It is an effective inhibitor of browning and prevents the familiar browning of fruit and vegetables after they have been peeled. That is why some people can eat hot chips at home, but react violently to them in a restaurant. It is almost universally used for this purpose in restaurants and takeaway outlets, by processors who handle potatoes and other vegetables that tend to brown, and on salads in salad bars. Three of the four known deaths in the United States have been attributed to sulphite sprayed on salads, and one from potatoes that had been dipped in sulphur dioxide.

Sulphur dioxide has been known for many years to provoke asthma among those who cannot tolerate it. Among the most common sulphur-containing foods that commonly trigger an asthma attack are natural fruit juices, soft drinks and cordials, wine and cider, sausages and sausage meat, pickles, dehydrated fruit, potatoes and potato crisps, and, absurdly, some broncho-dilators which are expressly manufactured and prescribed for asthmatics!

When one group of asthmatics were tested with sulphite, in various forms, about 25 per cent were found to be hypersensitive to it. Some 30 per cent of asthmatics report a history of reaction to pickled onions (which contain sulphite) and up to 90 per cent of these react adversely to being tested with sulphite. Cask wines, which are packaged in flexible plastic containers (which, as we shall see in Chapter 20, cause problems in their own right) are likely to contain more sulphur dioxide than bottled wines, because they need greater protection against oxidation.

Victims of sulphite intolerance suffer many symptoms. One patient given a test meal of peaches dusted with sulphur dioxide felt sick, vomited five minutes later, and forty minutes after the test was still cold, clammy, pale and depressed. Even after her stomach had been emptied by vomiting, she continued to have severe stomach cramps and deep depression for the rest of the day.

Sulphite is a very difficult substance to get away from because it is used in the processing of twenty-two different categories of foods as well as in a wide range of drugs. Some of its applications are hardly life-preserving: it is often used to give asparagus a more attractive colour, for example. There is not a single application for which there is not an equally effective alternative. The only disadvantage of the alternatives is that they are more expensive.

Of the non-fatal reactions to sulphite that have been reported in a number of surveys, 80 per cent were associated with restaurant food and 20 per cent with various foods eaten at home, including wine (particularly cask wine), dried fruits and tinned seafoods. Sometimes the nature of the food itself provides a safeguard against excessive use of sulphur dioxide, and even though there is no safe minimum level of exposure, the more it is eaten, the greater the risk of trouble ensuing. Sulphur dioxide is widely used by prawn processors, for example, to eliminate a fault known as blackspot, but if they are too heavy-handed with the sulphite, the prawns become bleached and tough, to the point where they are almost inedible. With some food and wines, as well, there is a limit to the amount of sulphur dioxide that can be used before the taste of it becomes obvious.

Paper test strips are available for the sulphur-sensitive. These indicate sulphur dioxide levels in the range 10 to 500 milligrams per litre, which is a useful range. The strips are not expensive and will detect, for example, sulphur dioxide in mashed potatoes, a frequent source of trouble. Conducting a chemical experiment with your hostess's potatoes in the middle of dinner might take some tactful explanation, but the test strips can save a lot of very unpleasant symptoms.

Anti-oxidants These are substances that are put into food to prevent oxidation, or the effect on certain foods of contact with the oxygen in the atmosphere. It is particularly important for edible oils and fats, which turn rancid when they are exposed to oxygen and can make anyone eating them very sick.

A second role of anti-oxidants is in keeping individual ingredients in many processed foods separate, thus preventing an unpleasant-looking homogeneous mess inside the tin. Sugar is widely used for the same purpose, and not simply as a sweetener, which explains why sugar is so often listed among the ingredients in foods where you would least expect to find it.

Vitamins C and E are natural anti-oxidants, but the two chemicals that are most widely used are butylated hydroxyanisole (BHA) and butylated hydroxytoluene (BHT). The more we learn about both of them, and particularly BHT, the more intolerable it is that manufacturers are allowed to continue using them.

BHA raises the lipid and cholesterol levels in the blood and is associated with an increased risk of breakdown of vitamin D levels. It is banned from all foods intended for babies and young children (with the single exception of its use as a preservative in vitamin A). Its uses are so varied that it is found not only in many foods but in the polyethylene film that wraps them. It is used extensively in margarines and vegetable oils, cream cheese and dried, mashed potatoes.

BHT is a much more sinister product. It is still widely used overseas in foods as varied as chewing gum and cereals, but in Australia it is now rarely found, except in nuts. Like BHA it is also used in the manufacture of polyethylene film.

BHT has all BHA's side effects and more. Toluene (the "T" in BHT) is mainly a coal tar derivative, and this adds a lot of people to the list of potential victims of ecological disease for which it is responsible. Most alarmingly, a Danish report claims that BHT increases tumour formation in rats. One series of experiments showed that pregnant animals fed on BHT revealed an alarmingly high incidence of babies born without eyes. BHT suppressed the activity of three important blood enzymes, caused enlargement of the liver and only metabolised with great difficulty into less toxic substances in the body.

Sequestrants In chemistry sequestrants bind substances, so that they cannot react. As food additives, sequestrants also remove minute traces of metals that are always present in the environment and which cause food to deteriorate by speeding up the oxidation process and by discolouration. Sequestrants attach themselves to these trace metals and remove them so that they can do no harm. To this extent, sequestrants rightly belong in the category of preservatives.

Citric acid is a common — and natural — sequestrant as are glycine, an amino acid and EDRA (salts of ethylenediaminetetra acetic acid). They are all used in salad dressings, margarine, cheese, tinned meat, mayonnaise, lard, soup, shortening and aerated and alcoholic drinks.

Fumigants Fumigants are important compounds in food handling and storage, present in grains, dates and other dried fruits. The most important fumigants are methyl bromide and hydrocyanic acid. Residues may survive right through the food chain.

Benzoic Acid Benzoic acid occurs naturally in many edible berries, including raspberries, and is also prepared synthetically. It is an antibacterial, antifungal preservative, which works by inhibiting bacterial growth. Its main application is in cordials, soft drinks and fruit juices, but it is widely used in products as varied as bread, sausage meat, chutney, soup, sauces, pressed meats and the syrups that milk bars use for flavouring milkshakes.

It has been reported to cause neurological disorders and asthma sufferers should avoid it.

Propionic Acid Propionic acid is a naturally occurring fatty acid and is also produced commercially by fermentation as a preservative for flour products. Manufacturers correctly state that it is non-toxic (it works by inhibiting micro-organisms), but regular exposure can certainly lead to intolerance.

Sorbic Acid One of the most widely used natural preservatives, sorbic acid is particularly effective when the risk of mould growth is high. It occurs naturally in some fruits, but is also manufactured synthetically. Occasionally it is a skin irritant, but its main side effects are the result of intolerance in those who are specifically sensitive to it.

Other Preserving Methods As well as these specific preservatives, salt and sugar are both used for lowering water activity and so preventing or at least slowing down bacterial growth. (Sugar has recently been proved to reduce infection in wounds, and honey is even better.) Freezing and refrigeration do not destroy micro-organisms, but again prevent or slow down bacterial growth. Meat and milk must be placed in the refrigerator as soon as possible after purchase because the low temperature prevents the constantly present micro-organisms from multiplying.

3. AESTHETIC AGENTS ■

Aesthetic agents are the chemicals and occasionally the natural substances that are put into food to make it more attractive to the customer. They usually have little or nothing to do with the quality or nutritional value of the food, and they are not a key part of the manufacturing process. They include sweeteners, acidulants, alkalis and buffers (chemicals that have the ability to maintain the acidity or alkalinity of a food at the required level, even when other acids or alkalis are added during manufacture). But by far the most important (and evident) aesthetic additives are those that flavour and colour food, and none of the chemicals used in food processing collectively cause as much concern.

Flavourings Flavourings are a nightmare for clinical ecologists because they are usually a highly complex mixture of many chemicals and nobody except the manufacturer knows what those chemicals are. Flavourings are excluded from all labelling requirements on the specious grounds that they are trade secrets. Only very rarely do manufacturers reveal even to government health authorities what their flavourings contain.

Not all flavours are elevated to the height of state secrets. Some are simple, single-substance additives, while others, though synthetic, are chemically identical to flavour compounds that have been found natural in foods. Citral, for example, is the main flavour ingredient of lemon oil. It is extracted and used as a flavouring agent, but it can also be synthesised. Chemically the natural and the artificial products are identical, so that from an intolerance point of view, it does not matter whether the flavour additive is derived from a lemon or is synthetic.

Producing a desired flavour synthetically is a very complicated science. A relatively straightforward raspberry flavour, for example, that has to survive high temperatures during processing in an acidic environment, is likely to need at least seven quite distinct chemicals to achieve the desired taste.

When the ingredients are known, it is very difficult to single out one of them as the cause of intolerance; and it is much more difficult if the symptoms are triggered by a combination of more than one of them. Clinical ecologists identify harmful substances by a process of elimination, testing until they find those that are responsible for a reaction. At the best of times, it can be a long business. Without any information or help from manufacturers — paranoid that a competitor might stumble upon their flavour's secret ingredients — it can be almost impossible.

MSG — *the Chinese Curse* Sometimes confused with flavouring agents are the flavour enhancers and modifiers, which are not flavours at all, but chemicals that are used either to strengthen or weaken the taste or smell of a food, without giving it any flavour of their own. By far the best known of these is monosodium glutamate (MSG). The Chinese, appreciating the meaty flavour that MSG draws out of food to which it is added (in reality it probably works on the taste buds, not on the food itself), have used it for centuries in their cooking. Chinese food is still the best known and certainly the most abundant source of MSG. Chinese foods are particularly worrying, not because the Chinese have any monopoly on MSG (it is now so prevalent that it is impossible to list all the products that contain it), but because Chinese food contains such very large amounts of it.

The symptoms experienced by the very large number of people who cannot tolerate MSG are so well documented and so clearly shown to involve Chinese food that they are known collectively as Chinese Restaurant syndrome. They include heart palpitations, headache, dizziness, nausea, an overpowering desire to go to sleep whatever the time of day or the place, weakness in the upper arms, pains in the neck and migraine.

Cases have been reported where victims' breathing has been so affected that they have needed resuscitation; and sometimes frightening asthma-like symptoms occur. Now there is evidence that MSG can trigger "severe, life-threatening asthmatic attacks in sensitive individuals". And symptoms, including paraesthesia (a tingling, burning sensation and aching in the shoulders, upper arms and face), have been so strong that doctors have mistaken them for coronary heart disease.

MSG is very difficult to avoid today. Quite apart from Chinese (and all other oriental) restaurants, it is everywhere on supermarket shelves, in products as varied as fish fingers, noodles, canned soups, gravy mix and almost all meat-flavoured, or meat-containing, products and sauces. Soy sauce, described by one doctor as "not much more than a black dye consisting of MSG in a concentrated solution", is tipped on to a wide assortment of foods by Australians. It is also used to improve the flavour of tobacco. Travelling on the plane from San Francisco to Denver in the United States, aptly to attend a meeting in clinical ecology, I was given a packet of peanuts with my drink. In that modest little bag there were no less than ten added ingredients, including MSG (if Australian labelling requirements were as strict as American, I am sure that the same information would be revealed on some packaged peanuts in Australia).

Fluid retention is yet another serious problem with MSG. I had one patient who put on more than 2 kilograms in weight during a Chinese meal! It is the sodium in MSG that causes retention of fluids (the amount of MSG in the ingredients has to be added to all the other forms of salt when working out the total salt content of any product). You cannot keep fluid in the body without sodium and you cannot get rid of it without losing sodium. Diuretics, which make you pass water, are actually making you lose sodium, or salt, which automatically takes the water with it.

MSG occurs naturally in a Japanese seaweed and a few other substances, but it is prepared commercially from gluten, a protein obtained from wheat or corn, and from sugar-beet pulp. In large amounts it may be toxic, quite aside from all the problems of intolerance reactions that it causes.

When it was discovered that MSG causes neurotoxicity (or poisons nervous tissue) in newborn laboratory animals, it was very rapidly banned from all baby foods, but there is still a great deal that we do not understand about it. It is therefore a bad substance to give to young children, whether they show signs of intolerance to it or not — and that includes allowing them to have Chinese food.

There are, incidentally, a few Chinese restaurants that do not use MSG at all in their cooking: they may not be easy to find, but if you like Chinese food and want to avoid MSG, it may be worth the hunt.

Colouring Agents   None of the food additives have come under such scrutiny and been so widely condemned as many of the food dyes. Critics of their continued use insist that they are merely cosmetics and that they have been implicated in so many illnesses and unpleasant symptoms that, like MSG, the risks far outweigh any advantages and they should be banned unless they are natural. In particular, the so-called azo dyes, which include most of the registered synthetic colourings, should be outlawed.

The food manufacturing industry, on the other hand, argues that the appearance of food is so important to people's enjoyment of it, and therefore to their willingness to buy it, that it *must* use colouring additives; that as nature is very short on colourings that can be incorporated in other foods, dyes must be synthesised. "Off" colours, they rightly insist, suggest bad food; and the act of processing often results in colours that are "off". Dyes also give uniformity to foods that would otherwise vary in colour, such as fruit juices made from fruit bought at different times of the year. Dyes also give food the colour that consumers expect it to have.

Fruit yoghurt is a good example of this. It would remain white, or a murky grey, if it relied solely on the natural fruit that it contains for colouring. But consumers have shown that they expect their strawberry yoghurt to be the colour of strawberries, so the natural product has to have its colour boosted with a synthetic red dye. The same argument is applied when sauces, soft drinks and most tinned and frozen vegetables are coloured artificially. (Fresh fruit and vegetables, like fresh meat and fish, cannot by law be coloured artificially in Australia, but this doesn't prevent suspected carcinogens like alar, which affect colour but are not food dyes, being sprayed on apples and other fruit. Alar has been proved to cause cancer in animals, but it can still be used legally to make young trees bear fruit sooner, to delay flowering (for frost protection) and to prolong the fruit's storage life, as well as improving its colour.

At the time of writing, there are forty-six permitted colouring agents available to processors in Australia, and twenty-six of these are natural, such as chlorophyll (code 140), the green in plants. The only other green dye permitted is a synthetic coal tar dye, green S (code 142). As more of the colours fall under suspicion, this total of forty-six will almost certainly decrease. All the synthetic dyes made from aromatic amines derived from coal tar are suspected of being carcinogens, and can also provoke asthma. These azo dyes, as they are called, adversely affect about one person in five of all those who are sensitive to salicylates (which of course includes aspirin), usually the middle-aged, and more commonly women than men. The reaction often takes the form of contractions of the bronchi, the tubes that allow air into the lungs and that are involved in an asthma attack. Other symptoms include rash, runny nose and eyes, blurred vision and, occasionally, shock.

Now that all colours have to be identified on the product by code numbers, it is much easier to avoid azo dyes if sensitivity is even suspected — though it is still impossible to do this with any foods that are bought unwrapped or unpackaged. The registered azo colours are as follows:

102	tartrazine	(yellow)
107	yellow TG	(yellow)
110	sunset yellow FCF	(yellow)
122	carmoisine	(red)
123	amaranth	(red)
124	ponceau 4R	(red)
155	chocolate brown HT	(brown)
151	black PN	(black).

In addition, there are three azo colours which are permitted in Europe and therefore would in all probability be accepted by authorities in Australia if there was any demand for them from manufacturers. These three are:

E128	red 2G	(red)
E154	brown FK	(the kipper dye)
E180	pigment rubine	(reddish).

Hyperactive children, in particular, should avoid all these dyes and in addition, six others that have been implicated in hyperactivity. Four are synthetic:

127	erythrosine	(red)
132	indigo carmine	(blue)

133   brilliant blue   (blue)
150   caramel   (brown).

One is natural:

120   cochineal   (red).

There is one on the list of approved colours in Europe that has not yet been registered in Australia:

E104   quinoline yellow   (yellow).

Erythrosine (127) is the dye in the plaque-disclosing tablets used by dentists. As well as causing phototoxicity, or sensitivity to light, erythrosine can cause hyperthyroidism, or overactive thyroid, if large amounts of food containing it are eaten, because of its high iodine content. It is extensively used in products ranging from glacé cherries, Swiss roll and custard powder, to canned strawberries and Scotch eggs.

It is nearly forty years since Dr Stephen Lockey first published a paper on allergy to dyes that are used to colour and identify pills and tablets. He warned that artificial colours in drugs are one of the main sources of health problems in children and adults, a view echoed twenty-five years later by Dr Ben Feingold. Feingold proposed that there was a clear relationship between hyperactivity and learning disorders in children, and various chemical substances including salicylates, the preservatives BHA and BHT and, in particular, the commonest yellow dye, tartrazine. Tartrazine is a chemical that can provoke so many symptoms and is so often implicated in intolerance that it is folly to consume it knowingly. It is a measure of how foolish scientists can be that, until recently, one of the most prescribed drugs for calming hyperactive children — thioridazine (sold as Melleril) — was coloured with sunset yellow, a dye that is known to trigger hyperactivity! (Belatedly Sandoz, the manufacturers, did change it.)

How cautious we need to be with these chemicals, which are so often used with no more thought than an egg yolk, can be seen in the really disastrous food chemicals that are occasionally uncovered. Red dye no. 2 was one of the most widely used of all food dyes until it was found to be a very potent carcinogen in animals. It was quickly taken off the market, but the obvious questions about how it came to be available there in the first place, and the effect that it might be having on humans, were pushed aside and never properly answered.

Another red dye, amaranth, an azo synthetic coal tar dye, which is still frequently used for colouring foods, medicines and toiletries, regularly causes swelling of the lips, the tongue and the uvula, sometimes so seriously that patients are almost asphyxiated.

Tartrazine   Of all the synthetic food dyes, none provokes such concern as the yellow dye tartrazine (code 102). It is the commonest yellow and orange colouring agent, also used in green S (142), and it can be found in bakery goods, including icing and decorations, custard, toppings, flavoured milk, jams, jellies, soft drinks and indeed almost any food that is coloured yellow or orange.

Up to the age of 12, Australians consume an average 15 milligrams of tartrazine *each day* of their lives, and the amount consumed then reduces slightly as people get older. The incidence of intolerance to tartrazine is not less than 10 per cent of the population — perhaps 1.5 million in Australia alone! The difficulty in getting it thrown out of the marketplace is that there is no effective and commercially acceptable substitute that is not expensive. Another common yellow, for example, sunset yellow FCF (110) is unacceptable because it gives an orange colour; and natural carotenoid colours (the natural colouring in carrots) are insoluble in water, cost about ten times as much as tartrazine by the kilo, and have to be used at five times the concentration. It may yet prove to be a cheap price to pay.

The most common symptoms associated with tartrazine — apart from being linked, like all the azo dyes, with cancer in laboratory animal experiments — involve the skin, the gastrointestinal tract, the respiratory tract and the whole of the central nervous system: an impressive starting point for a product that is only put in food to please the customer. Like all azo dyes, it is cross-reactive not only with aspirin and other salicylates, but with other food dyes and other medications. Intolerance of it is likely to be closely linked with intolerance of any of these other substances.

4. TEXTURISERS AND STABILISERS ▮

These are substances that aid various stages of food processing and help to give food the consistency that is required. Many of them

ATTEMPTED SUICIDE OR TARTRAZINE?

Judith was a victim of tartrazine, although she didn't know it until it was almost too late. Married with two children, she was being treated by me for depression and what we call an inadequate personality, with poor self-image. She didn't think much of herself, which inevitably exacerbated the symptoms of her depression.

I knew that in the past she had taken an overdose and been put into hospital, so it wasn't altogether a surprise when her husband called frantically to my rooms to say that she had done it again. She was rushed by ambulance to a nearby teaching hospital and was deeply comatose for more than four hours. When she finally awoke spontaneously, the hospital staff were mystified: her blood and urine tests were normal and a gastric wash-out showed no evidence of any overdose. The only clue we had to go on was a bottle of prescribed tranquilliser with forty-nine of the original fifty tablets still in it.

All the evidence suggested that Judith had not tried to commit suicide but had suffered a violent reaction to some food or chemical, and we began to test

her. Foods proved negative, or insignificant, and we were making little progress until the almost full bottle of tranquillisers, yellow and innocuous-looking, were brought to my attention. There was nothing in a single tablet that could have provoked such a reaction, but the yellow colouring was almost certainly tartrazine and I had no illusions about the devastating effect that this can have on those sensitive to it.

I gave Judith a minute dose of highly diluted tartrazine under her tongue and the effect was dramatic. She rapidly appeared to become extremely drunk, she could not walk properly, see properly or talk except with slurred, almost unintelligible speech, and this went on for three-quarters of an hour. Her tartrazine sensitivity had masqueraded as an overdose. She subsequently recalled that on two other occasions, including the previous "attempted suicide", she had taken other medications and reacted very violently. Both, on checking, were found to have tartrazine as their colouring agent. Many drug manufacturers are now removing it from their products, but many are not.

are natural substances. The main hazard comes from regular and frequent exposure to them in foods that we eat on a daily basis, such as bread.

Emulsifiers   These assist in the mixing of fats and water in preparations like mayonnaise, dough, ice-cream, processed cheese and meat products. They include lecithin (which comes from egg yolks), various glycerides and alginates from seaweed.

Humectants   These keep foods moist that would other-wise harden, such as many sweets, icings and fruit cake. The most commonly used are sorbitol and glycerine.

Thickeners   Thickeners may be vegetable gums, cellulose derivatives, or starch derivatives. Most thickeners are of plant origin, but there is a single approved non-organic thickener, called silicon dioxide (551), which has an unlikely origin for a food ingredient: it is the most common rock-forming mineral. Sand, for example, is composed mainly of small grains of quartz or flint, both of which are silicon dioxide. For the food industry, which uses them as both a thickener and a stabiliser, they are ground down to a fine powder, from which both a gel and a col-loidal, or gooey, form is produced. It is extensively used in the sweets and confectionary industries and in wine.

Stabilisers — Surface-active and Foaming Agents, and Gums   All the other substances in this category are stabilisers, performing specific roles in processing, but in particular, affect-ing the texture of the finished product. Surface-active agents, for instance, are the chemicals that ensure that a bottle of mayonnaise is always ready to pour and that it does not have a skin on the top; and stabilisers overcome the tendency of droplets in an emulsion to separate. The roles of stabilisers and thickeners often overlap.

5. PROCESSING AGENTS ■

In this final group of additives are the processing agents that are indispensable in modern factory production of food. *Aerators* are used in baked goods, taking advantage of the carbon monoxide produced from wild yeasts, or the action of cream of tartar on baking soda. *Propellants* are gases or volatile liquids that expel the contents of aerosol cans when the button is pressed. *Anti-caking agents*, or *free-running agents* prevent powdered and granulated foods from sticking and so allow them to run freely. Icing sugar, milk powder, cheese powder and salt are all common products that contain anti-caking agents. Most are inorganic silicates and

ICE-CREAM — A CHEMICAL CONCOCTION

An English magazine, Seed, ingeniously identified the ingredients of a typical cheap ice-cream and came up with the following:

Benzyl acetate: *used to give ice-cream its strawberry flavour. Also used as a nitrate solvent.*

Amyl acetate: *provides ice-cream with banana flavour. Used commercially as an oil paint solvent.*

Diethyl glucol: *a cheap chemical used as an emulsifier and a substitute for eggs. The same chemical is used in paint-remover and antifreeze.*

Aldehyde C17: *used to flavour cherry ice-cream. It is also an inflammable liquid used in aniline dyes, plastics and rubber.*

Ethyl acetate: *used to give pineapple flavour. It is also used as a leather and textile cleaner, and is known to cause chronic lung, heart and especially liver damage in leather and textile workers.*

Butylaldehyde: *provides nut-like flavour. This is also one of the most common ingredients of rubber cement.*

Piperonal: *widely used as a substitute for vanilla. It is also a favourite of exterminators for killing lice.*

Seed *suggested that an ice-cream might not be quite so appetising if you look on it as a mixture of antifreeze, oil paint solvent, paint remover, nitrate solvent, leather cleaner and lice exterminator! To be scrupulously fair to the ice-cream industry, which has been dragged screaming into the position where it must divulge all its awful ingredients on the label, there is some poetic licence in this, but not very much.*

Streets, *incidentally, produces an ice-cream which it very aptly calls Crazy Rainbow. It would be difficult to find a more awful concoction for anyone chemically sensitive. Among the ingredients are cane sugar, the main item; vegetable shortening (a mixture of oils that are rarely identified because manufacturers change them according to current market prices, making it difficult for people to avoid oils of which they are intolerant); skim milk solids; glucose syrup (sugar is often listed under different names such as sucrose, glucose and lactose to give the impression that there is less sugar in a product than is the actual case); whey solids; mono- or di-glycerides of fatty acids; carrageenan (a seaweed extract used as an emulsifier); locust bean gum and guar gum (two other emulsifiers / stabilisers: guar gum is cultured in India as an animal food); flavours (who knows, except Streets, what these include?); DL-Malic acid (a food acid); tartrazine, carmoisine, brilliant blue* *FCF (all azo dyes on the black list for asthmatics, hyperactive children and indeed all humans who want to be healthy); and annato extracts (a vegetable dye, yellow to peach in colour, which is extracted from the seed coats of a tropical tree known as the lipstick tree); water rounds off the contents of this delectable party treat.*

phosphates, but cornflour, which is finely ground maize, is also widely used and corn-intolerant people may react to it. Bleaching agents, which whiten flour, also come into this category and are usually nitrogen oxides, chlorine, chlorine dioxide or benzoyl peroxide.

Many of history's great voyages of exploration were made in search of exotic spices as food additives. Marco Polo would never have travelled to the east had there not been an insatiable market for spices in Europe; and Hernan Cortes, as well as destroying the Aztec Empire, found vanilla there and introduced it to the Western world. The voyages of modern scientific exploration in the world of food have been less romantic, if not always less memorable. The picture of American scientists labouring away in their laboratories to produce a perfect four-legged chicken or a flawless pretend-potato, is indelibly imprinted on the mind.

ANTIBIOTICS, HORMONES AND STEROIDS ■
There is a very insidious form of chemical pollution of food that falls between the food additives introduced by processing and the contaminants, which are usually the residues of pesticides and herbicides. In a sense, they are additives rather than contaminants, in that they are put directly into food — except that the food is still alive.

Contaminated grain that gets into livestock and then moves along the food chain to contaminate humans is a well recognised hazard. Less understood — at least by those who are not closely involved in the research — but potentially much more serious because it is so widespread, is the intensive use of antibiotics, hormones and steroids by farmers.

Antibiotics Few people are aware of the extent to which antibiotics are used today in agriculture. In the United States, nearly half the total annual production of antibiotics is fed not to sick people, but to farm animals, mainly cattle, poultry and pigs. Antibiotics are particularly in demand where animals are kept in close confinement and where the danger of disease spreading through a herd or battery is very high. But that is only a part of the story because antibiotics are not used only for this purpose.

For reasons that are still not fully understood, antibiotics bring a number of side effects that are very appealing to farmers, and very unappealing to consumers. When they are given in "sub-therapeutic" doses (doses that are smaller than needed to treat disease) they accelerate an animal's growth and weight. The obvious commercial attraction of this is that it results in an increase in "feed efficiency", or the amount of meat produced per kilogram of feed consumed during the animal's life. The prevention of disease has sometimes become almost a secondary consideration.

The highly undesirable side of this coin is that this whole-sale use of the same antibiotics that are commonly used to treat humans is producing antibiotic-resistant bacteria. That would be serious enough if it went no further than the animals, but it has the same effect in the humans who eat their meat, drink their milk or use their eggs. When any antibiotic is used to excess — and the threshold is often surprisingly low — the bacteria at which it is targeted are likely to develop resistance to it and adapt to it. That is why doctors are concerned that antibiotics should be used as sparingly as possible.

Most farmers, indifferent to the problem or probably for the most part ignorant of it, refuse, on the grounds of economy, even to switch to more expensive antibiotics that are not used by humans. There is a wide range of them available. Instead, they persist in using such familiars as penicillin and tetracyclines.

For the humans at the other end of the food chain, it is serious enough to find that they have unwittingly developed re-sistance to normally effective and safe antibiotics. They usually find this out only when the antibiotics that have been prescribed for them or their children — who are likely to be the main milk drinkers in the family — do not work. Most people find it very disturbing even to suspect that their food arrives contaminated with pharmaceutical drugs — processing usually leaves them unscathed — without having to run the gauntlet of unknowingly eating antibiotics whose main purpose was to increase a farmer's profitability. In extreme cases it can be disastrous, even fatal, for those who are intolerant of penicillin and tetracyclines to consume them in their food.

This exposure can also result in the development of allergy and of severe anaphylactic reactions when an antibiotic is prescribed for a patient who has never before been prescribed that antibiotic. We see it, for example, with patients who react violently to penicillin the first time it is prescribed, because they have drunk milk from cows treated for mastitis with penicillin.

Antibiotics have been used in this way since 1949 and the Australian Consumers Association has claimed widespread evidence of their improper and sometimes illegal use in pigs, cattle and chickens in Australia. Its analysts found residues of tetracycline well above the approved maximum Australian and World Health Organisation levels in five out of fourteen red meat samples and two turkey samples. In every commercial chicken sample tested, bacteria were found that had become resistant to antibiotics used in human medicine. The response of the producers is invariably that they are using only antibiotics prescribed by veterinarians. Perhaps they are, which only reinforces the need for sweeping legislation to control the practice.

Hormones and Steroids No less worrying are the growth-promoting hormones that farmers use to speed up the growth of animals and poultry. Again, rapid growth to marketing weight means less feed and greater profitability; and again, this is causing serious health problems to humans. In Puerto Rico, chicken containing steroids (fed to chickens by local intensive chicken farmers to speed growth) resulted in bisexual development in children who ate it. Breast tissue developed so grossly that kindergarten children were as physically developed as adult women. Only when this was shown in Western nations in a powerful television documentary was there the first public stirring of outrage at such practices and the first real awareness that this might also be happening in their own countries.

A Puerto Rican physician who treated a number of infants

with abnormal breast development related 97 per cent of these cases directly to weaning on to formula made from locally produced milk that came from cows given steroid treatment. There is growing evidence that oestrogen (which is the hormone that develops and maintains female characteristics in the body, and was the hormone implicated in the Puerto Rican cases) and the metabolites of oestrogen play a role in the development of cancer, in addition to their other dangers.

The use of artificial hormone growth promotants in the beef industry has been totally banned in much of western Europe since 1988. Australian cattlemen still spend more than $6 million a year on them.

Even fruit doesn't escape, though few people are probably aware of it. Grapes, for example, are given a dose of a growth hormone called gibberellic acid to blow up the fruit to the desired dimensions for many overseas markets.

Alarming Reactions   It came as no surprise, therefore, to clinical ecologists when intolerance reactions were also found to be occurring on an alarming scale as a result of exposure to these same drugs. Those who cannot tolerate penicillin, tetracycline or any other antibiotic will inevitably suffer a reaction if they encounter these in their food. The prestigious American journal *Annals of Allergy* reported the case of a 14-year-old in the United States who had a serious anaphylactic reaction four times after eating meals containing beef (anaphylaxis is a violent allergic reaction that occurs occasionally, notoriously after the second or subsequent injection of snake antivenene, which is made in horse serum). The obvious assumption was that she was intolerant of beef, but after extensive testing, it was found that the trigger was not the meat at all, but streptomycin, which was present as an antibiotic residue in the beef.

Much greater care needs to be taken. In Australia the antibiotic Carbadox is a veterinary drug intended for the treatment of diseases in pigs, particularly swine fever, but used extensively and effectively to promote growth in pigs. Carbadox residues in pork would probably have remained an ever-present threat to the chemically sensitive for years, had not testing overseas established that it was also causing cancer in laboratory animals, and that it was potentially dangerous to people using and handling it on the farm, as well as to anyone eating food containing the residue.

The National Health and Medical Research Council

(NHMRC) reacted by removing the maximum residue limits permitted, which effectively prevents it being used at all because it means that no level of residue is considered safe. But it decided at the same time that this would not be enforced until the end of 1986, some six months later. The NHMRC was presumably not influenced by any pleas from farmers that they first be allowed to use up existing stocks, but a six-month moratorium certainly had that effect.

Setting the "Safe" Levels Organisations such as the World Health Organisation, the Food and Agriculture Organisation in the United States and the NHMRC in Australia set what are known as "maximum residue levels" for many chemicals. These are the maximum concentrations of pesticides, for example, that are legally permitted to remain in food. They are determined by a number of factors, particularly by what is known as the LD_{50} test, which establishes the amount of the chemical that kills half the test animals in a particular study, within a certain period. It is also a test that is coming in for increasing criticism.

These organisations also set Allowable Daily Intake Levels which are the maximum permissible levels of a chemical that should be ingested or inhaled each day, regardless of the residue levels in the food itself.

These two controls are important in reducing the risks particularly of pesticide residues, many of which persist right along the food chain and are almost impossible to eradicate. Where the controls fail is that they take no account of individual susceptibility, and most importantly, of the special vulnerability of children, the sick and the malnourished. Instead they assume an "average" person to be well-fed, healthy, adult and male. Even among this group, which by definition must include well under half the population, many well-fed, healthy, adult men have a much lower than average threshold of tolerance for various chemicals and foods. Averaging is a risky business when health and lives are at stake.

It would be much safer if a chemical that kills even one laboratory animal were automatically assumed to be a risk to humans until proved otherwise, but this doesn't happen. Some countries have legislated to ban antibiotics commonly used by humans from being routinely administered to livestock (Britain did so in 1971), but the agricultural and pharmaceutical lobbies are very powerful and they have succeeded in delaying similar legislation in most other countries, including Australia, unless a product has conclusively been shown to cause cancer or birth defects. Even then, this discovery is all too often made long after the product has been released on to the market as "safe as long as the directions on the packet are adhered to", the standard let-out for the pharmaceutical industry.

Many European countries are now severely restricting or banning the use of hormones as a growth aid in livestock and this is intended to come into effect in 1988. An official of one of the most powerful agricultural organisations in Australia, confirming that there were no plans for similar action to be taken in this country, described the European decision as "silly".

UNINTENDED ADDITIVES — TRAPS FOR THE UNWARY ■

There are traps for the unwary and the sensitive in the most unlikely places. Marion knew that she was chemically sensitive when she came to me. Plastics and vinyls, particularly the softer plastics, left her wheezing and gasping for breath. What she could not understand was why tinned salmon seemed to have the same effect on her, which ostensibly contained nothing but fish and salt. She had already established that the salt was sea salt placed back into a brine and vacuum-evaporated to remove impurities such as sand and dirt.

After a great deal of prompting, Seakist Foods, the manufacturer of the particular brand of salmon that she had been eating, provided the explanation that she needed — and it was one that had never even crossed her mind. The problem lay not with the salmon at all, or with any ingredient added by the manufacturer. It was the lining on the inside of the tin, the golden-brown coating that prevents the metal from bleaching the colour of the food, that was causing Marion's breathlessness and wheezing.

If you can taste a difference between any tinned food and its fresh equivalent, it is almost certainly because of some chemical additive or contaminant in that food. The lining on the inside of tins leaves no taste at all, yet it can have a very significant effect on the health of anyone intolerant of it.

Seakist described the lacquer on the inside coating of their tinned salmon as follows, which will be of great interest to anyone sensitive to any of the ingredients involved:

> *220 gram tin of Ally Pink Salmon* (the brand that caused the trouble for Marion): the inside of the tin is roller-coated with V-53 enamel, a modified, aluminised vinyl dispersion material;
> *440 gram tin of Ally Pink Salmon*: the tin is roller-coated with V-74 enamel, a heat-reactive aluminised phenolic material.

To be fair to Seakist and all the other manufacturers who treat the inside of their tins, there has never been any suggestion that the processes are harmful to anyone except those who are chemically intolerant. But that still leaves a lot of people who suffer as a result of it. At the very least, the information ought to be freely available without having to be squeezed out of a manufacturer, so that people can avoid these chemicals.

Another supplier of Ally Pink Salmon has advised that the interior tin coating is a water-based baked-on vinyl, which is a standard metal tin coating. Until only a few years ago, most coatings had a petroleum solvent base, but this has largely been replaced by water-based coatings. The change came not from any concern for consumers, or from any fears about the effect of the petroleum solvent leaching into the food, but because the evaporation of the solvent during the baking process was posing a serious hazard for workers.

IRRADIATION ▌

To many people, there is no more sinister method of processing food than irradiating it. The United States Food and Drug Administration looks on irradiation as a food additive, not a process, but it is much more. It sterilises, pasteurises, disinfects, inhibits enzyme processes such as sprouting (even low levels prevent wheat sprouting) and destroys any infestation of pests. It delays ripening, extends the shelf life of foods, including foods that normally deteriorate very rapidly and have to be thrown away, and destroys infections and fungi, as well as bugs.

Irradiation technology has been in use for a long time (for more than fifteen years in Australia), mainly for sterilising medical and surgical equipment. The irradiation of food is a much more recent development, but by mid-1986, more than twenty countries had already approved some food irradiation. Few countries find the idea more appealing than Australia, and few parts of Australia more so than Queensland and other tropical and sub-tropical regions.

For more than thirty years, Queensland fruit farmers, plagued by fruit fly as well as other pests, have relied on ethylene dibromide (EDB) to rid their product of it. It was an essential method of processing, because without it much of Queensland's fruit crop, for example, would be unsellable outside the state. Now EDB has been banned in the United States and is being phased out in Japan, as evidence grows that it is linked with cancer. The unavoidable residues in the Queensland fruit may be dangerous. (In Australia ethylene gas is also widely used for ripening bananas and other fruit.)

The perfect solution for Queensland's growers seemed to be irradiation, which not only destroys fruit fly but comes with other appealing fringe benefits such as much longer shelf life and delayed ripening. Indeed, in Australia, not only fruit and vegetables, but cereals, poultry, herbs and spices could all be irradiated, with substantial benefits for the producers and retailers.

Radiation Plants — "A Major Health Risk" Bitterly opposed to the new technology are cancer specialists, many other scientists and a growing number of ordinary people who are fearful that irradiation is being introduced without any certainty that it is safe.

The danger in irradiating food comes not from any risk that the food itself is radioactive. The danger of radioactivity is confined to the devastation that would follow if one of these radiation plants, which are being planned for construction in highly populated city suburbs, runs amok. The accidents at Windscale in Britain, Three Mile Island in New York, USA, and Chernobyl in the USSR are some of the more publicised mistakes that have occurred, but there have been numerous others.

The company promising to bring its technology to Australia, Radiation Technology, operates three plants in the United States. In one of them it accidentally irradiated a worker with the equivalent of 20,000 chest X-rays in about twenty seconds; and in two other mishaps, it contaminated the air and the water. In 1986, this same company, which at the time of writing is being held up by the Australian fruit and vegetable growers and by Queensland government officials as the paragon whose word and experience are beyond reproach, has just had one of these three plants closed down by American health officials as "a major health risk" to its employees.

The Nuclear Regulatory Commission charged that Radiation Technology by-passed the safety locks within the plant; failed to maintain irradiated pool depths at the required level; allowed excessive radiation levels in unrestricted areas; failed to provide required training to employees; failed adequately to evaluate the radiation dose to which workers were being exposed; and failed to evaluate material being sent for disposal in ordinary garbage. The commission's order said that "There was a pattern of wrongdoing so pervasive that [we] no longer had a reasonable assurance that the safety of Radiation Technology's employees would be protected".

The transportation of cobalt to and from the plant is another reason for concern. (Brisbane is planning to build its first irradiation plant next door to the markets.) In mid-1986, Australia does not even have uniform laws from state to state for moving radioactive materials (and the quantity involved is unprecedented). The average cancer therapy unit needs about 4000 to 6000 curies to operate: the average food irradiation plant requires between one and three *million* curies. To transport just four radioactive cobalt rods, each about the size of a pencil and about 2000 curies, requires massive 3 tonne containers with several layers of steel, lead and aluminium: for the irradiation plant, up to half a million curies will be regularly shuttled back and forth through the suburbs and into the densely populated parts of our cities. For irradiation to be cost-effective, it must be carried out in very close proximity to the markets, which almost invariably will mean in built-up areas.

What Irradiation Does to Our Food   The risk of an accident occurring sooner or later, either during transportation or in the plant itself, must be a real one even in the most disciplined complex. Radiation Technology, which is acknowledged to be one of the leaders in the industry in the USA, and seems set to dominate the industry in Australia, has hardly set an example that would give anyone much confidence. Equally real is the fear that the process itself is not safe for those who will eat irradiated food.

To start with, irradiation destroys many vitamins and this is of concern to dieticians and to anyone who recognises the importance of proper nutrition. Vitamins A, B, C, E and K are particularly radiation sensitive (40 per cent of vitamin A is lost). We simply cannot afford to lose this much nutrition in addition to the losses that already occur in home and factory processing. But at least we can supplement the vitamins in our food when we know there is a deficiency. There is a very much grimmer prospect, however, associated with irradiation: the mutagenic, chromosome-changing effect that it has on food. The instant that food is irradiated, millions of chemical bonds are shattered. When they recombine, as they must, new chemical compounds may be formed. The larger the dose of radiation, the greater is the number of these new compounds, or radiolytic products, and it is these that are at the very core of the controversy over irradiated foods.

The rays of caesium 137 can be used to irradiate food, but the most common source is cobalt 60, which kills virtually everything living in or on the food, and changes the nature of the substance being irradiated. The big problem is that we don't know whether these changes are harmful and particularly whether they can cause cancer, which is the greatest risk. Some studies have shown that the process may be potentially very dangerous. Irradiation causes an overproduction of aflotoxins, for example, which are naturally occurring fungi that are extremely carcinogenic. For the most part, however, we simply do not know what is happening. All legislation has been based on the premise that because irradiation has not been shown to be dangerous, it can therefore be declared safe. The truth is that most of the studies carried out have not found any cause for concern. The NHMRC points to research such as that carried out at the Lucas Heights plant of the Atomic Energy Commission, where there is a colony of rats now in its forty-eighth generation, and each generation has been fed on irradiated food without ill effect.

As every scientist involved in cancer research knows only too well, however, you cannot dogmatically declare that a substance is not carcinogenic to humans because it has not been proved to be a carcinogen to animals in laboratory conditions, or because a few astronauts and prisoners have eaten it, apparently without ill effects. There are no short cuts. The only worthwhile test to determine the incidence of cancer production is to feed 100,000 people on irradiated food, and then monitor them over ten to fifteen years against a control group of another 100,000 matched people who are not given irradiated food. Then count the cancers.

The reason why it is so difficult to be precise about the safety of food that has been altered by irradiation is that you might produce one or ten or a hundred or a thousand different chemical constituents, any number of which may have a carcinogenic effect, albeit a small one, on those who are individually susceptible to contracting cancer. In addition, any of these constituents may react with any of the others to produce yet another carcinogen; and the combined effect of all these carcinogens in a human (though not necessarily in a rat or a guineapig) may be needed to induce a cancer. It is impossible to analyse chemically the hundreds of thousands of possible permutations. (It is also a profoundly important reason for withdrawing any chemical from circulation as soon as it is linked with cancer in even one laboratory animal.)

It may take twenty-five years to complete a study of a large sample of people, but that is surely not a very high price to pay before subjecting the entire population to irradiated food which they will probably not even be able to avoid. Will every tomato, every potato, every orange carry a little label warning that it has been irradiated? Will every menu in every restaurant have a little skull beside items that have been irradiated?

Irradiation may in the end prove to be as safe as its advocates maintain; but if that proves not to be the case, we will have paid a price too horrendous even to contemplate. There must be a moratorium while we find out.

11 Some Troublesome Foods

Any food, eaten frequently and regularly, can result in intolerance, or food addiction, in those who are specifically sensitive to it. Probably 80 per cent of us react adversely to some food or food chemical, usually without being aware that this is the cause of the unpleasant symptoms that we dismiss as part of modern living. Only when we understand the link between food or chemicals and those symptoms, and then take steps to remove them from our personal environment (in the case of food, by stopping eating it), do we realise how much they have affected our health and the quality of our lives.

There are some foods, however, usually because they are so prevalent, that present special problems, or are frequently implicated in intolerance and the resulting illnesses and symptoms. High on the hit list of such suspect foods is caffeine, and particularly caffeine in its most popular form, coffee.

COFFEE ▌

Nerida drank forty cups of coffee a day and insisted that she needed every one of them to function in what she thought was a normal manner. To her friends and her associates at work, however, she was so hyped up by the coffee that for much of the day she was practically incoherent. Such is the potency of caffeine.

In moderation, caffeine probably poses no serious or lasting health hazards for the majority of people, except for its remarkable propensity for triggering intolerance reactions. In small amounts it can safely keep people alert and even working more efficiently. Some doctors even maintain that it has positive uses. Unfortunately, the stimulating effect decreases with increased intake. The trouble is that a great many people drink coffee in amounts that are very far from small. A high dose of coffee, with its potent combination of food (the coffee bean) and drug (caffeine), is considered to be anything more than 200 milligrams, or two cups, a day; and caffeine abuse is taken to be more than 500 milligrams, or five cups, a day. The coffee industry believes that at least 25 per cent of the adult population is drinking *more* than five cups a day.

Caffeine is found naturally in coffee, tea, cola and cocoa: it is therefore present in Coca-Cola, Pepsi Cola and some other popular soft drinks, and in chocolate. It is also a stimulant and a drug that affects all parts of the cerebral cortex and central nervous system, causing anxiety, tremors, gastritis, irritability, agitation, insomnia, headache and, in very large doses, cardiac failure.

Two Cups a Day Too Many Even small amounts of caffeine (less than two cups of coffee a day) can cause wakefulness. Its effects on sleep are probably better documented than any of its other undesirable side effects. Taken before bedtime, coffee usually makes it difficult to get to sleep. It increases the amount of dream (REM) sleep early in the night, but reduces REM sleep overall. This means that the quality and restorative powers of sleep are affected adversely.

Drinking more than two cups a day for some people, and more than six cups for most people, can produce the condition known as caffeinism, which is caffeine poisoning or addiction, characterised by withdrawal symptoms that include headaches, tremors, nervousness, irritability and jittery legs. Depression is another common feature of high caffeine consumption. The drug also affects the heart and causes blood vessels to narrow, forcing the heart to pump harder to force the blood through them. At high doses, it causes tachycardia (abnormally rapid heartbeat) and raises blood-sugar levels by inhibiting the metabolism of glucose.

Because of caffeine's effect on the kidneys, it is a diuretic, provoking increased urination and with this the loss of essential nutrients. (It was because of its effect on the kidneys that caffeine was taken out of most over-the-counter pain relievers, in which it was widely used in association with aspirin.) Some animal studies suggest that there is even an association between excessive caffeine intake (anything over 600 milligrams, or six cups, a day) and complicated deliveries and birth defects. This has still to be confirmed in humans, but most health-care professionals now recommend that pregnant women avoid, or at least limit, their coffee and tea consumption.

Coffee and Cholesterol A report in the *British Medical Journal* in June 1984 described a study of 14,581 subjects, linking coffee to increased cholesterol. The study found that drinking more than six cups a day increased the serum cholesterol concentration even in otherwise healthy people. There is also a growing suspicion that high levels of caffeine, particularly in coffee, may be associated with cancer of the bladder, kidneys and pancreas. Caffeine has long been known to be capable of causing cellular change.

In addition to all these very compelling reasons for treating any caffeine-containing substances with great caution (coffee in particular because it is so high in caffeine), coffee is a very potent drug of addiction. It is one of the most popular drinks in the world and, at the same time, one of the most insidious and subtle forms of addiction, affecting many millions of people. We have already seen why so many people need their first cup of coffee in the day before they can function properly; and that the all too familiar weekend headache is often a withdrawal symptom triggered because the coffee is drunk later than usual (see Chapter 5).

More people are probably made chronically ill because of their habitual use of this drug than from any other substance. If coffee was introduced today, it would almost certainly be available only on prescription. Numerous studies have confirmed the problems associated with caffeine, many of them double-blind studies using nasogastric tubes so that the patients are unable to taste or smell the foods or chemicals they are eating. In spite of this, coffee, tea and cola drinks are usually treated as harmless and enjoyable beverages. Doctors rarely question their patients about their total caffeine consumption, when they are trying to make a diagnosis; and to a degree, the far greater publicity properly attached to abuse of other drugs has drawn attention away from coffee as a health hazard.

Where is the Caffeine? Caffeine is rapidly absorbed into the bloodstream and reaches the peak of its effect in about an hour, before wearing off very rapidly after three hours, even in those who are not addicted to it.

By far the heaviest concentration of caffeine is in coffee. A cup (150 grams) of filtered coffee, for instance, contains up to 150 milligrams of caffeine, compared with about 45 to 50 milligrams for the same amount of tea brewed for five minutes (the longer the brew, the more the caffeine); 47 milligrams in a 300 gram bottle of Coca-Cola and, worryingly (because it is marketed as a health product), substantially more in Lucozade; 20 milligrams in a 30 gram chocolate bar; and 15 milligrams in a typical caffeine-containing cold tablet. Certain migraine suppressants include caffeine, such as Cafergot which contains 100 milligrams of the drug in each tablet, so that in a normal dose of two tablets there is an immediate introduction of 200 milligrams. After that, even a single cup of coffee takes the patient above what is for many people a "safe" dose.

Decaffeinated coffee is not, in spite of the name, entirely free of caffeine. Even though the caffeine content is only a modest 3 milligrams in an average cup, that may still be sufficient to trigger reaction symptoms in those who are sensitive to caffeine. In addition, there is something in the chemical caffeine-removing process that makes this kind of coffee intolerable even to some people who can drink ordinary coffee.

Relieving the Withdrawal Symptoms As with any addictive substance, withdrawal symptoms are usually relieved, once adaptation has occurred, by taking more caffeine. Severe headache is the symptom that is most often experienced, although masking will often make the association between any symptoms and the caffeine difficult to pinpoint. It is the familiar problem in ecological illness: it is often the *absence* of the substance causing the trouble that results in the headaches and other symptoms and illnesses.

I have had a disturbing number of patients who have given up their jobs because their headaches have become so unbearable that they can no longer tolerate working. They have had neurological examinations, been seen and assessed by psychiatrists, admitted to hospital for brainscans and diagnosed, at the very least, as having severe migraine.

Children and the Elderly Vulnerable Children and the elderly are particularly sensitive to the stimulating effect of caffeine. As with all drugs, the effect of the dose is directly related to body weight and size, so that a can of Coca-Cola is likely to have the same stimulating effect on a child as four cups of coffee on an adult, a high dose. Children slip all too easily into caffeinism through a combination of cola drinks and chocolate, and paediatricians are becoming increasingly troubled by the incidence of headache, irritability and nervousness in many children, caused entirely by cola and other soft drinks and chocolate in its numerous forms.

Tolerance to caffeine decreases with age, so that the elderly are increasingly sensitive to it. Sleep disturbance is likely to be more pronounced with advancing years if coffee or tea are drunk within two or three hours of going to bed.

WHEN CAFFEINE TAKES OVER

Donald had been a successful businessman, running his own company. He had been forced to give up his business because of the severity of his headaches. For three years before he was finally referred to me, he had been unemployed, and for a year of that time he had been virtually housebound, convinced that he was going mad. His wife was equally certain that there was an organic explanation for his pain, if only it could be found. And she was right!

For as long as he could remember, Donald had been drinking up to twenty cups of coffee a day, yet not one of the bevy of physicians and other doctors who had examined him with almost microscopic thoroughness had thought to ask him about this. I advised him to give up coffee — nothing else — and after a few days of very stressful and painful withdrawal, all his headache symptoms disappeared. At his last examination, he had been symptom-free for one year and had set up his business again.

Another patient, Linda,

felt almost constantly nauseous and, to her horror and revulsion, actually vomited in public when she was out to dinner. Nor did this very distressing situation improve when she began to take large amounts of anti-emetics in an effort to quell her nausea. By the time she was referred to me she was understandably on the verge of severe depression. Her history revealed one striking fact: she drank tea with almost the same abandon as Donald had consumed coffee. On my advice, she immediately eliminated it from her diet. Without any medication, the nausea and vomiting disappeared, as did the agoraphobia that was adding to the misery of her life.

In both Donald's and Linda's cases, supportive psychotherapy was given to help restore their confidence in themselves. As we shall see a little later, counselling of this kind, together with diet, supplementary nutrition, exercise and instruction in how to recognise and avoid intolerance in future are all important.

It is not only the caffeine that causes the trouble. Coffee can be hazardous for some people in its own right. The coffee bean itself stimulates acid production in the stomach (which is why ulcer sufferers are warned against it). In addition, both coffee and tea, as well as cola drinks, interfere with iron absorption. Most vegetarians, and anyone else with a marginal iron status, should avoid any of these for at least an hour after meals.

Pure chocolate, which is related to caffeine and coffee, is an extremely complex chemical product, containing up to 30 per cent fat and 50 per cent sugar and containing little else in many cases. It is another food—drug substance (cocoa and caffeine). It is often implicated in food intolerance and should be given very sparingly to children.

EGGS ■

Egg sensitivity is very common, and cross-sensitivity between eggs and chicken also occasionally occurs, where intolerance to one results in an adverse reaction to the other as well. (Occasionally we see this same cross-reactivity between beef and cow's milk.)

The presence of eggs is obvious when they are cooked and eaten as an egg dish, but they turn up in many processed foods and in home cooking as ingredients that cannot be recognised as eggs, either by appearance or taste. Salad dressings, Ovaltine, many soups (particularly soups with noodles), packet cake mixes, some hamburger minces, tartare sauce and macaroni are only a few of the foods that include eggs.

If you are intolerant of eggs and buy your bread and cakes from a small hot-bread bakery, ask if there is dried or powdered egg, as well as fresh egg, in the product. These are sometimes overlooked, but to the intolerance victim, they are just as unsafe as scrambled egg on toast. Eggs, incidentally, can be replaced in cakes with gelatine. One tablespoon of gelatine, dissolved in cold water, with a cup of boiling water added, is the equivalent of three eggs. So too is a tablespoon of golden syrup in 300 milli-litres of warm milk.

FISH ■

Unless you happen to be an Eskimo, you wouldn't imagine that anyone would eat fish regularly and frequently enough to acquire intolerance to it. It happens, though, and this isn't the only problem associated with fish. Once again, it is chemicals that get into the picture and are responsible.

Fish would seem to be one of the few foods that are almost tamper-proof by humans, but that isn't correct either. In a confidential memorandum written in January 1986 as a briefing for another officer, a senior officer of the New South Wales Fish Marketing Authority listed some examples of just how contaminated some of the fish is that we eat regularly. "Tasmanian and presumably other scallops", he wrote, "are sprayed with polyphosphates to enhance and retain colour. Prawns from Moreton Bay in Brisbane are treated with sodium metabisulphite to preserve them from bacterial agents ... Fillets — in normal circumstances are sprayed with preservatives: only use fillets if the supplier can personally guarantee otherwise."

The memorandum went on to warn that although no admission should be made that in-shore fish come from polluted waters and are therefore unsafe, "Nevertheless, off-shore fish would be better (as in much better), e.g. mackerel, tuna, kingfish, snapper, deep sea bream (morwong)". The writer described shark (flake) as "probably OK" and concluded with a recommendation that "allergic people" should preferably use whole fish (i.e. not fillets) with clear, bright eyes, bright red under the gills and with no obnoxious odour".

Whenever a chemical is being regularly ingested, there is the risk of chemical intolerance developing. Sodium metabisulphite is a frequent cause of intolerance reactions, and the other substances, such as the polyphosphates to "improve" the scallops' colour and the preservatives sprayed on the fillets, are no better.

Fish farming, or aquaculture, is being increasingly exploited by large fish processors. Apart from the obvious economies and convenience that a well-managed fish farm offers, the fish can be fed pelleted food containing any additives that the processor chooses to add. With some fish, pink colouring can be added for example, to improve the appearance of the fish when it is dead. The majority of trout supplied to restaurants come from freshwater fish farms and their main drawback is that freshwater trout are pale, insipid-looking things compared with their salt-water relatives. A process which even partially overcomes this handicap by making them pinker has obvious commercial appeal.

It is generally illegal to add chemicals to a so-called "fresh" fish to preserve its shelf life, but there is no control on the food that is given to them while they are still swimming around at the farm. Some reared fish are fed in part on grain-based meal, which can become a hidden reactant for anyone sensitive to grain — hidden because whatever most consumers expect their fish to consist of, it is unlikely to include bread. Furthermore, because farms are particularly vulnerable to being wiped out by an epidemic, there has been considerable research into the use of antibiotics, and these inevitably remain in trace residues to be ingested by the consumer.

FRUIT AND VEGETABLES ■

Intolerance of fruit and vegetables is common and stems from two distinct sources. Some sensitive people are unable to eat certain fruits or vegetables, particularly citrus and members of the cabbage family; and there is an even larger group of people who react not to the food itself, but to the chemicals to which the food has been exposed at various stages of its production.

Multiple fruit sensitivity was common enough to have been a puzzle for a long time to clinical ecologists, because susceptible patients seemed to be intolerant of fruit right across the board, and not of individual food families, as one would expect. The explanation, in most cases, was intolerance of the multiple chemicals in the fruit.

Spraying fruit and vegetables is a commercially necessary evil. Without it, people would rarely see produce grown outside the area where they live. Most "fresh" fruit, particularly in the cooler states of Australia and in cooler countries, comes from some distance away or from overseas, and may have been stored for weeks, if not months. For example, bananas are picked in the tropics before they are ripe and are then shipped and stored at a controlled, even temperature of less than 13°C, before being ripened by exposure to ethylene gas. This is the gas that is given off naturally by ripening fruit, but when it is applied artificially to fruit to *make* it ripen, it is so strongly suspected of being a major health hazard that it has either been banned or, at the time of writing is on the point of being banned, in almost every Western country (one of the arguments in favour of allowing irradiation of food to replace it, see Chapter 10).

Unlike bananas, oranges are picked when they are ripe and they are normally shipped and stored at a lower temperature than bananas, about 3°C in dry air, with a raised carbon dioxide level.

Their skins have to be protected from mould infection, often by wrapping them in chemically treated paper. Even though the orange has been picked, its cells are still alive and absorb these and any other chemical molecules with which they come in contact.

There is a peculiarly acrid smell that is sometimes associated with fruit and vegetable markets, which can be traced to the crates that are used for packing citrus fruit. This smell comes from the crates themselves, which are impregnated with fungicides. All boxes and containers used for transporting fruit and vegetables are routinely sprayed to control mould as well as insects.

The most frequently "unsafe" vegetables for the intolerant are the large-leafed varieties, such as cabbage and spinach, which are usually the most heavily contaminated because they have the largest leaf area to attract and hold chemicals.

Among the fruits, peaches, apples and cherries are probably the most hazardous because they are the most commonly contaminated. Up to fourteen different sprays are used on apples between the end of blossoming and the arrival of the fruit in the shop. In fact, by the time they reach the consumer they may be saturated with chemicals, many of which are capable individually of causing intolerance in the susceptible let alone what their synergistic effect might be.

So heavily is much of our commercial fruit and vegetables sprayed, that it is almost impossible to say which particular spray is causing which symptoms in a patient. Once the fruit has been sprayed, it is usually impossible to remove the chemical entirely, especially if it is a pesticide or herbicide applied in a petroleum-based solvent. Air passes readily through the skin of fruit, taking with it the spray ingredients, which are then incorporated into the pulp itself. Stewing fruit boils off some of these chemicals (although some patients are made sick by the vapour): rubbing an apple to make it shine appealingly, or washing it, does little to make it any more chemical-free.

It is often mandatory for producers to use methyl bromide for fumigating dates and many dried fruits as a condition of taking them across state boundaries, or from one country to another. Almost all dates contain a small, sometimes troublesome, residue of this chemical. Sulphur is also widely used as an antifungal measure, as well as for its even more common use of keeping salads looking fresh and potatoes from turning brown after they have been peeled. Many people react to sulphur, sometimes so violently that we have to suspend testing.

In addition to those already mentioned, other fruits that are likely to have been heavily exposed to chemicals include: avocados (particularly in certain states, including Victoria), pears, pawpaw, plums, peaches, nectarines, apricots, all berry fruits (including strawberries, raspberries and loganberries) as well as leafy vegetables. Citrus fruit causes less of a problem than most fruit from the point of chemical contamination (but is probably responsible for more intolerance in itself) and bananas are usually safe, apart from gassing to ripen them.

Some fruits and vegetables are sold with a coating of wax, particularly apples, which are often so thickly waxed that the wax can be scraped off with a finger nail. The wax is safe from a toxicological viewpoint, but is responsible for intolerance. A number of formulations are used, many of them based on petroleum-derived paraffin wax, which gives good control of water loss, but poor shine; and carnauba, a natural wax, that gives an attractive lustre, but has poorer control of water loss. Wax also retains malic acid in apples, which is the property that gives them their flavour. There are also some natural food-grade waxes that often contain milk casein in a water solution and so pose a threat to the milk sensitive. There is no way of telling by taste, appearance or smell which formulation of wax has been used, nor is it correct that peeling an apple removes all traces of the wax, as fruiterers sometimes recommend to anyone who objects to it. You can prove this easily by peeling a heavily waxed apple and then dipping it in boiling water. Droplets of wax will still usually rise to the surface.

Another common practice that contributes to the contamination of food is the indiscriminate spraying of fruit and vegetable counters in shops and supermarkets to control insects, flies and mould. This practice is even more widespread in the wholesale markets.

All these chemicals are present before we even begin to consider the chemicals that are added during processing, when the fruit or vegetables are not sold raw. Even potatoes don't escape. They are treated with sulphur dioxide after peeling and then, if they are to be frozen, often coated with methyl cellulose to ensure that they harden when they are fried, to produce a crisp outer

THE CASE OF THE ELUSIVE APPLES

Establishing the cause of intolerance in fruit and vegetables seems to require the skills of a seasoned detective. One of my patients had become acutely depressed and asthmatic, to the point of believing that he needed psychiatric help, before he was referred to me. From his history and his answers to the questionnaire, I strongly suspected food intolerance, but none of the foods that he had listed as regularly and frequently eaten tested positive, and there was no indication that he was chemically intolerant when I tested for the common troublemakers.

It was only by a process of elimination, which took many months, that we finally hit upon an explanation. The villain turned out to be apples — but not the apples in his own garden, which had produced no reaction when we tested them after a five-day fast. The troublesome apples were some that were sent regularly as a present by his brother in Queensland. As we subsequently discovered, they were packed in crates that had been sprayed with a fungicide for which I hadn't tested. It was this fungicide, transferred to the fruit itself, that was the source of all my patient's troubles, even though the crates themselves never left Queensland, and my patient lived in New South Wales.

It is unusual to find only a single intolerance in people whose symptoms are as severe as this. We might have missed it altogether if he had not been keeping a diary of every food that passed into his mouth for a month and precise details of where he had obtained it. It is important for everyone who suspects food intolerance to do this.

shell with a tender, moist interior, as the advertisements promise. It might do interesting things to the taste, but it is very unwelcome to the unsuspecting customer with intolerance to methyl cellulose.

In theory it is quite easy to establish whether patients are being affected by a chemical in the food, or by the fruit or vegetable itself. By allowing them first to eat an organically grown sample, free of pesticides, herbicides and all the other contaminants that accumulate in the commercial products, we can see if they tolerate the fruit or vegetable in its own right. If that proves negative, we repeat the test with the same food bought commercially.

In reality, and particularly in cities, it is very difficult to find fruit and vegetables that can be guaranteed to be free of contaminants. People who can eat only chemically-free foods know well that they are often difficult to find, and invariably expensive to buy, unless they are home grown.

MEAT AND POULTRY ■

Just like any other food, meat can cause intolerance if it is eaten regularly and frequently by anyone with a specific intolerance of meat, the two essential factors in any food addiction. Intolerance of one red meat tends to predispose people to be intolerant of all other red meats, but not usually white meats as well.

Pork seems to be particularly implicated in intolerance and the symptoms are notorious for mimicking a great many disorders. It has been responsible for impaired hearing and tinnitus (ringing in the ears), dizziness and loss of equilibrium, headache and migraine, and numerous other reactions. Pork is also a difficult meat to avoid, because as well as appearing in obvious forms, such as pork chops and bacon, its derivatives turn up in numerous unlikely products. Pork farmers pride themselves on producing an animal in which nothing is wasted, from its bristles to its trotters, so perhaps we shouldn't be surprised to find it in everything from salad dressing and cake mixes, to cheese dip and soap. Because of its use in lard and shortening, it turns up in fried foods and pastries; it is in potato chips, many instant foods including mashed potatoes; non-dairy creams and ice-cream; jellies, some processed cheeses and cocktail dips; and glue.

I know of a colleague who reported a patient who was highly intolerant of pork: it made her weep and brought her out in hives. She studiously discovered all the uses to which pork is put and avoided them all — or all except one. Her symptoms refused to go away completely, although they were much improved when she began her boycott of everything that contained any pig products, so he went back to her history. He took her through every moment's activity in her typical week and it was only a meticulous process of elimination that led them to an activity that she performed each day at the office. Her last task before she went home was to put the stamps on the day's mail and post it on the way to the train. There was the cause of her problems: the glue on the back of the stamps contained a pork ingredient.

It took a good deal of legwork to establish that, but once they suspected the truth and she began to use a sponge to wet the glue, instead of licking it, the last of the symptoms vanished. Just occasionally they still come back, probably because she has unwittingly come into contact with some by-product of this very ubiquitous animal.

A much greater problem associated with meat, however, for many people is one that we have already discussed (Chapter 10): the chemicals that either deliberately or inadvertently get into the tissue of animals before they are slaughtered. Red meat, white meat, poultry and even farm-reared fish are all vulnerable. Since the end of the Second World War, an array of synthetic hormones, tranquillisers and particularly antibiotics have been given to farm animals, either to promote growth or to prevent disease. Traces of all these chemicals are likely to remain after slaughter, as are the herbicides and pesticides that enter their bodies in the food they eat.

Poultry are given drugs to stimulate appetite as well as to control bacteria and prevent disease. When they go for slaughter they are tranquillised to reduce flapping (they hang by one leg on a conveyor belt) — not for any humanitarian reasons, but because the stress affects the quality of the flesh.

To a considerable extent, an intolerant reaction to meat can be greatly reduced by cutting off all the fat *before* cooking. It is no use waiting until after the meat has been cooked, for by then the contaminants will have spread throughout the food. Even this, though, may not be sufficient for those who are hypersensitive to any of the chemical residues.

Dr Richard Mackarness has described an appalling case of a 21-year-old girl, a music student, who had been ill for eight years with depression, lack of concentration, loss of libido and an inability to sit still or read comprehendingly. She had attempted suicide and was overweight. Before Mackarness first saw her she had been shunted around from doctor to doctor, through hospitals and clinics, been treated with psychotropic drugs, electric shock and group therapy, before being finally consigned to a hostel for mentally disturbed adolescents, where she cut her wrists. Mackarness tested her, found that she was severely intolerant of chemicals in many of the foods that she ate, especially

MARK'S UNCONTROLLABLE VIOLENCE

Typical of those who react to chemicals in meat was Mark, 5½, who was hyperactive and suffered bouts of uncontrollable violence. His doctor recognised that this violence might be ecologically caused and referred Mark to me.

Testing revealed that his unsociable behaviour was indeed being triggered by many processed foods, but especially by red meat and poultry. We tested him first on chicken that had been bought in the supermarket and the reaction came swiftly. He went into an almost uncontrollable rage, clawing at the nurse, screaming at the top of his voice and generally threatening to tear the ward apart.

When the reaction had worn off, he was challenged with chicken again, to the considerable alarm of the same nurse, but this time it was a free-range chicken that had been given no chemicals since it hatched and had eaten only chemical-free feed. Mark ate his test meal, unaware that the chicken was any different from the first one. There was no reaction at all.

After waiting for two hours in case there was an unexpected delayed response, the nurse brought in what appeared to be yet another identical piece of chicken except that, unknown to Mark, this time it had been taken from the first bird. The reaction was even more rapid than the first time and we witnessed the same wildly hyperactive response. Then we challenged him with red meat from two sources, and again obtained the same two reactions.

The problem, of course, was the chemicals and particularly the hormones, in both the chicken and the beef. On a diet that was as near as possible unprocessed and unrefined, avoiding all meat (he had no access to any meat other than in the supermarket and the butcher's), he remained well and symptom-free. Only when he inadvertently ate a food containing a chemical that he could not tolerate, nearly always in a restaurant or at someone else's home where there was no way of knowing, did any of his symptoms recur — almost the perfect double-blind proof of his intolerance!

in meat, and altered her diet appropriately. Her symptoms disappeared and, with counselling to help overcome the trauma of what she had suffered in the previous years, she made a complete recovery.

I am sure that every doctor using an ecological approach to the illnesses of their patients, could tell a hundred variations of this case. What possible justification can there be for treating such a girl for so long without even apparently considering that all her symptoms might be nothing more than reactions to something in her environment? For at least six years before she was eventually referred to Richard Mackarness, it must have been known that there was nothing organically wrong with her. If just one of all those doctors who saw her had had any understanding of clinical ecology, things might have been so different for her.

MILK ■

Cow's milk is the single most important cause of food intolerance. Books have been written on the havoc that it can cause, and most paediatricians immediately suspect cow's milk intolerance or allergy as being responsible for many otherwise unexplainable disorders and symptoms.

The problem in a nutshell is that cow's milk was designed for small calves and not small people. Its sole purpose in nature, which it does highly efficiently, is to take a 40 kilogram baby cow and bring it up to about 900 kilograms within nine months: a man begins life at about 3 kilograms and takes eighteen years to reach about 70 kilograms.

The milk of each mammal is structured exactly to meet the needs of its young and not the young of any other species. Humans are no exception. The mother's milk production matches her baby's needs so perfectly that when a baby is born prematurely the milk has different concentrations of protein, sodium and chloride than when it is born at full-term. This means that the milk is exactly suited to the needs of the baby at that moment to give it the greatest chance of surviving and thriving.

Breastfed babies acquire a great deal of immunity against illness and disease, not only when they are very small when it most matters, but right into adulthood. Cow's milk, on the other hand, is a mucus-producing, acid-forming substance, practically devoid of vitamin C, with three times the amount of sodium as human milk — just what a calf requires!

Heart specialists worry that cow's milk contains disturbingly high amounts of fat and cholesterol. A British study, reported in the journal *Archives of Disease in Childhood*, reached the conclusion that 40 per cent of children are sensitive to cow's milk. Other papers have described the damaging effect of cow's milk on psychiatric patients, many of them suffering for years from confusion, poor memory, detachment and paranoia, invariably accompanied by fatigue. Yet these patients, 80 per cent of them in one study, made a significant and sometimes complete recovery from their symptoms when cow's milk was removed from their diets and they received appropriate counselling.

In the case of psychiatric illnesses brought on by intolerance to foods or chemicals, the "treatment" of patients over many years has so damaged their personalities and affected their behaviour, that skilled counselling is usually also required to restore normality, once the food or chemical has been withdrawn and a healthy diet imposed.

Symptoms of Cow's Milk Intolerance In most instances, the symptoms of cow's milk intolerance affect the skin, the gut and the respiratory tract. If the skin is the target area, the symptoms tend to develop comparatively quickly, but can last for seventy-two hours or more, much longer than most food reactions. Nevertheless, during testing, there is almost always at least an initial reaction within four hours, as with other food intolerance. The symptoms usually include an eruption and an urticarial or hives reaction, often around the mouth, although it can be generalised. In children intolerant of milk, the skin symptoms appear after only relatively small amounts have been drunk.

If the reaction occurs in the gastrointestinal tract, the main symptoms are likely to be vomiting or diarrhoea, and quite frequently both. Children who vomit as the first symptom tend to develop the symptoms in a relatively short time, after consuming only a small amount of milk. If diarrhoea appears first, comparatively large amounts of milk have usually been drunk and the reaction takes longer to appear, sometimes even days, although again there is nearly always an initial reaction that announces the intolerance.

Finally, if the trouble is in the respiratory tract, the symptoms take longer to develop than on the skin, but last for a shorter time, and larger amounts of milk have to be drunk. In one study, about 20 per cent of children, who were all milk intolerant, coughed and wheezed and developed runny eyes and a runny nose as significant symptoms of their intolerance.

Other more bizarre symptoms have been recorded. Dr Theron Randolph reported the case of a woman who was arrested for apparent drunken driving, when he knew that all she had consumed was a glass of milk in his surgery (it was before the days of breathalysing). When the police stopped her, she exhibited all the signs of being drunk. Some people feel punch-drunk two hours after drinking milk, and behave in traffic as though they are immortal.

Perhaps some of the lethal drivers on the road today had one glass too many — of milk. The encouragement of the Milk Board to "Make it milk and make it home", as one of their slogans said, would be bad advice for such a sufferer.

Babies and Young Children The reason why children react so often and so badly to cow's milk is mainly because they drink a great deal of it, and because they have usually been drinking it every day of their lives since before they could walk. In infancy, as we have seen, the protective immune mechanisms of the body are still easily disturbed. Intolerance often develops very young and the reaction becomes masked, so there is no longer obvious cause and effect. What happens is that one or more of the proteins in cow's milk pass through the permeable wall of the gut, where they are met by a brisk and destructive response from the immune system. Of the five main proteins in cow's milk, the one that causes the most trouble is beta-lactoglobulin, a protein that is not present in human milk. Casein is another of the proteins that is a frequent cause of intolerance reactions.

For intolerance to develop in babies, it is not even necessary for them to be drinking cow's milk themselves. Babies can become intolerant or allergic (in the true sense of the word) from the cow's milk that the mother drinks and that she passes on to her baby in her own milk. Many breastfeeding mothers eat plenty of yoghurt and cheese and drink a lot of cow's milk, thinking that this is good nutrition and that the consumption of cow's milk will aid their own milk production. In part they are right, for it is foolish to deny that cow's milk, for all the problems it causes, is very nutritious for those who develop no intolerance of it, and it continues to play a vital role in feeding the malnourished in many deprived parts of the world. However, mothers may also be passing on to their babies the food of which they are the most intolerant. There is evidence that some babies even come into the world intolerant of cow's milk, predisposed to a lifetime of intolerance, because of the cow's milk their mothers drank during pregnancy.

Colic, the painful intestinal cramps and spasms of the bowel that affect babies and are so mortifying to their mothers, is frequently a reaction to cow's milk. If the baby is being breastfed and is drinking no cow's milk directly, the mother should stop drinking milk herself. This is often the only treatment that is necessary.

Because masking can take place at such an early age, parents often mistake the signs. They do not understand that the once-a-week attack of colic is the result of the baby drinking cow's milk three times every day. If cow's milk used to make a baby ill when it was first introduced into his diet, but the mother persevered because she thought it was good for the baby and eventually the vomiting stopped and now the child cries when he doesn't get his milk, then ninety-nine times out of a hundred the child is intolerant of cow's milk, and masking has already occurred. The baby is a milk addict and, if a lifetime of problems of intolerance is not to develop, he must be weaned off the cow's milk as a matter of urgency.

Masking can also have occurred in the mother so that *she* has no idea that she is milk intolerant. If she knew, she would immediately be warned that there was a better than average likelihood that her child would also develop cow's milk intolerance.

Pasteurisation Virtually all commercially available cow's milk is subjected to pasteurisation and homogenisation. There is a lot of confusion about whether these two processes improve or worsen the situation so far as intolerance goes. Pasteurisation partially sterilises milk, while homogenisation emulsifies the fat droplets in milk, allowing them to disperse in the rest of the milk. The cream doesn't separate, which is why you rarely see the layer of cream that used to be at the top of the milk bottle.

These processes remove some of the greatest dangers associated with cow's milk, which has a very short safe life if left untreated. Until pasteurisation, in particular, became available, dairy herds had to be kept in the city because there was no way of transporting the milk safely from country areas into the towns and cities where it was most needed. For many people, pasteurisation made milk available for the first time and its impact on nutrition was enormous. Despite all its undoubted benefits, pasteurisation also affects and inactivates some very important substances that are in cow's milk, including the thirty-five natural enzymes in raw milk, enzymes that are essential for the full and sufficient digestion of the milk. One of the most important enzymes destroyed is lipase, the enzyme that breaks down fat. If pasteurisation did wonders for nutrition, it was disastrous for intolerance.

Interestingly, it appears that relatively primitive people who drink their milk straight from the cow, without pasteurisation or homogenisation, do not suffer from milk-activated disorders in the way that Westerners do. The only other factor that might be implicated is the routine testing of every dairy cow for tuberculosis in most Western countries: minute traces of the tuberculin vaccine remain in the milk and have long been suspected of being involved in intolerance.

One of the most significant studies into the possible effects of pasteurisation on cow's milk and on those who drink it was carried out more than forty years ago by Dr Francis Pottenger. Pottenger used cats for his experiment, so the results cannot necessarily be extrapolated for humans, but his findings nevertheless raised the most alarming possibilities, which have never been adequately countered.

The cats were divided into three groups. One group was fed primarily on raw cow's milk (that is, milk that had been neither pasteurised nor homogenised); the second group on pasteurised milk; and the third on evaporated cow's milk and condensed milk. Pottenger continued this experiment over four generations of cats, or at least that was his plan.

All four generations fed on raw milk thrived, but the other two groups began to deteriorate rapidly. Even by the second generation, there was a high incidence of stillbirths, spontaneous abortions and miscarriages, and the survivors had many problems that included gross anatomical defects, abnormalities in their neuro-muscular coordination and neuroses, as well as eczema and calcification of the tissues. Even anatomical differences between the sexes became less apparent and homosexuality manifested itself. The third generation was even further depleted and showed no interest at all in even attempting to reproduce. There was no fourth generation. The second and third groups had become extinct.

Now one would be very rash to argue from this that drinking cow's milk can make humans homosexual and lead to their fairly rapid extinction, but it must be equally foolish to dismiss the Pottenger experiment as having no significance at all for humans. In particular the dairy industry cannot insist that the benefits of pasteurising cow's milk are achieved without even the possibility that there are undesirable side effects.

Ethnic Background and Lactase Deficiency   Ethnic background plays a role in determining how well children, in particular, handle cow's milk. A recent study by the University of Sydney's School of Public Health and Tropical Medicine investigated 109 children in two inner Sydney suburbs, looking particularly at possible lactase deficiency and its effects. Lactase is an enzyme that breaks down lactose, a sugar in milk, into glucose and galactose, another simple sugar. The study found that 40 per cent of the children had a serious deficiency of lactase, which inevitably predisposed them to have trouble with cow's milk; but intriguingly, they also found that the ethnic background of the children was very significant.

People who are not of Anglo-Celtic origin, it appears, do not produce lactase after weaning, or they produce it only in very limited amounts. In consequence, they are unable to break down any milk or milk products that contain lactose.

The problems of lactose malabsorption, which must greatly increase the chance of intolerance developing, were found to be worst in children of Asian origin (Vietnamese, Chinese, Indonesian and Filipino in this study), 93 per cent of whom were deficient. Among Greek children, 56 per cent showed malabsorption and were unable to absorb lactose efficiently; the figure from other Mediterranean and Middle Eastern countries, including Italy, Spain, Portugal and Egypt, was 41 per cent. On the other hand, only one (3 per cent) of the thirty-two Anglo-Celtic-descended children showed evidence of lactose malabsorption.

The study, published in the *Medical Journal of Australia*, went on to reveal that 57 per cent of those children who showed a lactase deficiency reported symptoms of intolerance from cow's milk, compared with 29 per cent of those who could absorb lactose. In other words, based on the findings of this study, non-Anglo-Celtic children are roughly twice as likely to develop milk intolerance as the Anglo-Celts, nearly a third of whom will suffer from milk intolerance anyway.

The most common symptom of intolerance was abdominal pain, reported by thirty-two of the forty-four children who reacted; the mothers of non-Anglo-Celtic babies who suffer from colic must have even more reason than most to suspect cow's milk before anything else. If the mother is also drinking cow's milk that she cannot absorb properly, the problem can only be intensified. Eleven children suffered diarrhoea and seven of these demonstrated lactose malabsorption.

The reason for this discrepancy is probably that Anglo-Celts have a much longer history of consuming cow's milk than the other races and adaptation saw to it that they were able to produce sufficient lactase in their systems to control the lactose levels that would be acquired from drinking it. Asians tend to use soya products for the same purpose, Middle Eastern peoples use tahini, a ground sesame paste, and Southern Europeans traditionally get their calcium from cheeses which are made from milk curd and do not contain lactose.

The importance of these findings is that they demonstrate the need to put much more care into planning the nutritional requirements of youngsters in schools in essentially Anglo-Celtic societies. Much more work clearly needs to be done along the same lines with Aboriginal children who have no tradition of consuming cow's milk. There were no cattle in Australia until five cows and two bulls arrived in 1788 from the Cape of Good Hope. In addition, it shouldn't be overlooked that nearly a third of the children who *could* absorb lactose still suffered reactions to the cow's milk the school provided for them.

Goat's Milk — Not Always a Suitable Alternative
Goat's milk, incidentally, is frequently not a suitable alternative for those who cannot tolerate cow's milk. In particular, it should never be fed to babies under six months, except with a doctor's agreement. Most of the enthusiasm for the alleged benefits of goat's milk comes from the goat industry, the farmers and the retailers who market goat's milk. The *British Medical Journal* recently reported evidence that the salt content of goat's milk is much too high for young babies whose kidneys may not be able to handle it. As a result, some babies fed on goat's milk by unsus-

pecting parents have developed a dangerous condition called hypertonic dehydration.

It is true that goat's milk appears to be tolerated by some children who cannot tolerate cow's milk. From the point of view of allergy and intolerance, it is different, but if there is lactose intolerance, the lactose of goats is handled no differently from that in cow's milk. Neither is there any significant difference in the protein content of goat's milk and cow's milk, so that the change from one to the other is often a pointless exercise.

Goat's milk also poses worrying questions about quality control. At the time of writing, it does not need to be pasteurised in most states of Australia. Farmers have resisted pasteurisation strongly on the grounds that the level of production simply doesn't warrant the expense of setting up pasteurisation plants. They argue that in any case pasteurisation destroys much that is good in their milk (which is irrefutable), and that their existing precautions are adequate, which is very questionable. The risk of bacterial infection is just too high to take *any* risks with milk.

A Difficult Food to Avoid   Milk can come in many guises. Anything with the prefix "lact-", such as lactose, is a milk, and many so-called non-dairy products, including non-dairy creamers, contain milk by-products or fractions of the milk proteins. They may therefore cause the same reactions as milk. Powdered artificial sweeteners often contain lactose, as well as saccharin which is derived from coal tar, a combination that causes many intolerance problems. Many people who know that they or their children are intolerant of dairy products, buy margarine instead, little realising that most margarines contain milk. Only the occasional brand does not contain milk and this is stated on the label.

On the other hand everything that looks like milk is not necessarily milk. The thick shakes in many takeaway restaurants are not called milkshakes for the very good reason that they are not made with milk. Instead, they use pig fat or the fat of some other animal to achieve the same effect. Their customers could more accurately go up to the counter and order a glass of vanilla or strawberry flavoured, sweetened pig fat.

Excluding all cow's milk from an infant's diet may not be easy, particularly in those developing countries, or in poorer Western families, where it plays a vital role in nutrition. Avoiding milk for long periods may cause nutritional problems that are even more severe than the ecological disorders that come from consuming it. In most families in Western countries, however, cow's milk can be used very sparingly without any risk. In most situations a mother would be strongly advised to avoid giving cow's milk to young children, especially under the age of six months.

For adults who cannot tolerate milk, it is even more difficult to avoid it. Go into any restaurant and you have to be suspicious of every course, from the bread roll through to the dessert and the final after-dinner mint. The list of foods that contain milk — or may contain it — is almost endless. It is a very hard food to get away from.

Kosher breads (challah) and some Italian and French breads are made without milk, but almost all popular supermarket brands of bread and bakery lines have cow's milk in them, or cow's milk derivatives. The only way to know is to read the label or, in the case of unwrapped bread, to ask the baker and hope for a truthful answer.

American allergist Dr D. W. Brown Jnr suggested that to be safe, people who cannot tolerate cow's milk ought to ask, every time they go into a food shop or a restaurant, "Do you use butter, oleo-margarine, cream, cheese of any kind, fresh milk, buttermilk, dried milk, powdered milk, condensed milk, evaporated milk or yoghurt in this food?" It is likely to be met with a glazed look from most shop assistants and waiters, but it is an indication of how difficult it is to avoid milk.

Because dairy products are processed in many different ways, not all of them contain the five main proteins in cow's milk. If you suspect dairy products, therefore, without knowing which one is responsible for intolerance, test them individually by exclusion in the following order. They are listed in descending order of the intolerance problems they usually cause.

- Hard cheeses
- Ricotta (a soft cottage cheese made from whey)
- Cream
- Butter
- Milk
- Yoghurt

Probably because it has been "reprocessed" by the yoghurt bacteria, yoghurt is far more digestible than milk and has far less problems than those associated with cow's milk protein. Cream, on the other hand, brings a host of problems with it, most of them associated with its very high fat and cholesterol content, in addition to the normal problems linked with cow's milk. Of course, these products must not only be avoided when they come straight from the packet or the carton, but also in cooking.

Although any cheese made from cow's milk must be suspected until it is proved safe, there are a few that are especially troubling for many people, including cheddar — by far the most popular cheese. There are so many different methods of making cheese that tolerance of one or two may be possible when all the others have to be shunned. I have one patient who can tolerate any cheese except parmesan. As soon as even a trace turns up in the cooking, she immediately breaks out in severe dermatitis. Even the smell of parmesan causes itching and redness of the skin.

Parmesan, camembert and blue vein all contain monosodium glutamate (MSG) naturally, so that in addition to triggering milk intolerance in some people, these cheeses also bring with them all the problems associated with MSG.

A tip that is claimed to help people who find it difficult to digest any dairy products without suffering headaches, sore eyes, or any of the other common symptoms of milk intolerance, is to take 1000 milligrams of alfalfa (which is available in tablet form) immediately after any meal or snack containing milk or indeed any animal fat. There are no possible undesirable side effects from consuming alfalfa. But the best solution is to avoid cow's milk altogether whenever possible.

WHEAT ■

Along with milk, wheat is probably the leading cause of food intolerance in the Western world except for the United States, where corn replaces it. Like milk, wheat first enters our systems when we are very young. From about the time we are toddlers, our gastrointestinal tracts are almost never free of it for the rest of our lives. (See "The Problem with Amanda, p. 81.) The food intolerance it spawns is compounded by the innumerable chemicals that are either added to it or contaminate it between the time the first seeds are sown until it appears on our table in any of its familiar forms.

It has been suggested that corn products cause more problems than wheat products, but this is probably because, to separate different parts of the kernel, corn is often soaked for several days in sulphur dioxide, a chemical that is notorious for its involvement in intolerance. However, kilo for kilo, wheat causes just as many problems as corn.

Wheat includes everything that is made from the wheat grain, including wheat flour, wheatgerm and bran. It is used in obvious products such as bread and cakes (even most rye bread and pumpernickel contain wheat), pies and doughnuts; but also in less immediately identifiable products such as frankfurters, chutneys and artificial cream.

Establishing beyond doubt whether intolerance is the result of the wheat or one of the chemicals is often very difficult and time consuming, but it is usually not necessary. If white bread results in a maladaptive reaction and masking, then avoid white bread. The culprit may well be one of the bleaching agents used to whiten flour, but it may equally well be the flour itself, the anti-oxidants or the thickeners, or any of the other additives used by bakers.

The following list of common products that frequently contain wheat includes many where the presence of wheat would not normally be suspected.

- Foods prepackaged or thickened with flour, batter or breadcrumbs
- Small goods, e.g. devon, sausages, meat pies, tinned meats and fish in sauce
- Vegetables, tinned in sauce
- Commercial vegetable salad
- Wheatmeal porridge, semolina, etc
- Wheat breakfast cereals
- Wheat flour, wheat starch
- Macaroni, spaghetti, vermicelli
- Malted milk and other malt products
- All commercial breads
- Commercial baking powder
- All desserts containing wheat flour or wheat starch
- Cakes and biscuits
- Ice-cream cones and wafers
- Custard powders, packet puddings and pie fillings
- Pastry mixes

- Artificial cream
- Soups, gravies and stews thickened with flour or noodles, etc
- Packet or tinned soups
- Commercial sweets and cream-filled chocolates
- Pretzels
- Spreads and pastes
- Commercial sauces, relishes, chutneys, salad creams, etc
- Wheat germ
- Beer, gin and any drink containing neutral grain spirits.

A disease that is peculiarly associated with wheat but also with other grains and notably rye, is coeliac disease. It is a bowel condition that is usually seen in children. One of the important functions of the intestine is to remove the nutrients from the food that we eat and pass them on to the various body systems. For some still poorly understood reason, there is an immune reaction to wheat gluten in particular (gluten is a mixture of certain proteins in wheat and other cereal grains), which impairs this absorptive function.

As a result, the child may have diarrhoea or greasy stools; growth and weight gain may slow down, muscles become weak and the abdomen swell up. This child is likely to become lethargic and bad-tempered. The symptoms commonly appear before the second birthday, after solid foods, especially cereals and foods that contain flour, have been introduced into the diet.

Many diseases, of course, produce these symptoms, but what singles out coeliac disease is that the symptoms rapidly disappear once gluten has been removed from the diet. The problem is that it is a difficult disease to diagnose with certainty without taking a biopsy, and this usually has to be done; and it is very difficult to ensure a diet that contains no gluten. Avoiding the obvious sources such as bread and biscuits is easy enough, but countless manufactured and processed foods also contain it. And as if this isn't enough, gluten is present in many pharmaceutical drugs — even those likely to be prescribed for the relief of the disease that is caused by gluten! Appendix VII lists the bewildering array of drugs which at the time of writing contain gluten. It is very unlikely that most general practitioners will be aware that the drugs they are prescribing contain gluten, so check this list if coeliac disease is a problem in your family.

Apart from the difficulty of avoiding foods that contain

gluten, treatment is relatively simple: once all wheat and rye gluten has been removed from the diet, the symptoms disappear. Until that occurs, coeliac children (only comparatively rarely does coeliac disease first appear later in life) need to be treated as sick children. They need rest and great understanding because they can be very bad-tempered and difficult to handle. Gluten may well have to be avoided for the rest of their lives.

WATER, AND THE FLUORIDE DEBATE ■

Most people think of water — if they think of it at all — as a neutral, harmless substance that is purified with chemicals to make it safe to drink, but in every other way is the same, whether it comes out of a tap in the city, or from a mountain stream. Unless they have drunk water free of any added chemicals, they will have no idea just how much the taste is altered for the worse by chemicals.

Unfortunately for many people, water is very far from being inert and harmless. The numerous chemicals that reticulated water supplies contain, which are either put there deliberately, or are contaminants, affect many of those who are chemically sensitive and it is the most difficult of all the substances that we ingest to avoid.

It was to prevent the spread of infectious diseases, such as typhoid, that cities in the United States first began adding chlorine to drinking water in 1912. It was so effective in stopping the spread of infection that nobody showed much interest in the findings some twenty years later of two allergists who proved that chlorinated drinking water was causing asthma in an alarming number of their patients. We know now that chlorine is a common cause of many more symptoms than only asthma in people who have general sensitivity to chemicals. Some patients with extreme sensitivity do not even need to drink chlorinated water to be seriously affected by it. Breathing the chlorinated vapours emanating from a swimming pool may be enough to trigger the symptoms; and a few people become sick even standing over a bath containing chlorinated water.

Water "purification", however, involves a great deal more than simply adding chlorine to the water. Most treated municipal water supplies also include benzene, toluene, carbon tetrachloride, dichlormethane and bromo-dichlormethane and most controversially, significant quantities of fluoride, ostensibly put there to improve dental health. In addition, most water is contaminated even before it is treated, and normal treatment cannot remove this contamination. Traces of pesticides and herbicides in particular are invariably present in drinking water. They run off into streams and rivers and into reservoirs, or filter through into the subterranean water table; or they fall into the water as airborne residues.

Industry pollutes the rivers and the water supply with detergents, formaldehyde, phenols, phosphates, hexachlorophene and innumerable other chemicals, usually in legally permissible levels, but levels that may be very harmful to people sensitive to them in doses as low as a few parts per billion. The treatment plants then add *their* chemicals to all the others. More than 350 organic chemicals have been detected in water in areas of the United States and it is very doubtful, if a similar exercise were ever conducted in Australia, that the findings would be any better.

It is important not to get the problem out of perspective. Water treatment is essential and the contamination level by chemicals is usually low. But if water is drunk regularly every day, whether straight from the tap, in processed foods cooked in it, or in the form of purchased fruit juices and other drink, this frequent and regular consumption immediately makes it a candidate for causing ecological illness. As always, there must be individual susceptibility — not everyone reacts in the same way to the same substances — but probably because there are so many chemicals in water, my experience is that tap water is a very common source of trouble. When patients are tested for food intolerance or chemical sensitivity of any kind, pure water is invariably used, such as deionised water, and never water out of the tap.

Filtering is often sufficient to make town water drinkable for patients who are not too intolerant. There are a number of commercial filters on the market that remove up to 95 per cent of chlorine and 99 per cent of most other chemicals. It is the remaining traces of these chemicals that cause the trouble in the most sensitive patients. The price of these filters depends very much on the level of efficiency that is required and the amount of water that is needed. They vary from only about $25 to more than $500 for an average domestic-size unit.

Even after town water has been through the treatment

PEGGY'S PERPLEXING SYMPTOMS

The case of 7-year-old Peggy shows how perplexing intolerance to the chemicals in water can be. Since she was 1 year old, Peggy had suffered from unpleasant ulcer-like eruptions in her mouth. As well as being very painful, they were associated with what her doctor called "constitutional symptoms", by which he meant that when the ulcers were widespread, she felt unwell and lacked energy.

When she was 18 months old, she was first treated with two different antibiotics, which were no help, but a blood test done at the time revealed that her neutrophils, white blood cells, were low. Neutrophils play a key role in the immune system's defence against infection. This discovery prompted her doctor to have her admitted to the children's hospital in the city where she lived and she was given a barrage of tests for a host of diseases, particularly immunological disorders. Nothing was found.

Her next port of call was to a paediatric gastroenterologist who produced a list of things that may have been wrong with her, some of them downright rare and obscure. She was treated with a drug called Tegretol for a form of

neuralgia, which was one of the diagnoses on the paediatrician's list and although it did nothing for her "neuralgia" (not surprisingly, because she didn't have neuralgia), there was a marked reduction in the severity and duration of her ulcers. When Peggy's family doctor reported this to the paediatrician, he said bluntly that he didn't believe it and that the improvement must have been in the imagination not even of Peggy, but of her parents.

Eventually, as the last resort, she was sent to me. The paediatrician had got tired of little Peggy with her recurrent illness that didn't respond to any of his treatments, and he put her into the neurotic basket. Only the refusal of her own family doctor to believe this — and the diligence and patience of so many family doctors is wonderful — prompted him to keep going and he sent her to see me. Seven years had now elapsed since her symptoms were first observed and except for the fluke benefit of the Tegretol, there had been not a trace of improvement.

Her doctor wrote perceptively that he was sure Peggy was ingesting some chemical that was triggering her lymphocytes to release substances that were poisonous to her cells, though he had no idea what might be involved. The effect of this, he reasoned, on the mucus in her mouth was to cause the ulceration and when it entered her circulation, it resulted in the other symptoms.

Peggy was tested for food intolerance soon after she arrived. She reacted quite strongly to several foods, which were subsequently left out of her diet. By far the strongest reaction came, however, when we tested the contents of a bottle that she had brought with her — taken from the water supply of the city where she lived. It was the chemicals in this water that were responsible for all her symptoms. There was no point trying to identify which particular chemicals were responsible because they were inseparable from the water.

She returned home, went on to a diet that excluded the foods to which she had reacted, and drank only deionised water which was as pure as she could reasonably make it. From then on — and five years have gone by now — she was free of her ulcers, her lack of energy and all the other symptoms. Just occasionally a single ulcer would make an

appearance, almost certainly because she ate vegetables or other fresh foods washed in the city water when she went out. Except, that is, for one relapse.

Because it is rare to find chemical victims who are vulnerable to just one chemical (and of course, Peggy might have been reacting to several of the chemicals in the water), I wasn't surprised when I received a letter some two years later telling me that Peggy had slipped back and suffered an apparent relapse during school term. Her mother, by now a shrewd detective, as all chemical victims or their parents must be, suspected that there was a link either with the duplicated material that the school used, or the ink itself.

Without needing to see Peggy, I prepared special desensitising drops based on the different chemical substances that were likely to be used in the school, including spirit duplicator and ink. Peggy's treatment consisted of putting one drop of this solution under her tongue each morning and evening. From the first day, everything was brought under control again and at the time of writing, has remained that way.

plant, it may still be exposed to chemical contamination. If the water is hard, for instance (which means that it has high levels of mineral salts), it is difficult to use in washing, so it is softened with chemical water softeners. Most people can tolerate softened water, but there is a minority who are made ill by it.

Tank water sometimes causes problems in country areas, usually because the source of the supply itself is contaminated, and usually again by chemicals. (Dead creatures in the water, like possums that have fallen into the tank, are not implicated nearly so often as many town-dwellers believe.) The use of sealing agents inside the tank, often bitumen, can also contaminate the water for anyone sufficiently sensitive to petrochemicals. As in all chemical intolerance, it is not necessary for the bitumen to be present in toxic quantities: the slightest trace leaching into the water may be sufficient. If the tank is fed by water that runs off a recently treated or painted roof, chemicals from the treatment or the paint will go striaght into the water. The same will happen if the roof has been contaminated by the residue of agrochemical sprays or other atmospheric fallout.

Not many people today would knowingly use lead paint anywhere near anything that comes in contact with food or drink, yet lead is still widely used in soldering copper pipes that carry water. This too inevitably leeches into the water supply, which is drunk by members of the family for twenty years or more. Again the dose that is being received will certainly be much less than anything considered dangerous by toxicologists, and it may never result in any of the classic symptoms of lead poisoning. But for those who are intolerant of lead in any amount, the result may very well be ecological illness and any of the symptoms of chemical intolerance. There are entirely satisfactory substitutes for lead that can be requested when the plumber is doing the job.

The minerals in bottled water present no problem except in the most extreme cases of chemical intolerance, and indeed mineral water is frequently ordered for those who cannot take tap water. Even naturally, in spring water and bore water, organic chemicals are present in low concentrations, principally benzene, toluene and chlorine.

THE BITTER FLUORIDE DEBATE ■

Nothing that is added to water causes such bitter debate as fluoride. Those who support fluoridation of the water supply argue that it is one of the most significant advances in dental health care and that the dramatic fall in the incidence of caries, or tooth decay, supports this. The opponents, who are equally vociferous, claim that it does not have anything like the benefits that have been claimed and that the incidence of caries has fallen at much the same rate in cities and countries where the water is not fluoridated, largely because of improved health care and diet and an understanding of the causes of caries. Many clinical ecologists have noticed substantial reductions in plaque on the teeth of children they are treating, presumably because of the stress placed on diet and the reduction of sugary foods. Above all they insist that it is wrong that whole populations should be compulsorily exposed to a chemical from which there is no practical escape, whatever benefits it is supposed to bring short of preserving life. An increasing number of authorities have taken this approach, and Sweden, West Germany and Holland have all ended their fluoridation programs. Most other European countries had never been sufficiently satisfied to introduce it in the first place.

There have been some very prominent turncoats. The former chairman of the New Zealand Fluoridation Promotion Committee and one-time principal dental officer in New Zealand's Health Department, John Colquhoun, believes that New Zealand's original enthusiasm, which resulted in mass fluoridation, was completely misplaced in the light of later evidence. "We dentists made a big mistake", he said in a lecture in 1987. "We overrated the benefit of fluoridation and ignored genuine evidence that, for some people, even the low levels of fluoride used in fluoridation, are a health hazard."

There is little argument that fluoride does protect teeth from decay. That is not the point of the dispute. Where fluoride is found naturally in drinking water, at one part per million or less, it gives protection without any apparent adverse symptoms. This may explain why some communities in less developed countries have a very low incidence of caries while others, often with similar diets and socioeconomic conditions, equally poor oral hygiene and geographically not far away, have a very high level of the disease. In the few studies that have been done, natural fluoride has been found in the drinking water of those with healthy teeth, but not in that of the group with a greater incidence of tooth decay.

However, at a level of only two parts per million, fluoride

can cause yellowing of the teeth, and at greater concentrations symptoms of fluorosis, or poisoning by fluoride, begin to occur. Tablets of 1.1 milligrams are usually prescribed for children under 2 years old, and double this strength for children up to 10 years. If a child is taking sodium fluoride tablets at a strength of 2.2 milligrams, in addition to drinking water, even occasionally, that contains fluoride (either naturally or as an additive) and brushing his teeth with a fluoride toothpaste, he will be substantially overdosing.

In November 1985, the *British Medical Journal* reported a link between fluoride and anorexia, even in children, and recently American chemists discovered that fluoride attacks the centre of an important body enzyme and renders it inactive. It is now strongly suspected that fluoride can also change the proteins that control the genetics of cells in the same way that it changes this enzyme. Theoretically, cancer may result from this. The antifluoride lobby argues that all mass fluoridation programs should be stopped immediately, and not after further studies have confirmed whether or not this hypothesis is true.

Fluoride is certainly a major cause of ecological illness. In one busy practice, some 1200 patients with a history of intolerance to a variety of chemicals were tested to see if they reacted to fluoride. More than 30 per cent were found to have a significant positive reaction to sodium fluoride (the form in which it is added to water supplies).

Most of the support for continuing the fluoridation of water has, understandably, come from dentists. I am not a dentist and I have no special expertise that allows me to speak authoritatively about teeth, but I am a physician and I am concerned about any substance that threatens the health and well-being of my patients.

It seems regrettable, to say the least, that almost all the decisions to continue fluoridation have been based on the demands of dentists and what John Colquhoun says was "the low-standard scientific work" that allowed fluoridation to be accepted in the first place. There are very few dentists whose qualifications entitle them to speak with authority about the general health of their patients, let alone of the whole community, and this seems to me to be far more fundamental than the increasingly questionable claims that it is the only means available of reducing the level of rotten teeth.

PART TWO

Fasting, Testing and Treatment

12 *What Your Doctor Needs to Know*

If you consult a doctor who takes an ecological approach to sickness when it is warranted, one of the first things that you will notice is that he or she will take a very comprehensive history that is much more detailed than you have probably been accustomed to with your family doctor. This is for two reasons.

In the first place, there are no visible indications in ecological illness, apart from the symptoms themselves, that anything is wrong: there are no "easy" tests as there are, for instance, in true allergy, where the immunoglobulin IgE is elevated and can be measured. Doctors cannot look down the answers on a questionnaire and cry "Eureka!" when they come to cornflakes or broccoli, for example, and know that these are responsible for a patient's migraine.

Secondly, to the doctor skilled in treating intolerance, the patient's answers will often give important clues that will lead to suspicion of the involvement of a particular food or chemical. Remember that regular and frequent exposure to a food is a prerequisite for intolerance, and this normally means that the food is eaten at least once every four days.

The typical questionnaires that I use are included in appendixes I to IV at the end of the book, and you can use them yourself to establish, for example, the foods and chemicals that should be suspected because of the frequency with which you eat them.

When the doctor takes your history you will also be asked about your background, your previous illnesses and the health of your parents. History tends to repeat itself and, as we have seen, particularly where allergy is concerned, problems that affected your parents may affect you, or more often are likely to predispose you to have any intolerance or allergy.

The questionnaires, which are normally filled in at home and not during the consultation, require very detailed answers to questions about every food that is eaten regularly and frequently, and about your total environment, meaning where you live, work and play. The doctor also looks for stressors in the patient's life, which can remorselessly add up until the critical threshold has been passed and illness takes over.

Because masking will probably have ensured that there is no obvious link between the cause and the effect of the intolerance symptoms, some of the questions that the doctor asks may seem quite irrelevant, but they may be the very ones that provide the clue to tracking down the cause of the trouble. For the same reason, patients are asked to keep a careful diary throughout their treatment, so that the doctor has a complete picture of what is happening.

With a full history taken, we can begin trying to identify the cause or causes (for there are often more than one) of the symptoms or the illness.

THE CHALLENGE TEST ■

There have been many attempts at devising methods of testing for food intolerance but, with a single exception, they have all turned out to be unreliable — and in spite of the fact that two or three of them are still quite widely used.

Only one method, known as the challenge test, has been shown to be consistently reliable, not only in proving the existence of intolerance, but in pinpointing the foods or chemicals that are responsible for it. Criticised by scientific purists for being cumbersome and scientifically clumsy (which it is), it continues to have one unique virtue. It works!

It is called the challenge test because it involves challenging the body's system in a particular way to try and provoke a reaction that will prove the existence of intolerance. The steps that are involved can be neatly summarised in three words: *suspect — eliminate — reintroduce.*

Because there is usually no way of knowing in advance if intolerance is responsible for illness and symptoms (the phenomenon of "masking" removes any obvious cause and effect, and no pathology or other tests show anything amiss), the best that we can start with is a suspicion that intolerance is involved. That usually isn't difficult, given that up to 80 per cent of all the cases seen by GPs that fail to respond to orthodox medical methods of diagnosis and treatment do involve intolerance.

The challenge test relies on a very peculiar phenomenon

that is common to all addiction. If you avoid an addictant for long enough to get it right out of the system, and then re-introduce it shortly afterwards, there follows a very swift and often heightened reaction, even if the dose was extremely small.

Even if the symptoms were previously chronic and masked, so that days passed between the actual ingestion of the addictant food and the reaction, they now become acute and immediate. Cause and effect are revealed so that we know beyond doubt that this particular substance is responsible for at least some of the intolerance reactions.

We put this to work in food intolerance (chemical intolerance also responds to the challenge test, though in a different way, as we shall see shortly), by first avoiding the suspected foods for at least five days. If they provoke a reaction when they are reintroduced, we know they are implicated and we can avoid them in future. It is marvellously simple!

We avoid them for five days because it takes up to ninety-six hours for many foods in our typical Western diet to pass through the digestive tract. In theory it ought to be possible to identify the troublemakers by eliminating from our diet during those five days only those foods that are eaten regularly and frequently enough to be implicated, and this is sometimes done. But the best results are obtained by eliminating all food for the five days.

There is only one way to do this and that is to fast — to go for five days without consuming anything except water. And that causes a good deal of quite unwarranted misapprehension.

13 The Truth About Fasting

IS FASTING SAFE?

Almost without exception, the first question that patients ask when I suggest that they fast is whether it is safe to go for so long without food. And almost without exception, I can assure them that contrary to the predictions of doom and disaster made by some of my colleagues, fasting is not only entirely safe, but highly beneficial!

That pre-eminent faster Mahatma Gandhi, who elevated fasting to something close to a cult, not only enjoyed it immensely, but found it spiritually uplifting. "Fasting", he wrote, "relates not merely to the palate, but to all sense organs. Thus all fasting, if it is a spiritual act, is an intense prayer or a preparation for it. It is a yearning of the soul to merge in the divine essence . . ." That might not be quite how most people embarking on a fast would describe it, but there is no doubt that fasting is a cleansing, uplifting experience with some very unexpected benefits thrown in.

Over the centuries, many great people have fasted and remarked on the acute sense of well-being, even euphoria, that they experienced. Jesus Christ fasted for forty days and nights just before starting his public ministry. Perhaps it was a therapeutic cleansing fast to prepare himself for the rigours of the next three and a half years of his life.

For all that, many people have to overcome a very real psychological barrier before they can bring themselves to fast. Their concern is not only that fasting will leave them without enough energy to function normally, but that it may be positively harmful.

The Fear of Starving   In our society there is certainly a deeply ingrained cultural and psychological fear of going without food. Unconsciously — and sometimes consciously — many people equate fasting with starvation, and starvation with death. When planes crash in remote areas, survivors frequently report that almost immediately they experienced an overwhelming fear of dying from starvation, far more powerful than that of dying of exposure or even from lack of water — and this in spite of the fact that humans can survive for at least ten times as long without food as they can without water. After three days with nothing to drink, they are likely to be in serious trouble.

In large part, this is because of the way in which most of us were brought up. From our earliest years, food was something we ate according to the time on the clock, not because we needed it. Among the first words many people heard as children were "Eat up everything on your plate", often accompanied by something along the lines of "Think of all those starving children in Africa who would be thankful for it!" We were too young to retort with the only sensible answer to that kind of nonsense — "Then wrap it up and send it to them!" Instead, all too often we perpetuate it with our own children.

Thus the regular intake of food quickly became one of our greatest priorities. Many survivors of the German concentration camps, where true starvation and death from it were rife, have described how their greatest reward for surviving was the opportunity to have unlimited food.

WHAT IS FASTING? ■

What, then, is fasting? The first thing to establish very clearly is that fasting is *not* starvation.

The derivation of the two words gives us a clue. "Fast" comes from an Old English word, *faestan*, which meant "to abstain". Starvation comes to us from *steorfan*, another Old English word and a derivation of the Teutonic word *sterben*, which meant "to die".

Fasting is a constructive process by which the body cleanses itself and, when it is denied any sustenance, nourishes itself from its own reserves. Starvation, on the other hand, is destructive and dangerous. It is the method by which life is maintained in extremis by breaking down vital tissues and organs and feeding on them, and it doesn't begin until the body has consumed its spare resources and still continues to be denied food. Fasting is beneficial, but starvation may result in permanent harm, including brain damage and sometimes death.

So how do we know the difference? Subjectively, we always know the difference. Starvation is unpleasant and usually painful, with a clear sensation that something is very wrong. Fasting is never like that and, in the great majority of cases of testing for food intolerance, lasts no longer than five days. Nobody should embark on any fast of longer than twenty-four hours without first telling their doctor (for various other reasons). The doctor is the best person to give the reassurance that it is completely safe in individual cases.

The actual mechanism of fasting is among nature's greatest triumphs of ingenuity. During fasting the body draws nourishment from tissue and other sources in the reverse order of their usefulness. Mainly this nourishment comes from fat, but also to a much lesser degree from muscle tissue, which provides protein. Even toxic waste products are broken down and yield energy during the process of being eliminated.

The first to go is excess fluid. Fluid retention is very common in intolerance, but it is fat that is the primary source of fuel during fasting. Only when the fat stores have been used up does the body begin to draw on other vital tissues. All the organs may sacrifice safe and very limited quantities of their own substances to maintain the blood, heart and brain in a normal condition.

Whether fasting is undertaken for its own therapeutic sake, or as a prelude to food testing, it serves a very valuable purpose. The amount and the quality of the food that most of us eat today ensure that our elimination organs, particularly the kidneys and liver, are constantly overloaded. Every year, the average adult on a typical Western diet eats so much refined carbohydrate, particularly sugar, and fat that we sometimes seem more like walking garbage bins than anything else.

It isn't simply a question of putting on too much weight that is the worry, although it does no harm to remember that we can become fat by eating just 1 or 2 per cent more calories (or kilojoules) than we need every day. Four and a half kilograms (10 pounds) of fat is about 146,500 kilojoules (35,000 calories), or put another way, it takes only an extra slice of bread and butter each day to put on 4.5 kilograms of surplus weight each year.

As a result of this overindulgence, toxic waste accumulates throughout the body. Fasting reverses this process, and all the energy that normally goes into digestion is now channelled by the body into speeding up the process of elimination. It is very good for us.

Changes occur in the body during a fast that actually make

it easier for us to perform normally. Because the body cannot metabolise fat fully when it is the only source of fuel, fractions of fat called ketones remain. (Acetone is one of these ketones.) This leads to a condition called ketosis, or acidosis, which is a reduction in the alkalinity of the blood, and which in turn reduces the appetite and so makes it easier to fast. Nature is very ingenious when it is asked to assist in a process that it recognises as beneficial!

The ketones are subsequently excreted in the urine and also on the breath, which explains why the breath of a person who is fasting has a characteristic smell, which has been compared to that of fresh hay.

WHEN IS A FAST NOT A FAST? ■

This isn't such a silly question as it looks. The word "fast" is used for a great many situations that are not true fasts at all. Doctors often refer to overnight "fasting", for instance, when they mean that they don't want their patients to eat anything before a pathology test or an operation, but this isn't a *true* fast.

By definition, a fast means total abstinence from all food, and commonsense tells us that means abstinence for at least twenty-four hours.

Some of the best-known so-called fasts are positively unhealthy and that certainly includes the annual "fast" by Moslems during Ramadan when no food may be eaten during the hours of daylight. What happens more often than not is that they observe the obligation during the day, but in the evening they cram themselves with as much food as they can force into their stomachs to ward off hunger pangs the next day.

The only thing that can be consumed during a true fast is water. The black coffee or tea that are allowed by some are ridiculous things to take when the object of the fast is to clear the system of all foods and addictive substances. Apart from being a frequent cause of intolerance themselves, they stimulate the central nervous system at the very time when tranquillity is most needed.

There is a very practical reason for avoiding the low-kilojoule foods that are sometimes approved during a regular cleansing fast. When all food is denied, the brain loses the "memory" for food quite quickly and for much of a five-day water fast there is no sensation of hunger at all. Even the smallest amount of food, however, whether it is low-calorie or not, immediately stimulates the brain and results in a sensation of hunger.

HOW LONG CAN I SAFELY FAST? ■

There is no definite rule as to how long a fast can be maintained. Some people shouldn't fast at all, except under medical supervision (see below); most can comfortably fast for at least five days (the normal length of a fast leading up to a food challenge); and a few can fast for an astonishing length of time without any ill effects. Your doctor will tell you which category you fall into.

Fasts of more than 200 days have been undertaken under strict medical supervision (usually to lose excessive weight), and have been reported in the medical literature. Grossly obese and pathologically overweight people have enormous reserves of energy stored in their fatty tissue.

My longest-fasting patient, a 160 kilogram, 23-year-old woman, lost 80 kilograms in a closely supervised fast that lasted for 240 days. For all that time, she not only consumed nothing but water (and in the later days some vitamin supplements), but at the end of it she was still feeding off her own fat supplies and was not near starvation.

Her case was especially interesting because she continued to work full-time shift work throughout the fast! Her job was in a teaching hospital and the medical staff there constantly monitored her condition, with regular pathology tests, to ensure that she was in good health. She experienced no loss of energy and felt fine.

The truth is that the body tolerates a fast much better than a feast. People who protest by going on a hunger strike are usually not only safe (as long as they take care not to continue for so long that they begin starving), but they probably come out of it, like Gandhi, feeling a lot better than before they started.

CONSULTING A DOCTOR ■

There is a very important question that we need to dispose of before going any further, and that is when it is necessary to consult a doctor before undertaking a fast and a challenge test. There is unfortunately no doubt that there are still some doctors who look on all fasting as a dangerous fad, and on the whole question of food addiction with, to put it kindly, a good deal of scepticism.

The irony, of course, is that these same doctors are usually willing enough to subject their patients to interminable drug therapy, surgery, even electric shock treatment, in preference to the far less traumatic procedures involving only rest and abstinence that clinical ecologists advocate. To the reactionary doctor, these are "unscientific", better left to the unqualified fringe practitioners, or better still, ignored altogether.

The truth is that they simply don't know anything about it, in most cases, because it was not part of their medical training. It seems wrong to suggest that patients who are the victims of food intolerance should go to this kind of doctor, but that is what I must recommend if there is no alternative. Let me make it clear from the outset that no responsible doctor can ever advocate that a patient become involved in self-diagnosis, let alone start treating himself, without medical approval. Always consult a doctor first, which nearly always means a family doctor or another general practitioner. Some patients, of course, will already have seen a great deal of their doctor by the time they become aware that some environmental factor might be responsible for their ills.

Even if you have what appear to you to be the most trivial symptoms, such as an occasional, but regular, low-grade headache, still go to a doctor before embarking on a fast or challenge test. You might suspect that it is caused by something you are eating, or something in the environment at work or at home — and you may well be right — but only a doctor can eliminate other more serious causes. Although intolerance and ecological illness are very common, so too are infection, poisoning, psychological upset, tumours and true allergy! The cause of your chest pain may be the beef soup you ate last night, but only a doctor can confirm that it isn't pneumonia.

Those who are trained in medicine are indisputably the best qualified to diagnose demonstrable or organic illness, as well as true psychological and psychiatric illness. It is also certainly true that, although the great majority of people can fast and be challenge-tested without the slightest risk, there are also a small number of patients who must not fast except under close medical supervision.

It is very foolish for anyone thinking of going on a long fast for the first time (that is anything longer than thirty-six hours without any food, except water) to assume that they almost certainly do fall into a safe category. This isn't drumming up business for my profession, but a quick and safe precaution that, apart from anything else, is very reassuring.

I never treat any patient on the assumption that he or she is suffering from environmental illness, until I am satisfied that all the conventional methods of diagnosis have already been explored and have revealed nothing. I might be 99 per cent sure that the cause of the trouble is ecological, but that is nowhere near good enough.

Let me give just one example. Epileptic-type seizures are sometimes encountered as a symptom of environmental illness, and doctors experienced in this kind of disorder can often be fairly certain that this is the cause of the fits. But however much a doctor might suspect that this is the case, it would be the height of irresponsibility not to first study these patients neurologically to exclude brain tumours and any of the other demonstrable causes of epilepsy. (If it is environmentally induced, of course, it will not be demonstrable, for example, by skull X-ray, electrocardiograph or brain scans.) If these organic illnesses are not managed and treated properly, they may even be fatal.

Even when the neurologist has excluded other factors, a doctor must be constantly on guard, because a brain tumour can produce epilepsy-type seizures even before the tumour is large enough to be identified by any but the most sophisticated diagnostic machinery, which may not have been available.

With all this in mind, the clinical ecologist can begin treating his epilepsy-prone patient, exploring the environmental options. Indeed, there are cases of epilepsy that are caused by food and chemical intolerance and are very simply treated by removing a single item from the patient's diet.

Go to a doctor as soon as you suspect that you are suffering from some form of food or chemical intolerance, explain the symptoms and get the doctor's reassurance that all is organically well. Sometimes a doctor will be able to eliminate organic or psychiatric illness at the first consultation; sometimes specialist tests will be ordered, most frequently from a pathologist. This is entirely proper. It becomes worrying only when the doctor begins to order repeats of tests that have already proved negative at least once, without first exploring the possibility that intolerance may be involved.

Don't be afraid to ask your doctor, if he doesn't bring it up himself, if he thinks that food or chemicals may be at the root of the trouble. You have every right — once all the obvious causes have been eliminated, and whether the doctor believes in it or not — to demand a drug-free approach before undertaking a course of ever stronger, more insidious drugs. You have got the law of probability on your side, because you know now that once everything else has been eliminated intolerance is likely to be to blame.

Attitudes within the medical profession are changing, albeit slowly, and an increasing number of doctors are questioning the wisdom of refusing to consider anything that we were not taught at medical school. And there is a steady rise in the number of doctors who understand, even if they don't yet actively practise, the ecological approach to illness as an adjunct to more orthodox methods.

I have had many doctors call me and say, "I want to supervise a fast, or do a challenge test. Can I call you if I get into difficulties?" Of course, I welcome this. It almost invariably means a lifelong convert!

Your doctor may well be interested in exploring this avenue, even if he or she has never brought the subject up during consultation.

HOW TO DEAL WITH THE OBSTINATE DOCTOR ∎

The real difficulty comes when you find yourself faced with a doctor who adamantly refuses to have anything to do with a fast, probably adding that it is dangerous; and who openly ridicules ecological illness. And we have to face it, there are some horses that will never even sniff the water, let alone drink it, no matter how often you lead them to it. Berating the horse achieves nothing but high blood pressure — usually yours!

My advice when this unfortunate situation occurs is never to have a stand-up argument with the doctor. There are some people who just take unkindly to being offered what they see as gratuitous advice about how to do their job, and this certainly isn't unique to doctors.

Instead, end the consultation, decline any offer of further referrals to specialists and, if you know a doctor who is likely to be more understanding, take your business there. There is no reason why you should persist with a doctor who isn't offering you the service you want, any more than with a plumber or an accountant.

I know that many patients find it extremely difficult to go against the advice of their doctor, but it is *your* body and the final choice is yours and nobody else's. You simply don't have to put up with horror statements like "I can't find anything wrong with you, but take these drugs and see if they help".

All ethical drugs — the drugs that can be obtained only on prescription — have unwanted side effects. Look again at the example in Chapter 1 (page 8) for reassurance on that point. And don't self-medicate with the products that are so readily bought over the counter in chemists or even in the supermarket.

Frankly, there are many informed naturopaths who are following the same methods of fasting as clinical ecologists. Compared with medical practitioners, they are generally only minimally qualified and they are not competent to diagnose illness; but once a doctor has ruled out organic or other causes, the supervision of a naturopath may be preferable to being on your own.

Even if the doctor refuses to give you any support with the fast or the challenge test, at least he will be aware of the background to your case in the unlikely event of your needing help to cope with the withdrawal symptoms. He cannot refuse to give you that help. The most likely situation that would arise would be such symptoms as severe migraine or vomiting, both of which can quickly and easily be treated by any doctor or hospital casualty department.

A NOTE OF CAUTION ■

There are a very few people, particularly patients suffering from certain illnesses, who must not fast except under strict medical supervision. This is not because the fast in itself is unsafe (except in rare circumstances such as malnutrition when there is a danger of it developing into starvation, or when certain drugs are being taken), but because the withdrawal symptoms that may be experienced can be harmful.

This is the case particularly with asthmatics, where withdrawal may include worsening of the asthma. As asthma in some cases can be fatal (asthmatics are rarely able to scuba dive, for example), it is important that asthmatics are not exposed to any situation that may make the asthma worse. They must fast and be tested under direct medical supervision (which means as an in-patient) to ensure that help is immediately available if the withdrawal proves too distressing or threatening. That does not mean that asthmatics should never fast, because there is ample evidence that food intolerance may play a significant role in the asthma itself. They must just fast cautiously.

For the same reason, epileptics and markedly debilitated patients, as well as diabetics and people suffering from severe hypoglycaemia, must also fast and be tested under constant medical supervision; neither should patients receiving treatment for any of the more severe mental disorders embark on a fast of longer than twenty-fours without close medical supervision.

Patients suffering from any condition for which medication is being regularly taken must seek medical advice before starting a fast, particularly to find out whether these drugs should continue to be taken or can safely be omitted. Although we often find that medication can be safely reduced, or left out altogether, nobody should *ever* take it on themselves to stop taking a prescribed drug.

The reason why special caution is needed with these patients is that an acute reaction, either during testing or as a withdrawal symptom during the fast, may worsen the symptoms that are being treated; also, the effect of some drugs is heightened when they are taken without any food.

To put the risks into perspective, only two cases of death occurring during fasting, both in the United States, have been published in the medical literature. Both involved patients who were taking prescribed drugs and who, in my opinion, should never have been allowed to fast in the first place. Both had a history of severe congestive heart failure and both were being treated with multiple drugs including, most significantly, the drug digitalis, which is prescribed for failing hearts.

Unlike most modern pharmaceutical drugs, there is a very thin line between the useful therapeutic dose of digitalis and the dangerously toxic level, and the patient's body weight is critical when setting the correct dosage. In prolonged fasts (and both deaths occurred during an extended fast), as the body weight steadily reduces less medication is required to give the desired therapeutic effect.

If, as appears to be the case, these two patients continued to be treated with the original level of digitalis, they could well have been killed by the digitalis, not by the fast. To put patients such as this on to anything but a closely monitored fast, which should have included strict control of any medication they were taking, makes as little sense as telling patients with chronic heart disease to sprint round a sports oval to tone up their muscles before heart surgery.

There is a concept known as "lean body mass", to which doctors attach importance when deciding if a person is fit to fast. It is the condition that exists when all the energy stores in the fatty, or adipose, tissues have been used up. Such a person is invariably thin and the pinch test confirms that there is minimal fatty tissue remaining under the skin.

Fasting should never continue beyond this point, because there is no longer any unused energy available in the form of fat. This means that vital tissue, such as muscle, will be burned up as fuel. It is the start of starvation.

Thin people are understandably concerned about whether they are too thin to fast, and the doctor's approval is as reassuring as it is important. If a full fast isn't possible for them, there is an acceptable alternative in what is known as a mono-exclusion diet, which allows a single food, selected because it has never formed a part of the regular diet and so cannot be implicated in addiction (brown rice is often used) to be eaten while everything else is excluded. The mono-exclusion diet prevents further unacceptable weight loss, even though it is not quite as effective with most patients as the full fast.

Proper explanation and reassurance from a doctor before starting a fast and challenge test are always invaluable in creating a calm, relaxed experience. It has been claimed by some writers that fasting itself is stressful and adds to the total stress load. My experience is that with the right reassurance fasting is extremely restful, especially if the fast is supervised by a sympathetic, experienced person, or is carried out in a supportive environment such as a hospital. Nor should this be surprising. Fasting relaxes the nervous system and eases the anxieties that account for symptoms such as sleeplessness.

In 1987 I published in the *Medical Journal of Australia* a survey of patients who were critically evaluated from a biochemical point of view: the results confirmed the safety of short-term fasting.

CHILDREN AND FASTING ▮

Children should never undertake strict fasting, except under direct medical supervision and, in particular, a water diet lasting for more than a day may be harmful. In part this is because children's lean body mass is such that they have no fat reserves to draw on. There have been tragic cases of misguided parents putting their children on to water diets, with fatal results.

The preferred alternative for children is also the mono-exclusion diet; and the fast normally lasts for three and a half days instead of the five days usually recommended for adults. This shorter time is because food passes through the gastrointestinal tract faster in children. (Withdrawal symptoms in children, where they occur, also seem to last for less time than in adults.) At the end of mono-exclusion diets, patients are taken off the one food they have been allowed before the challenge test meals are given.

14 Managing the Fast

Once a doctor has given approval to a patient to fast, there is no reason, as far as the fast itself is concerned, for the fast to be undertaken in a hospital or under close supervision. Normally fasting is not only beneficial and safe, but very enjoyable. I fast for one day each week, and three or four times a year I also go on a three- or five-day fast. I never fail to feel invigorated by it.

We seem to have forgotten that the body has very considerable healing powers of its own. The fast cures nothing, but it does effectively remove from the body many of the substances that cause harm, and this in turn allows the body to get on with the business of curing itself.

Every creature in the world except humans, it seems, stops eating when it is ill. Generations of doting human mothers, on the other hand, have almost force-fed their sickly children with the threat that they must eat, no matter how awful they are feeling, "to keep up your strength". Few old wives' tales could more profitably be banished to the realm of folklore where they belong than this one.

So the fast is not something to approach with trepidation. It is also very fortunate that when it is a prelude to testing for food addiction, it does not always have to be conducted in hospital, because we don't have seven million spare hospital beds in Australia! (Remember that the health of perhaps about half the population is affected by food and chemical intolerance.)

COPING WITH THE WITHDRAWAL

When problems do arise, they are nearly always because of unexpectedly severe withdrawal symptoms, and occasionally there is no doubt that these can be disconcertingly severe.

It is important to understand withdrawal *before* embarking on a fast, to put the problem into proper perspective. Withdrawal symptoms are an unavoidable reaction when giving up any addictant, whether it is heroin or potato. Although most people experience only mild symptoms when food is the addictant, a few do suffer badly. This withdrawal phase is *absolutely normal* and has to be passed through on the way back to normality. A severe reaction usually means that the symptoms were also severe, and just knowing this can be reassuring.

Many patients, who do not understand withdrawal, experience the symptoms and feel worse than they did before they began fasting. Understandably they think that the fast itself is responsible and even believe that it is actually harming them. It can also be disturbing to doctors who have no experience of fasting, and as a result they encourage their patients to end the fast prematurely (and the patients need no second bidding). What they don't know is that the withdrawal lasts for only a short time (although it can admittedly seem much longer), and that usually by the third day patients have passed through it and emerge feeling better than they have for months, and often years.

Withdrawal symptoms can be present from the very beginning of the fast. If the fast is started in the morning, the body has already been without food overnight and this may be enough to trigger the first withdrawal symptoms within hours. As we have already noted, this is why so many people have a Saturday morning headache, because they drink their first cup of coffee later than usual. Even when the symptoms do not appear quite so rapidly, they are usually well established by the end of the first day or the beginning of the second.

Common withdrawal symptoms include headache and migraine, nausea and sometimes vomiting, muscle and joint aches and pains, weakness and tiredness. Oddly, they are not necessarily the same symptoms that have been experienced as intolerance reactions, so that the *reaction to*, say, cheese may have been migraine and lethargy, while the *withdrawal from* cheese provokes weepiness and acute anxiety.

Other patients experience a heightened form of their familiar symptoms, with perhaps a worse headache or more uncontrollable lethargy, but in fact any of the symptoms associated with ecological illness may be encountered (see p. 216).

Nausea, which is a feeling of sickness, is a very common withdrawal symptom, as are headaches; and occasionally a patient suffers a violent and alarming attack of what is known as projectile vomiting that may even become continuous. An injection of a drug like Stemetil is all that is needed to control it, but this must be administered on a doctor's instructions. Severe migraine can also be effectively controlled in the short term by drugs such as pethidine. It is to cope with quite rare situations such as these that medical help should ideally be on hand when fasting and challenge testing are carried out. In most cases, though obviously not with projectile vomiting, it is usually possible to make your way to a doctor's surgery or a hospital out-patient department, but it is still important for a doctor to know in advance about the fast and the test so that he is aware at once of what he is treating.

If the withdrawals that start in the first twenty-four hours are mild (and I must emphasise that they usually *are* mild), the rest of the fast will normally present no difficulties. If withdrawal symptoms are severe from the start, even among those who are not so obviously at risk as asthmatics and diabetics (who should not be fasting at all without medical supervision), then the rest of the fast ought to be conducted under supervision.

By the end of the third day, most people are feeling much better, and by the end of the fourth, they are usually feeling brighter and fitter than they can remember feeling in years. After five days, with all the foods and food chemicals cleared out of their systems, most are quite euphoric about how well they feel. All their symptoms have usually disappeared, if food or food chemicals were responsible, including sometimes very severe mental symptoms, and the effect on the patient is often very moving.

If the symptoms persist beyond the fifth day, even though greatly reduced, it may be worth extending the fast. With some patients, seven or even ten days may be needed for all the withdrawal symptoms to take place and pass. This additional fasting must always be done with the specific approval of a doctor, though again not necessarily in hospital.

If the symptoms continue after ten days it is most likely that some other factor is involved, usually chemical intolerance to one or more substances in the environment — either at work, in the home or in the ambient atmosphere. I normally test for the main chemical groups during food testing. If these tests prove positive and neutralising drops do not remove the symptoms (see Chapter 26), the patient is a likely candidate for the Environmental Control Unit, where further testing can be carried out in a chemical-free environment.

A useful antidote to withdrawal symptoms and to many of the symptoms of intolerance (and a handy answer for a hangover) is a simple mixture of sodium and potassium bicarbonate, in a ratio of two parts of sodium to one of potassium. Five grams of the mixture should be taken in 200 millilitres of warm water and repeated as necessary.

Patients in hospital or a clinic are often given even speedier relief by breathing carbogen, which is a 5 per cent carbon dioxide and 95 per cent oxygen mixture. It is inhaled through a mask. (Sometimes, in intensely chemically sensitive patients, even the normal plastic face mask is unsafe and special ceramic masks have to be used.) I have also found that hypnotherapy helps some patients through withdrawal.

WHERE SHOULD WE FAST? ■

Fasting is normally undertaken at one of four different levels of supervision. First, maximum control is exercised in the Environmental Control Unit, where even the air has been cleaned. Secondly, fasting can be carried out in a hospital or clinic — sometimes in a special ward where some effort is made to keep the atmosphere as chemically clean as possible.

Thirdly, it can also be done under medical supervision at home. This usually means a daily house call from the doctor or visit to the surgery, or at least having a doctor who is aware of what is happening and who is no further away than the end of the telephone. Finally, of course, fasting can be conducted without any skilled supervision at all.

Some patients, as we have seen, must always fast as in-patients. Others need at least close medical supervision, including those with particular diseases such as asthma, diabetes, mental disorders, severe hypoglycaemia, and those who are very old, very young, or emaciated. Ideally almost everyone should fast and be challenge tested as an in-patient of a hospital or clinic. Only there can weight and blood pressure be regularly monitored and blood-glucose levels checked frequently. Symptoms of food intolerance reactions are often expressed through a change in blood-glucose, which can itself cause many problems.

In a hospital, trained people can also observe the patient continuously and closely, reporting signs that even the patient may not be aware of and that may give a clue to a reaction.

But we know in reality in-patient care in a hospital or clinic is simply not an option, except for a very small percentage of people. The hospital system could not cope with it. In the United States, some 90 per cent of all clinical ecology treatment is given on a part-time basis, meaning that the patients do it at home.

Because the conditions that exist in a hospital are ideal, we will use them to explain just what you can expect when you embark on a fast that is to lead up to a challenge test. Not all the services available in hospital will be available at home, but we should strive to get as close to the ideal as possible.

No-one should ever be under the delusion that fasting is easy, particularly the first time it is undertaken. From the very earliest age, we are so conditioned, as we have already discussed, to eating three times a day that suddenly going without food can be quite disturbing — even when we feel so much better doing it!

One of the practical reasons for preferring to do the fast in a hospital or clinic, when that is possible, is that most homes are far from being the ideal setting for a fast where important requirements are peace and quiet. Just as it is very difficult to be the life and soul of a party on an exclusive diet of water (and often deionised water at that!), so is it very hard to fast when you are surrounded by other people eating normal meals — especially if you are still having to prepare those meals!

Fasting takes a lot of willpower and the temptation to cheat can be very great. As with any addiction, the subconscious is usually working overtime to ensure that you don't deprive the system of its addictant, and smelling and handling food, quite apart from watching other people eating it, does nothing to make the fast any easier. One mouthful of the wrong food (which is likely to be the food you find most irresistible), meaning an unsafe food taken without thought, can undo all the good of the fast.

THE FAST ■

The approach I usually adopt to a fast that is the prelude to a food challenge is to go into it cold turkey. The patient just stops eating. At other times, especially before a prolonged fast undertaken for its own sake, it may be more comfortable to wind down gradually on the food intake in the days immediately before beginning the fast. Some people, for example, eat only fruit on the third and second days before the fast, and then only fruit juice on the day before it.

Thursday evening is a good time to start a five-day fast if you are not going into hospital or a special unit. It shouldn't be too difficult to get through Friday, Day One, even if withdrawal symptoms begin before you leave work. If people know what you are doing, their interest and your martyrdom will help ensure that you don't weaken!

If there are going to be withdrawal symptoms, they are most likely to appear on Day Two, which is Saturday, when you should be able to cope with them without the added stress of having to get through a day's work at the same time. By Sunday evening, the symptoms will have largely abated; and by Monday, when you go back to work, it is already Day Four and you will probably be feeling on top of the world and not even hungry.

There should be no need to change your lifestyle unless the withdrawal symptoms are troubling. You can go to work and lead a normal social life (except for the problem of being jolly on a glass of water!) as long as you bear in mind the following tips and cautionary remarks.

Water helps to relieve the hunger pangs that sometimes occur at the start of a fast, without stimulating the taste buds and provoking a sensation of hunger later on. It is not true, however, as some writers maintain, that as much water as possible should be drunk to sluice out the system. Two litres a day is quite sufficient to flush out toxins and waste materials, and to keep you from becoming dehydrated.

Another fallacy is that if you drink water, some of the fluid is retained and increases your weight. Much of the water we drink is eliminated not only via the kidneys but also through tens of millions of tiny pores in the skin, as well as on the breath.

The water that is drunk should preferably not be tap water, which is usually heavily chlorinated, fluoridated and contaminated (in an ecological sense) with other chemicals. It also tastes extremely unpleasant to many people who are fasting. Instead, mineral water, fresh spring water or deionised water, which is the equivalent of distilled water, should be drunk. Very cold water should be avoided.

A mild laxative, such as sugar-free milk of magnesia, is sometimes given after the last meal and may be repeated on the second day to speed up the elimination process and clear the gastrointestinal tract. Once the bowel has emptied, further evacuation activity ceases, even during prolonged fasting. Some patients find this troubling, but it is entirely normal.

Because the aim of a fast is to rid the body completely of all foreign substances, it may be possible to suspend taking prescribed drugs (though never without a doctor's approval — normally that of the doctor who prescribed them). Self-medication with aspirin and paracetamol (Panadol, for example) can safely be stopped during the fast, and *should* be stopped. Most of the symptoms that they are being taken for, particularly pain, will disappear during the fast anyway.

Don't take vitamins or mineral supplements during the fast unless they are specifically prescribed by your doctor. Even if they contain no harmful colours or other additives, anything that goes into the stomach apart from water, including pills, might trigger hunger pangs and make the fast more difficult.

It goes without saying that smoking should be avoided when fasting, but if patients find that this is too intolerable, I insist that they at least keep it to the barest minimum. If they are fasting in hospital, or in a chemical-free unit, smoking of any kind is forbidden because of its effect on the other patients.

To embark on a fast and continue smoking is really nonsense, and the fast may be the ideal environment for making a worthwhile start towards breaking the habit. Normally, I wouldn't allow a smoker anywhere near someone who is fasting, because of the smell (which means the presence of outgassing molecules) that always lingers on the breath, skin and clothes of a smoker.

It should not be necessary to lie in bed throughout the fast, and doing that is likely to make a person feel weak at any time. Even in the hospital setting, the patient is up and dressed, although bed rest is always allowed.

Try to avoid getting out of bed or standing up too quickly. With loss of weight, there is generally a reduction of blood pressure, and changes in postural position can produce dizziness through what is known as postural hypotension, when the blood pressure drops after a sudden change in body position from lying to sitting, or sitting to standing.

Exercise is beneficial and a daily walk of up to three hours is ideal, making sure that the pace is within your capacity. Don't force yourself to keep walking if it makes you unduly weak, or if symptoms such as breathlessness or palpitations occur. It is *sustained* activities that have to be avoided — no long-distance running or strenuous jogging, no energetic football matches or squash. A leisurely game of tennis or an easy swim in unchlorinated water, though, are often well tolerated and add to the sense of well-being.

The daily walk should not be in places where there is traffic pollution and it should stay well clear of heavy outgassing such as those areas of supermarkets that are set aside for detergents.

Exercise, incidentally, does not necessarily stimulate the appetite, as many people believe. In fact, a period of moderate exercise actually dampens it. The body burns up calories (kilo-joules) faster when we exercise, but it may continue to burn them up at an accelerated rate for as long as twenty-four hours after the exercise stops.

Keep warm during the fast. You may find that you feel rather cold when everyone else is warm. Put on a jumper but avoid extremes of heat (or cold), like huddling over a fire. Hot baths or saunas can leave you feeling weak, while extreme cold is an unnecessary additional stressor while your body struggles to keep warm.

Bad breath is a common problem during a fast but disappears when the system has been cleared out. I recommend that patients avoid commercial brands of toothpaste, which are heavily chemicalised, and use instead baking soda or sea salt. In most cases, brushing without anything is adequate.

You may be asked to give frequent handwriting samples during the fast, because it is a surprisingly good indicator that food or chemical intolerance is present, and it is particularly useful with children. The nervous system is often affected during withdrawal, and this in turn alters the handwriting, sometimes reducing it to an illegible scrawl. For the same reason, writing is also sometimes tested during the challenge test.

EXPECT TO FIND CHEMICAL SENSITIVITIES ■

In any intolerance, it is rare for there to be only one substance involved, certainly by the time most of my patients arrive at my rooms. The longer intolerance is allowed to persist untreated, the worse and the more numerous the symptoms become. There is also the likelihood that more than one food is involved, either producing different sets of symptoms or combining in a single synergistic effect. This is one of the reasons for recommending total fasting rather than an exclusion diet.

Another reason is that where there are associated chemical sensitivities, developing food tolerance may depend on the extent to which the chemical problem is also brought under control. During fasting for food intolerance, it is also common for chemical sensitivities to be heightened and, as we want the patient to be symptom free when testing begins, it makes sense to try to eliminate any factor that might complicate the picture. We achieve this more efficiently with a total fast.

One of the most difficult things to achieve at home is a lowering of the level of chemical outgassing. You can go some way towards achieving this by getting rid of the more obvious offending items, like aerosol sprays, tobacco smoke, detergents and perfume, but it is impossible to have a completely chemical-free environment in a normal home.

Even in special clinics, where a considerable effort is put into keeping the environment clean, dangers can creep up unsuspected. A thoughtless chemical spraying under the floor, a job often given to contractors who do it routinely on the same date each year, can cause havoc among chemically sensitive patients. A solvent marking pen, left open by mistake for only thirty seconds in one of my wards, was enough for the fumes to be wafted through the whole room by the breeze, seriously upsetting one chemically sensitive patient.

This happened on another occasion, not in a hospital ward but during a lecture. A visiting American doctor, who was himself a chemical victim, was speaking and he was supplied with a white board and solvent marking pen. He used the board to illustrate a point, but with disastrous results. For the next 20 minutes he gave a terrible lecture, which was all the more distressing because I had heard the same lecture before and knew how good he had been.

I happened to be chairman at that session and when he finished I discussed it frankly with him. Only then did the truth dawn on us both and, to his everlasting credit, he came back after a short break and used his own experience to illustrate just what chemicals can do. By now he was completely back to normal and speaking as well as ever.

If you are fasting and testing at home, it is obviously more difficult to keep to these suggestions, particularly if your family isn't sympathetic and doesn't cooperate. Even if they do cooperate but you are left to do the usual work while they go on eating and behaving normally, fasting can be very difficult.

Organisations such as the Allergy Association of Australia

(AAA) may be able to at least put you in touch with people who have been through the same problems, and their support and advice can be very reassuring. If a doctor is supervising the fast, make sure that at the end of it you tell him everything you experienced, even if you are not in daily touch with him. That means keeping a very detailed diary of all your symptoms and the time each occurred.

LOSING FAT QUICKLY ■

The rate at which you lose weight during a fast varies according to the amount that you were overweight before you began it, and of course, on the duration of the fast. Our bodies are mostly water and a 73 kilogram (160 pound) person, for instance, is composed of approximately 13 kilograms (29 pounds) of protein, 11 kilograms (25 pounds) of fat, 2.3 kilograms (5 pounds) of minerals, 450 grams (1 pound) of carbohydrate, 7 grams (a quarter of an ounce) of vitamins — and 45 kilograms (100 pounds) of water!

Rapid weight loss or gain is always caused by fluid loss or retention and, in many cases, when a person stops eating there is an initial and quite significant loss of water. As the scales don't differentiate between water and fat, weight loss at the start of a fast may be dramatic and very encouraging — up to 10 kilograms (22 pounds) in the first week in the case of an obese patient.

It is for this reason that fasting is sometimes said to be a useless way to lose weight, because as soon as the fast is over, the fluid returns immediately. In fact, fasting is by far the most effective way of losing weight safely — the trick is to ensure that the weight stays off once it has been shed. You can't blame the fast when that doesn't happen.

It is a common symptom in food intolerance for excessive amounts of water to be retained by the body, which is one of the reasons why so many people suffering from intolerance have a weight problem. What happens is that intolerance is often accompanied by increased permeability of the capillaries, so that these minute blood vessels tend to leak. Fluid gets out of the blood stream into the tissues, where it accumulates and the result is the condition known as oedema. If the leakage is excessive, the fluid produces lumps on the skin, or hives.

Once the retained fluid has been eliminated in the initial phase of the fast, weight loss slows down and is rarely more than 450 grams (1 pound) a day: it is now fat only that is being used up. To lose 1 kilogram (2.2 pounds) in weight, humans must burn up some 31,000 *more* kilojoules (7500 calories) than they consume. Most people who lead a sedentary life don't burn up more than this in a total of three days!

ENDING THE FAST ■

It is important not to terminate the fast too soon, when it is to be followed by a challenge test. During the withdrawal phase, there is sometimes a strong temptation to end the fast if the symptoms are unpleasant, and there is a natural tendency to want to begin testing before the withdrawal symptoms have been completely worked out.

If you begin testing too soon, however, far from effecting any kind of cure (even though this might appear to be what has happened, because the symptoms disappear) all you probably achieve is a recurrence of the old masking. Then you have to start all over again.

How we break the fast depends, as when deciding how to begin it, on whether it is to be followed by challenge testing, or whether it is simply a therapeutic cleansing exercise. With the latter, the most important thing to remember is that your eyes are likely to be a great deal bigger than your stomach. As soon as the fast is ended by eating even a small amount of food, the appetite is immediately re-awakened — and after five days without food, it is a very healthy appetite indeed! It is a desire that must be resisted.

If you give in to it, much of the good of the fast will be very swiftly undone, and you are likely to have a memorable stomach-ache into the bargain. I recommend only diluted fruit juices on the first day, then a gradual progression to salads, both fruit and vegetable, for another one or two days; and then small portions of a normal diet, eaten slowly and not gobbled. This is especially important if the fast lasted more than five days.

When the fast is followed by a food challenge, it is broken with one of the foods that is to be tested. If there is a fruit on the list, I generally recommend that it is eaten first. Then one by one, each food that has been consumed regularly and frequently enough to be suspected of causing intolerance is fed to the patient. Test meals usually consist of several spoonfuls of each food.

It is quite common for people to come out of the fast feeling so well and so free of their symptoms that they are unwilling to risk losing their feeling of well-being by deliberately eating a food that might put them back in their old condition. But they must persevere. All fasts must come to an end sooner or later, and the purpose of the whole exercise is to establish which foods must be eliminated so that the patient can feel good all the time, even eating a normal diet. That is the promise of clinical ecology.

15 The Challenge Test

It was long ago in the 1920s that an American clinical investigator, Dr Herbert Rinkel, discovered quite by chance the remarkable fact that if you omit from your diet a food to which you are addicted and then reintroduce it several days later, you will have an acute, swift and often exaggerated reaction (see Chapter 5). Masked intolerances are unmasked and the normal stimulation–withdrawal sequence of addiction which is usually spread over hours or even days when it is masked, becomes compressed into hours, and sometimes even minutes.

The foods chosen for testing are based on the answers to the questionnaire that patients must fill in. Those who want to test themselves, after a doctor has ruled out any other cause for their symptoms and illnesses, can use the questionnaires in Appendix II. Only foods that are eaten regularly and frequently (that is at least once a week) are tested, because only these can be responsible for food addiction. If you are uncertain where to begin, start with the most common troublemakers (assuming they are in your normal diet): milk, wheat, cheese, oranges and tomatoes.

Every patient has his or her own speed of reaction. Some are very quick to react to a food to which they are intolerant and within minutes they begin to experience the first symptoms; others are much slower. Interestingly, though, people tend to follow the same pattern each time, regardless of the food or chemicals involved. Almost without exception, however, some reaction takes place within four hours and usually within an hour, even if it becomes more severe afterwards. If there has been no reaction within four hours, it is safe to go on to the next food.

THE COMMON SYMPTOMS ▮

Although any symptom or set of symptoms that any organ or tissue is capable of evoking can be triggered by food and chemical intolerance, there are some symptoms that do recur much more frequently than others. The following check list includes those symptoms that should particularly be looked for during testing, because their presence is a strong indicator, in the absence of any other explanation, that intolerance is present.

GENERALISED
Dizziness, lightheadedness
Imbalance, staggering
Vertigo
Blackout
Going to faint
Chilly coldness
Warmth, hot flushes

JOINTS
Aches, pains
Stiffness
Swelling
Erythema (redness)
Unexplained warmth

MUSCLES
Muscle tremor, jerking
Muscle cramps, spasms
Pseudoparalysis, weakness
Tightness and stiffness
Aches and sore pains in:
    neck, trapezius
    upper and lower back
    upper and lower
        extremities

SKIN
Itching, local and general
Scratching
Moistness, sweating
Flushing
Hives
Pallor, white or ghostly

HEAD PAIN
Headache, mild or moderate
Severe migraine
Ache, pressure

Tightness, explode
Throbbing, stabbing pains

EYES
Itching, burning, pain
Lacrimation, tears
Infected, redness
Allergic "shiners"
Feel heavy

VISION
Blurring
Acuity decreased
Spots, flashes
Darker, vision loss
Photophobia, dislike of bright
    lights
Diplopia (double vision)
Dyslexia — difficulty in
    reading, transposition of
    similar letters, backwards
    writing or mirror writing,
    letters become small or
    large, words move around
Change in handwriting

NASAL
Sneezing, urge to sneeze
Itching, rubbing
Obstruction
Discharge
Post-nasal drip (watery
    secretion)
Sinus discomfort
Stuffy feeling

THROAT, MOUTH
Itching
Soreness, tightness, swelling
Dysphagia (difficulty in

swallowing), choking
Weak voice, hoarseness
Salivation, mucus
Bad, metallic taste

EARS
Itching
Full, blocked
Erythema of pinna (reddening
  of the ear)
Tinnitus (ringing in the ears)
Earache
Hearing loss
Hyperacusis (abnormal
  sensitivity to sound)

GENITO-URINARY
Voiding, mild urge
Frequency
Urgency, pressure
Dysuria (painful or difficult
  urination)

GASTROINTESTINAL, ABDOMEN
Nausea
Belching
Full, bloated
Vomiting
Pressure, pain, cramps
Flatus, rumbling
Bowel movement, diarrhoea
Gall bladder symptoms
Hunger, thirst
Hyperacidity

LUNGS, HEART
Coughing
Wheezing
Reduced air flow
Retracting, sob (breathing in
  sharply)
Heavy, tight
Not enough air

Hyperventilation (rapid
  breathing)
Chest pain
Tachycardia (rapid pulse)
Palpitations (rapid or
  throbbing pulse)
Premature ventricular
  contractions (PVC, extra
  heartbeats)

DEPRESSION
Withdrawn, listless
Vacant, dull face
Negative, indifferent
Confused, dazed
Depressed
Crying, sobbing

STIMULATION
Silly, intoxicated
Grimacing
More alert, talkative
Hyperactive
Tense, restless
Anxious, apprehensive
Fearful, panicky
Irritable, angry

FATIGUE
Tiredness
Generalised heaviness
Sleepiness, yawning
Exhaustion
Falling asleep

SPEECH, COMPREHENSION
Mentally sluggish
Concentration poor
Memory loss (acute)
Speech slurred
Stammering, stuttering
Speech paralysis, loss of
  speech

Reads aloud poorly
Reads without
comprehension
Hears without
comprehension
Maths and spelling errors

REALITY CONTACT
Poor contact
Surroundings unreal

Disoriented, catatonic
Stuporous
False belief, delusion,
hallucination, wandering
of the mind, false
perception
Suicidal, feel like hurting
oneself
Maniacal, very highly
disturbed

The reaction can last for a considerable time. Because of this and the need to wait for at least four hours to be sure that there is not going to be a reaction, we can usually give only three test meals a day. It can make the combined fasting and testing program quite lengthy and I always advise patients who want to undertake it in hospital to allow a fortnight.

The situation isn't quite as bad as it appears, even when testing progresses very slowly. Very few people eat more than thirty foods regularly from one end of the year to the next, so that ten days testing and five fasting is enough.

Many of these thirty foods, even though they appear to be different, actually share the same basic ingredients. Cakes, scones, biscuits, pastries, bread and Weetbix, for example, may appear to be different, but from an ecological point of view they are wheat, wheat and more wheat. Four other items are likely to be milk, butter, yoghurt, cream and cheese. These are also a single food type, which may simplify testing.

If a particular food continues to cause withdrawal symptoms after four hours — and sometimes reactions may not be at their most severe for twelve or even eighteen hours — it can confuse the picture if the next challenge is started too soon.

A doctor experienced in challenge testing may be able to distinguish between the end of one reaction and the start of the next. For anyone testing without such expert help, however, it is essential to wait until the last trace of the previous reaction has disappeared before going on with the next test, even if this means restricting the testing to one challenge a day.

Patients with skin or joint complaints may not be able to test more than one food every second or third day, because the reactions can take a long time to disappear from the joints. The reaction to cow's milk is sometimes also delayed. If milk is one of the suspected foods being tested (and it almost always is), allow two days for the full reaction to develop, provided as usual that there has been an initial reaction within four hours.

During prolonged testing, it is acceptable to go on to a mono-exclusion diet, which allows a single additional food to be eaten, invariably one that has never been eaten before with any regularity. At night, when testing for the day has finished, we can supplement this with foods that have been shown to be safe.

A common cold, or any other infection during testing, may confuse the results, so until the infection clears up, stay on a mono-exclusion diet or at least on foods that have just been tested and found to be safe. After the end of the fast, it will be approximately a month before the hypersensitivity begins to weaken and then lapses back into normal preadaptive intolerance, the first stage of addiction before masking occurs (Figure 2, p. 58). In preadaptive intolerance, consumption of an "unsafe" food is immediately followed by an unpleasant reaction, unlike masked intolerance, where there is rarely any obvious link between cause and effect. After that, the cycle of addiction remorselessly starts all over again.

THE STRANGE TURN-OFF ■

After establishing that a food is triggering a reaction, you have to be very careful not to eat it again too soon. After provoking a reaction, often with only a small dose of an "unsafe" food, you could reasonably expect that another dose, taken soon afterwards, would make those symptoms even worse. Instead, the reverse happens!

Far from exacerbating the reaction, you are likely to turn the symptoms right off. The first exposure triggers the withdrawal symptoms, the second masks the addiction. The addiction has not disappeared, rather the symptoms have just gone underground, where they become distanced from their cause: the patient once again has all the old symptoms and illnesses that prompted the visit to the doctor in the first place.

This characteristic of food intolerance, that it not only induces symptoms, but turns them off as easily, has few parallels in medicine. We put it to practical use, as we shall see, more often in chemical intolerance. By finding the weakest dilution of a chemical that triggers the symptoms, we can then dilute one further step to produce what is known as the turn-off dose and, with equal efficiency, switch off all the symptoms (see Chapter 26).

In food intolerance, it is usually more practical simply to avoid the offending foods rather than to bother with establishing a turn-off dose. If this approach is felt to be necessary (as, for example, when almost every food tested has been shown to cause intolerance), the turn-off dose is given sublingually before the food is consumed.

Very rarely a patient reacts so strongly to a substance being tested that he or she falls into a deep, even coma-like sleep. This is not dangerous, because the patient will always eventually wake up none the worse for wear; but it can complicate a carefully scheduled testing program. By putting into the patient's mouth a little of the same food that caused the reaction, we can turn off the symptoms and the patient rapidly wakes up.

If the fast and the test are not carefully conducted, the second exposure can easily occur by mistake. If this happens, it is necessary to remove that particular food from the diet, again for a minimum of five days, before re-testing. Unless this is done, the masking will inevitably become entrenched once more.

16 The
Alternatives
to Fasting

Although the five-day fast, which entirely rids the body of all
foods and food residues, is the ideal way to prepare the system for
food intolerance testing, it is not always an option that is available and we sometimes have to approach the problem from a different direction.

For some people, as we have seen, there are medical reasons
for not embarking on a long fast (in the case of children, the
elderly and those without lean body mass, for example). Others
find it psychologically too difficult to go without food for so long.
For these people, the alternative that I recommend is the mono-
exclusion diet, where all foods except one are omitted.

The one that is permitted is selected because it is not a part
of the patient's normal diet and as such cannot be involved in
food addiction. Brown rice is commonly used (especially with
children) and it is a useful food. It has no additives and it is
nutritious and filling. It is essential, of course, that no rice, in
any form, is a part of the regular diet.

If even this is too difficult to adhere to, then the next preferred alternative is an exclusion or elimination diet. This allows
a number of foods to be eaten, provided always that they do not
include any that the patient believes might be implicated in
the intolerance, together with a number of other foods that are
notorious troublemakers, particularly dairy products, wheat,
eggs, seafoods, nuts, peas and beans. These are all frequently
used in processed foods, all of which should be treated with great
suspicion during a fast.

With the exclusion diet, it is necessary to wait for much
longer than after a full water fast before beginning the challenge
test — usually between ten and fourteen days.

It takes considerably longer to withdraw when other foods
are being eaten, even though the challenge test itself appears to
be just as effective. Criticism is sometimes voiced that the exclu-

sion diet is often followed by no improvement. This, in my experience, is usually because other unsafe foods are still being unwittingly eaten.

One of the difficulties with following the exclusion diet is that it does require a degree of knowledge of food families, which are the botanical groupings of cereals, vegetables and fruits, as well as the zoological grouping of animals, birds and fish. There is frequently associated intolerance to foods belonging to the same food family as the problem food. Leaving cabbage out of the diet, for instance, even if it is known to be an addictant, may produce no improvement while you continue to eat brussels sprouts, which are very closely related to cabbage. Appendix V lists the commonest food families and it should be read carefully when preparing a suitable diet.

Another food classification is sometimes recommended, which is based on naturally occurring chemicals, such as salicylates, in different foods. Sensitivity to salicylates would require all foods that contain them to be excluded from the diet.

Any rigorous diet that is not devised skilfully by professional dieticians risks being inadequate for maintaining normal health. This is especially true with an exclusion diet that has to be adhered to for weeks. Multivitamin tablets (free from colouring) and approved "safe" nutrients, recommended by a dietician or a knowledgeable doctor, should be taken as a supplement.

AN EXCLUSION DIET ■

Dietitian Dr Anne Swain and immunologist and physician Dr Robert Clancy, both of the Royal Prince Alfred Hospital in Sydney, devised an excellent exclusion diet for Australians, which is equally useful as a basic diet and as an elimination diet leading up to challenge testing. As well as omitting all suspected foods, based on questionnaire answers, it prohibits especially foods and medicines that contain salicylates and benzoates, tartrazine, yeast and penicillin. These can be tested for separately.

In the basic diet recommended by Swain and Clancy (and adopted by fellow immunologist Dr Robert Loblay), lamb and chicken are used as sources of protein, fat and vitamins; and beef, after originally being excluded because of reported cases of beef-induced urticaria, is now also allowed. Butter and all dairy products are excluded, because they are a possible source of penicillin, still widely used to control infection in dairy cattle.

Margarine is excluded because of the addition of flavouring and because almost all margarines actually have butter products in them. Sunflower, safflower and olive oil are suitable.

Cereals present a problem. As a substitute for bread, Swain and Clancy recommend matzo, an unleavened crispbread that consists of semolina and water. Matzo is used by the Jews during Passover and is widely available.

Fresh pears are almost the only fruits that do not contain benzoates or salicylates, and they are also available preserved in tins with sugar and water syrup. Salt and pepper are the only condiments that are free of natural benzoates and salicylates. All aspirin-containing medicines, such as Aspro, Disprin or Alka Seltzer, are salicylates, and are prohibited in the diet; and so are medicines that contain tartrazine, the yellow food colouring. Salicylates are also found in toothpaste, cough lozenges, medicine and syrups; and in oil of wintergreen, which is in creams for muscle soreness, such as Dencorub and Deep Heat. Almost all toiletries have perfumes that contain salicylates and benzoates, and so need to be avoided in this diet.

In Chapter 10, we have seen some of the havoc that tartrazine can cause. As it is by far the most common yellow food dye, any yellow, orange or green medication, whether liquid, tablets or pills, should be avoided. (Your pharmacist can usually tell you the medicines that don't contain tartrazine.) If you are on a course of antihistamine tablets, ask specifically for those that are white, pink or blue. For the relief of pain, white codeine tablets are allowed; and Savlon antiseptic cream is one of the few permitted germicides because it is free from salicylates.

In summary, the foods that are allowed in the Swain-Clancy-Loblay diet are as follows, obviously with the additional exclusion of any foods suspected of being involved in intolerance because of the frequency with which they are consumed. EVERYTHING else is forbidden!

Meat: Lamb, chicken, beef
Vegetables: Lettuce, carrots and parsley (all free of natural
 benzoates and salicylates, but containing fibre, water,
 some vitamins and some minerals)
Fruit: Pears, fresh or tinned

Cereals: Matzo, plain flour, semolina (which is fine porridge made from hard wheat), rice, rice bubbles and rice noodles, Carrs water biscuits

Fats: Oils including sunflower, safflower and olive

Sugar: Sugar, golden syrup and honey (the diet is not concerned specifically with carbohydrate intake, and I believe these should be used very sparingly, if at all)

Miscellaneous: Salt, malt vinegar, pepper, gelatine

Beverages: Coffee, instant and ground (I don't recommend these because they are food–drug combinations and are a frequent source of intolerance problems. Tea, fruit juices — except pear — and all alcoholic drinks are forbidden because of their salicylate content.)

Many, however, do not improve on this exclusion diet, almost always, I believe, because they continue to eat food of which they are intolerant.

DOUBLE-BLIND TESTING ■

Clearly Swain and Loblay attach the greatest importance to avoiding salicylates and benzoates. They usually challenge double-blind, which means that neither the patient nor the person administering the test meal knows what it contains. Capsules containing salicylates and yeast, for example, are used to avoid any psychological overlay, for instance the bias of the patient who says, usually subconsciously, "I know I can't tolerate eggs; I have eaten an egg; therefore I must react in a predictable way".

It is always a possibility that this kind of subconscious reaction will occur. In my own supervised testing we constantly check pulse and blood glucose, and observe changes such as flushing or dark rings under the eyes, to help separate true intolerance from reactions induced by this psychological overlay.

With food, double-blind testing is possible only by using an intragastric tube to take the food directly to the stomach, so that theoretically there is no taste sensation. In fact, even with this technique, most patients do get a sufficiently strong taste to be able to identify the food. It is also an unpleasant procedure for the patient, and I normally never use it unless I suspect that the psychological overlay is so strong that it is interfering with the test. It may then be at least worth trying. The pure researchers, of course, who don't have to worry about the sensitivities of patients, would like to see every challenge test administered double-blind.

SOME OTHER WAYS OF TESTING ■

For all its imperfections, the challenge test is the most reliable and efficient way of establishing which foods (and chemicals) are responsible for the symptoms and disorders of intolerance. The fast itself, for the overwhelming majority of people, is safe, therapeutic in its own right and manageable at home with only minimal supervision.

This is not the only test, however, that is used for identifying food intolerance and, as you may well encounter one or more of the other tests, it is worth briefly explaining how they work. What most of them have in common is that they reveal only those foods to which a person has the *potential* to react adversely. The challenge test shows those to which a person actually *is* reacting, and that is a far more valuable piece of information for a doctor.

The RAST Test Probably the best known of these other tests is the RAST, an acronym for Radio Allergo-Sorbent Test. It involves testing for antibodies to specific substances in the blood and it is done in the laboratory as opposed to on the patient's actual body. Whenever antibodies attach themselves to the foreign substance that is being challenged, they are identified on a print-out.

As far as it goes, the RAST test is very efficient, particularly for sorting out allergies to pollens, grasses and danders. Otherwise tests for such allergies can be time-consuming and unpleasant for the patient. The traditional method of identifying these allergies involves making numerous skin pricks until there is a reaction on the skin. RAST requires only a blood sample to be taken.

The drawback of RAST in clinical ecology is that it identifies only those foods that trigger a production of antibodies — in other words, the true food allergies that make up only a tiny proportion of all food maladaptive reactions. For any reaction where there is no elevated antibody level, the test is useless, except that there is often an association between true food addiction and intolerance.

RAST also suffers from being comparatively expensive and very easy to abuse. The more substances you are testing for, the more expensive it becomes, because each substance has to be tested separately, even though all tests are done from the one blood sample. The opportunity for abuse by unethical pathologists and other doctors is obviously considerable, and stringent controls have been introduced to limit its use and so prevent abuse.

At the time of writing, only five RAST tests can initially be performed on a single day to qualify for Medicare reimbursement. These are generally one from each of the five groups, pollens, grasses, danders, housedust and food. If any of these prove positive, a further five a day are permitted.

Most doctors, while agreeing that the test needs to be rigorously controlled, think that the controls are too restrictive and that at least ten tests a day should be permitted, if one of the first five proved positive, to allow the laboratory to get through the number of possible allergens that are usually submitted, in a reasonable time.

There have been various refinements of RAST, including a very effective one known as the Fadel-Nailbuff modified RAST, which is claimed to be more accurate than basic RAST. But it still depends on the presence of specific antibodies for its findings. Even more sensitive is what is known as the IP assay of an enzyme called peroxidase. (Chemicals that end in "-ase" are always enzymes, which are catalysts formed by living cells whose job is to promote a chemical change of some kind.)

My own experience is that most of the positive findings of RAST tests, so far as food is concerned, can be picked up as reliably and a great deal more cheaply, in a properly taken history. A positive RAST does not mean that the specific sample being tested is causing the symptoms, merely that there has been exposure at some time in the past and that specific antibodies are present in the blood.

Cytotoxic Testing The word cytotoxic comes from the Greek *cyto*, meaning "cell", and the Latin *toxicare*, meaning "to poison". So cytotoxic refers to cells that are damaged by "poisoning".

The test was developed comparatively recently by an American husband-and-wife research team, William and Marian Bryde. It is a method of testing for food and chemical intolerance which relies on the damage that occurs to certain white cells in the blood when they come in contact wth an invading protein or molecule.

A sample of blood is taken and the white blood cells are concentrated. A drop of these cells is suspended in a solution and then placed on a slide, which has been treated with the substance being tested.

If a patient is sensitive to that particular food or chemical, the white cells appear abnormal under the microscope. Usually the white cells, the leucocytes, are the first to suffer damage, and the response of one type in particular, the neutrophil, is considered to be the best indicator of food hypersensitivity. (See Chapter 4 for more detail on the immune system.) The damage can vary from minimal, which is usually shown as 1 on a scale of 0 to 5, to the complete destruction of the cell which scores 5.

At a glance, one would imagine that in ecological illness cytotoxic testing is much more useful than RAST, because it doesn't depend on antibody levels. It is also much cheaper than RAST, although at the time of writing far fewer pathologists carry it out. It is certainly true that some patients who eliminate the foods pinpointed by cytotoxic testing as troublesome do well.

In reality, however, it turns out to be a disappointment. Even though someone is shown by cytotoxic testing to be sensitive to a particular food or chemical, this in no way means that he or she will actually suffer an adverse reaction after eating or inhaling the substance. Quite commonly there is a strong positive reaction to food that has never been eaten at all, and as we have seen, regular and frequent consumption is a prerequisite in food intolerance or addiction.

At the same time, in cytotoxic testing people respond positively to foods that they have eaten in copious quantities all their lives without any ill effect. What has more serious implications for their reliability is that the tests often fail to identify the foods and chemicals that *are* causing intolerance reactions, and often very strong reactions.

At best, therefore, the cytotoxic tests are a useful indicator that something may be causing intolerance, and the challenge test is still required to confirm this. In time a test similar to the cytotoxic test may be developed which will satisfy both the critics of the challenge test and its adherents. Until then, cytotoxic testing should be treated only as a guide.

The Coca Pulse Test Dr Arthur Coca was Professor of Clinical Medicine at Columbia University in New York and he has been a formidable force in furthering the cause of taking an ecological approach to many illnesses. Coca and I have shared the invaluable experience of at one time having been the medical director of a major pharmaceutical manufacturing company, which provided a unique insight into the drug-oriented medical practices of today. Both of us later moved back into the real world of clinical medicine.

Coca maintained, after many years of clinical experience, that our pulse accelerates in the presence of foods and chemicals that we are unable to tolerate (an abnormally high pulse means an increase in pulse beats of at least twelve per minute over the norm). A simple pulse test is often all that is needed to identify the source of food intolerance.

He developed a test that involves taking fourteen pulse measurements throughout the day, the first in bed immediately after waking, and the last, also in bed, before sleeping. In addition, four measurements are taken around the three main meals of the day, one (control) before the meal and the other three thirty, sixty and ninety minutes after the food has been eaten. The patient keeps a careful diary of everything he experiences. Fine tuning then takes place with what Coca called the Coca pulse-dietary system.

This system involves first establishing a control by taking the pulse reading a few hours after last eating the suspect food, and then carrying out food challenge tests, giving a small portion of a different suspect food every hour. The pulse is checked just before each of these meals and then half an hour afterwards. Again, according to Coca, any specific food to which the patient is intolerant is revealed.

The trouble with Coca's test is that I believe that only about 50 per cent of people are "pulse-responders". Many people show no significant change in their pulse rate, even when they are eating a food to which they are highly intolerant. I have had patients prostrate on the floor, so severe has their reaction been, while their pulse beats on with monotonous regularity at the same rate as before the test began.

I believe that an increased pulse rate in those who do respond in this way is a useful additional pointer to the existence of intolerance. In my own supervised testing, the pulse is always measured frequently. The main drawback is that there is no way of knowing whether a patient is not responding because there is no intolerance, or because he or she is simply not a pulse-responder. Once again, we have to fall back for confirmation on the challenge test, the one test that is almost never wrong.

17 *After the Test*

By the end of the challenge test, the patient should be feeling on top of the world, symptom-free and longing to begin living life to the full. That, after all, is what it is all about. If the testing was carried out in a hospital or clinic, the patient will probably have been there for about a fortnight and the initial wonder at being free of all those symptoms that he believed he would have to carry with him to the grave is now being matched by impatience to go home.

If the testing was carried out at home, there will certainly be the excitement of seeing the rest of the family reacting to this miraculous new person.

The first priority, therefore, is to ensure that none of the unsafe foods slip into the diet, either carelessly or by mistake. It will be necessary to exclude them entirely for a minimum of six months. After that they can be brought into the diet very cautiously, one at a time and never more often than once every four days. If there is even the slightest twinge to suggest that the intolerance is still there, abandon that food for another year. Then try it again in the same way, and if there is still a hint of a reaction, resign yourself to doing without it for life. If there is no reaction, the food can stay in the diet, but it must not be eaten more often than once every four days — *ever*. Too frequent exposure (once daily, for example) will result in the re-emergence of intolerance reactions.

SELECTING THE RIGHT DIET ∎

Apart from obviously avoiding unsafe foods, the choice of diet is not something about which most clinical ecologists are dogmatic. Clinical ecology is not another fad diet and I never lay down hard and fast rules about any diet that my patients must scrupulously follow.

On the other hand, any doctor adopting an ecological approach must be profoundly concerned that patients do eat a balanced, healthy diet. We are concerned with people as a whole, which is why we lay so much stress on the importance of exercise, particularly aerobic exercise, on relaxation and on counselling to help overcome any aspect of a patient's life that is a stressor. So the food that the patient eats is very important.

There are a few approaches to diet that I believe ought to be endorsed, and one or two that should be avoided like the plague. I endorse and recommend the eating habits recommended by Nathan Pritikin in his Pritikin Program, where kilojoules are for the most part supplied by complex carbohydrates, and refined carbohydrates are avoided. Fat, protein, salt, caffeine and alcohol are reduced or omitted. Also, Pritikin places great importance on exercise as an integral part of his program.

Two diets devised by Pritikin's close followers can be strongly recommended: that of Australian Ross Horne (*The New Health Revolution*, 1986) and the very clever vegetarian version of Pritikin by American husband-and-wife team, Dr John A. McDougall and Mary McDougall (*The McDougall Plan*, 1983).

DIETS TO AVOID ALL COSTS ■

There are some fashionable diets that I never recommend and I caution my patients strongly against using them, except on a short-term basis or as an exclusion diet in the course of trying to identify an offending food.

Much as I respect the work that my friend Richard Mackarness has done to further the cause of clinical ecology, I am certain that, in any situations except the two I have mentioned above, his so-called Stone Age diet, which is high in fat and protein, is unhealthy and undesirable in the long term. For precisely the reasons that I endorse Pritikin's low-fat, low-protein diet, I think the Mackarness diet is likely to do much more harm than good. The same applies equally to the high-fat and high-protein Atkins and less well-known Stillman diets, which are generally advocated on a long-term basis and lead to problems.

Amongst the other very real risks that these diets pose, they are likely to result in high levels of cholesterol, leading to the growth of plaque, or fat-like deposits, in the arteries and increasing the risk of arterial disease. That doesn't seem to me to be the basis of a healthy diet. The University of Cincinnati's Lipid Research Center found that for every 1 per cent reduction in total cholesterol level, there is a 2 per cent reduction in heart-disease risk. The last thing we should be doing is increasing fat consumption.

The Finns, with the fattiest diet in the Western world, have the highest cholesterol levels and the highest rate of heart disease; the Americans, with a diet only slightly less rich, are a close second on both counts; while the Japanese, whose diet is low in fat, have the lowest cholesterol and the lowest incidence of cardiovascular disease. These facts cannot be ignored.

PRITIKIN IS SO BORING! ■

Keeping to Pritikin can certainly be hard work. His diet is often criticised for being so boring that it turns people away from sensible dieting for the rest of their lives, or until a serious illness forces them back on to a diet — usually a Pritikin-type diet! But with imagination it can be made interesting and even if we follow only half the Pritikin diet because we miss many of the familiar foods too much, that is 50 per cent better than not trying to keep to Pritikin at all. Both Ross Horne and the McDougalls appear to have made Pritikin more palatable.

Pritikin modelled his diet, incidentally, on that of the countries where heart disease and the other degenerative diseases are virtually unknown, modifying it to ensure that it meets all the normally accepted recommended daily allowances of proteins, amino acids, essential fatty acids, minerals and vitamins. Tedious or not, it is a very good diet. I do feel, however, that some of the cereal grains should be replaced with extra fruit and vegetables.

Ideally, then, we are looking for a low-fat, low-protein diet, with a marked reduction in the protein and fats of animal origin, which includes eggs, butter and whole milk. Variety is important so that the food base should be as broad as possible, which is healthy in itself and reduces the chance of new food intolerance developing.

I am sure that this high-fibre diet, in the presence of low animal fat and low protein, is the reason why many degenerative diseases, such as diseases of the arteries and particularly coronary artery disease, are so rarely found in people who keep to it. Pritikin concluded that cholesterol is the principal factor in the onset of arterial closure, that fat is the secondary factor and that it makes little difference whether the fat is saturated or unsaturated. (Saturated fats are the ones that set hard when they are left to cool, like the fat left in the frying pan; unsaturated fats are oily fats, usually vegetable oils, that stay fluid when they are cooled.)

Conventional thinking has always been that saturated fats cause coronary artery disease as well as many other problems, because of their tendency to build up in the blood vessels. Unsaturated fats are claimed to give protection against heart disease. Pritikin maintains that to the contrary, they are as dangerous as each other.

ROTATING THE DIET ▪

The one proviso that I do make is that, as far as possible, the diet should be rotated on at least a four-day basis. Although foods shown to be safe by testing can be eaten every day, it is still best to avoid excessive regular consumption of them. Those foods not tested in the challenge testing, because they are not eaten regularly, can be eaten but must be rotated. The rotation diet is the best possible defence against new intolerances developing. The four-day rotation allows three full days between each food so that no individual food is eaten more frequently than once every four days. This equates with the ninety-six hours that is required for some foods to pass through the gastrointestinal tract.

The four-day rotational diet can be surprisingly complicated, because not only must individual foods be avoided more than once every four days, but so too must other members of the same food families because of the risk of cross-reactivity. Intolerance of tomatoes, for example, predisposes a person to be intolerant of other members of the tomato family, including potatoes, capsicum and tobacco.

Although a rotational diet is always to be recommended, we insist on rotation only if patients' intolerance is severe, which implies a high risk that further food intolerances may develop.

What the diet means in theory is that no member of any food family can be eaten more than once every four days. On day one, for example, any kind of citrus fruit — lemon, orange, mandarin, or grapefruit — can be eaten, but three clear days must elapse before they can be eaten again. If day one is Monday, then the next orange cannot be eaten before Friday.

A number of attempts have been made to simplify the rotational diet and make it fun for the family to follow. One of the most imaginative of these was the diet devised by Sally Rockwell, a nutritionist from the University of Washington in Seattle, who invented what she called the rotation game and cleverly colour-coded every item of food likely to come into a typical home. According to its botanical or zoological family, every food has a coloured label tied or stuck to it and you can eat only food of one colour on one day.

WORKING OUT A ROTATION DIET ■

It is most sensible to consult a dietician as soon as the doctor supervising your test explains in broad terms what diet you should follow. If you have tested yourself, still go to a dietician: no referral is needed. The dietician will prepare a suitable diet, taking into account your weight and individual nutritional requirements, as well as the need to go on to a rotational diet. It is difficult to work out your own four-day rotational diet without a dietician's advice because of the importance of keeping it balanced and of ensuring in particular the correct daily intake of vitamins and minerals.

In extreme food sensitivity there are occasions when the rotation diet has to be extended to seven days, which means that if citrus fruit is eaten on Monday, it cannot be eaten again until the following Monday. Sally Rockwell has a game for this as well, and also interesting menus for both the four- and seven-day versions.

The most common food families are included in Appendix V. Some may seem obscure, but it is important to know that if you are intolerant, for instance, of green beans and chocolate, switching to carob instead of chocolate may not provide relief. Carob and green beans are both legumes!

Food relationships in fruit, vegetables and all other plants depend on botanical characteristics that are not necessarily what most people think of. Onions and leeks are fairly obviously related, but asparagus is also in the same family — the lily family!

A few foods are not related, but are notorious for cross-reacting. Chocolate and cola drinks are common examples, even though cocoa beans and the cola nut are botanically unrelated. What this means in practice is that when intolerance develops to chocolate, cola drinks are likely to become a problem as well, probably because of common chemicals such as caffeine.

18 Treatment
of Intolerance
in Babies
and Children

We have already emphasised that children must never be put on a true fast, meaning a fast where all food except water is excluded, without the approval and daily supervision of a doctor, and ideally with constant supervision in a hospital or clinic. This is because growing children of normal weight have no reserves of fat. On a total fast they must be closely monitored to ensure that the fast doesn't slip over into starvation. Only a doctor is qualified to recognise the symptoms and treat them promptly and correctly if they arise.

In fact, fasting of this nature is very rarely necessary with children. Instead, as already mentioned, I normally put them on a mono-exclusion diet, in which the food eaten is one that has not been regularly and frequently consumed and which therefore cannot be involved in any addiction. Brown rice is the food that I favour. It is not most children's idea of the perfect diet, but it removes any risk of starvation developing. Oats is another useful food.

CONFUSING SYMPTOMS ▮

What situations lead up to the need for children to fast in the first place? There are no exceptions to the general rule that any food that can produce intolerance in an adult can have the same effect on children. The risk may even be higher because children tend to have a more restricted diet and eat less varied foods over the course of the week. And they are just as susceptible as adults to chemical intolerance. It is so common that once organic and other manifest causes have been explored and eliminated, intolerance is by far the most likely explanation for otherwise inexplicable disorders and symptoms.

I have had 4- and 5-year-olds referred to me who have been

diagnosed as brain-damaged, uncoordinated, hyperactive and generally ill, but they have been suffering from nothing more serious than intolerance to a food. I remember well the mother of one 4-year-old girl who was always ill and uncoordinated. She had been told by her doctor that she must "just make the best of it", whatever that was supposed to mean, because her daughter was never going to get any better. The only therapy that was needed to restore her to complete health, was to take eggs and all red-coloured foods out of her diet.

The initial acute symptoms become masked, as in all food addiction. Common among initial symptoms in children are ear troubles, bowel disorders, short attention span and poor school performance, excessive tiredness and depression, excitability, hyperactivity and that unmistakable give-away sign of allergy and intolerance, the pale, almost white face and the black circles under the eyes.

Babies and young children are particularly vulnerable to intolerance and allergies because their immune systems are not yet fully mature. Most symptoms disappear as the child grows older, or, more likely, they become masked and manifest themselves in different forms. Colic becomes hyperactivity, which becomes asthma, for instance. Others are clearly identifiable as they persist through childhood and adolescence into adulthood.

INTOLERANCE BEGINS AT BIRTH — AND EARLIER ▌

Intolerance can start very early, as early as in the womb. The individual susceptibility to develop intolerance can certainly be developed before birth, given the importance of heredity in pre-disposing people to become intolerant. But it can progress a step beyond this as well.

A mother who does not have cow's milk intolerance herself, for example, can still pass cow's milk intolerance on to her un-born baby, as well as to the baby she is breastfeeding, provided the baby has the individual susceptibility to develop cow's milk intolerance, which is always a requirement before any intolerance can develop. The baby is unable to cope with the residual traces of the cow's milk in its system, whether it gets there through the mother's blood or through her milk in its gut.

The problem of cow's milk in infants is often made worse because many mothers drink a lot of milk regularly in the belief

that they are going to give their babies strong bones. They may
be right but they may also be increasing the likelihood of intolerance to the milk developing. Drinking excessive amounts of
cow's milk should be avoided at any time (in normal circumstances it should never be introduced into a baby's diet until
at least six months old), and pregnancy and lactation are no
exceptions.

I believe, from patients I have seen, that babies may even be
affected by chemical outgassing while they are still in the womb.
Remember that it makes no difference how a substance gets into
the bloodstream, whether by eating, drinking, injecting or inhaling. Once in the mother's bloodstream, a substance can pass
to the baby. Babies of heroin addicts are at high risk of being
born heroin addicts too, and we know that there is no observable
difference between heroin addiction and food addiction in the
victims' systems.

HOSPITAL HAZARDS ■

If the mother is food or chemical intolerant, problems can arise
when she goes into hospital to have her baby. Most hospitals are
not geared for coping with intolerance, although the larger hospitals are more likely to have the facilities to prepare a suitable
exclusion diet: most dieticians are now well aware of the realities
of food addiction.

For the chemically sensitive, hospitals are overflowing with
outgassing substances calculated to make a mother's time there
miserable. It isn't the hospitals' fault. It is very difficult to clean a
ward without using a single substance that outgasses, and disinfectant is a hospital's lifeblood. More easily avoidable are such
practices as routinely giving new babies dextrose, even if the
mother is sugar intolerant (which predisposes the baby to be the
same). Many hospitals take unkindly to being told what to feed
babies in their care, even by the mother's family doctor, let alone
by the mother herself. Unfortunately it may sometimes be necessary for your doctor to demand it, if you are sufficiently concerned. My experience is that the medium-sized general hospitals
are the most obstinate. The big teaching hospitals are as coopera-
tive as they can be, while the country cottage hospitals have time
to make allowances for individual sensitivities.

Once you are home, make sure that outgassing is kept to an
absolute minimum in the baby's room. Don't use fly spray or any

other aerosol at *any* time: many of them are deliberately formulated to go on killing for days. Don't hang those chemical fly killers in the nursery for the same reason, and don't use any strong-smelling disinfectants, whose fumes will be inhaled.

If at all possible, kerosene heaters should not be used in the same room as the baby, whether they are lit or not. I know that for some families this is the only way of warming the baby's room, but the petrochemical fumes that outgas from these heaters can easily result in intolerance if they are there all the time, and leave the child with symptoms for life. At the very least, make sure that the heater is removed from the room at all times except when it is actually warming it.

By now it should not be necessary to point out that cigarette smoking is not only dangerous for the passive smoker, but can be counted on to increase the risk of both true allergy and intolerance developing. Don't smoke anywhere near a baby or a young child and don't let anyone else do it. The momentary embarrassment of asking someone to put out a cigarette (and I know many mothers whose fury at such thoughtlessness more than overcomes any feelings of embarrassment) is nothing compared to the proven dangers of smoking near young children.

Over the years, I have seen a number of cases where both a child under the age of two, still being breastfed, and the child's mother are victims of the same intolerance. The child's symptoms usually appear about an hour after feeding and they are not necessarily the same symptoms as the mother's. You cannot handle the baby's symptoms unless you first identify and avoid the cause of the intolerance in the mother. In some cases, where identification may take a long time, it is better for the mother to stop breastfeeding the baby. If she continues, there is a risk that the baby's own susceptibility to developing intolerance will become more ingrained.

THE BEST FOODS FOR BABY ■

It is always important for a woman to eat a variety of nutritious foods during pregnancy. Most doctors place the emphasis on nutrition and that is commendable; clinical ecologists are equally concerned about *variety*, so that the food base is as broad as possible. This in itself leads to good health and reduces the risk of food addiction.

In most situations, there is no substitute for breast milk. It is the perfect food for human babies. One of the main worries about most commercially available breast-milk substitutes (formulas) is that they are made from cow's milk, which is a habitual addictant. The alternatives often contain soy, which also produces intolerance in some babies, although it is much safer than cow's milk.

Goat's milk is rarely a satisfactory alternative to cow's milk (Chapter 11, p. 173); and skim and low-fat milk, from whatever animal, are unsuitable for babies for many reasons.

New foods should be introduced one at a time and wherever possible, delay the introduction of solids until the baby is at least five or six months old. Obviously, there are no hard and fast rules about this, and your doctor may have important reasons for introducing solids earlier. Introduce only one new food at a time and in small amounts, several days apart. Take particular care with the most common causes of intolerance, which in small children are likely to be cow's milk and dairy products, eggs, wheat, citrus fruits and peanut butter. Avoid them for nine months if you can.

These steps will minimise the risk of intolerance symptoms occurring without you being aware of it, and by leaving it until the baby is as old as possible before introducing solids, you will be giving the immune system and gastric system the most help in dealing with potentially "unsafe" foods.

CONFUSING SYMPTOMS ▮

Typical of the symptoms of intolerance in babies are the following, depending on where the reaction takes place. The three main target areas are the digestive system, respiratory system and skin. There may be several symptoms at the same time, from all three areas.

1. *Digestive System*: The stomach and intestine are affected and the symptoms may include nausea and vomiting, spitting up food, colicky behaviour including pulling away from the breast, stomach pain, diarrhoea, poor appetite and poor weight gain.
2. *Respiratory System*: This affects the nose, throat and lungs and the common symptoms are runny nose, sneezing, wheezing, asthma, recurrent attacks of bronchitis or croup, and a persistent cough. If the upper respiratory

tract is affected, we often see the familiar allergy salute as the child constantly rubs his nose, pushing it up to try and open up the airway — hence the crease across the end of the nose. Sticky eyelashes are another warning sign.

3. *Skin*: Eczema, hives and other rashes are common. Traces of eczema are often seen round the mouth and there is classic cracking at the base of the ears.

As in all intolerance, it is important to realise that these symptoms may all have other causes (true allergy is often implicated) and a doctor must eliminate these causes first. On the other hand, some of the symptoms may be part of normal baby behaviour and require no treatment at all. Your doctor will tell you — but remember that under normal baby behaviour he may include symptoms of intolerance that could be treated successfully by a doctor taking an ecological approach. No baby and no child should expect to have to live with symptoms that are uncomfortable on the grounds that they are "normal", unless they really are normal. If they are caused by food or chemical intolerance, that is not normal.

THE WORST CULPRIT ■

Cow's milk is the most common addictant in children, a mucus-producing, acid-forming food that is unnatural for humans to drink (Chapter 11, "Milk", pp. 167–176). If parents are not aware of the hazards of milk, it never occurs to them to link the daily doses of milk with any of the symptoms. How could it possibly be milk? they ask. Their child has been drinking it since she was a baby! Exactly! Milk for breakfast with cereal, milk mid-morning, a yoghurt for lunch, a glass of milk when she comes home in the afternoon, cheese with supper, a milky drink just before going to bed . . . There are many people who would recognise that sort of pattern in their own drinking habits quite as easily as in those of their children. It is the perfect prescription for intolerance.

As children reach school age, intolerance can cause a whole range of learning and behavioural disorders and that most difficult to live with syndrome, hyperactivity. Children who perform badly at school are usually considered to be poorly motivated, lazy, dull or stupid, without too much effort being expended on why they turned out that way. They may indeed be all those things, but they may equally well be intolerant of a food or chemical, and the poor motivation, laziness, dullness and stupidity are just symptoms of that intolerance.

Far too many children are put down in this way when they are simply reacting — unknown to themselves, their parents or their teachers — to something in their diet or their environment. Not infrequently it is something in the environment of the school itself, particularly outgassing chemicals such as floor polish or the strongly scented disinfectant that most cleaners seem to equate with cleanliness. If it smells clean, it must be right, is the argument. More to the point, if it smells of anything, it means that molecules of that substance are floating around in the air, any one of which can lead to intolerance when inhaled.

The relationship between nutrition and children's learning and behaviour has been studied for decades. Many authorities have noted the link between malnourishment and learning ability. Malnourished children tend to acquire language skills later than normal, and this affects their progress through the school system.

Lack of breakfast has been shown to affect children's attention span and concentration, their ability to get through the school day without being too fatigued and even their ability to socialise appropriately with their peers. Studies in preschool children have shown the same effect.

Some researchers are so convinced that if children have not had breakfast they will function at less than their maximum potential that they refuse to test them. Their reasoning is that they are interested in finding out the child's *full* potential. Starting the day without any food so reduces this optimal level that the tests would be meaningless.

FAT PARENTS, FAT CHILDREN ■

What we tend to forget is that malnourishment does not necessarily mean a lack of food. Increasingly in our affluent society malnourishment has come to mean overconsumption. The American Public Health Association, an influential body consisting of representatives from many health fields in both the United States and Canada, met in December 1979 with top experts in the field of nutrition to formulate objectives and concern for the 1980s. According to that meeting, the number-one problem facing health in developed countries would be not syphilis, drug abuse, television violence, or crime, but malnourishment caused by overeating. This is confirmed every day in my own practice.

Many children are already showing evidence of coronary artery disease and other degenerative diseases before they leave primary school. Unless the AIDS epidemic sneaks past it at the post, that 1979 assessment is as valid as we near the end of the 1980s as it was at the start of the decade.

Obesity must always be suspected as a symptom of food addiction, the result of compulsive eating. Children should never be obese, but look around some playgrounds and it seems as though every tenth child is too fat. Even in preschool there are obese children.

There would be some justification for it if the reason were biochemical, genetic, or the result of an enzymatic disorder, but only in the rarest cases is any of these the reason. Obese children are fat because of what they eat, or more accurately because of what their parents allow them to eat. Fat parents often seem to derive some comfort from seeing their children fat. It isn't the children's fault if they become fat.

Their obesity is the result of the ice-creams, pies, biscuits, fizzy drinks laden with sugar, lollies and packets of chips that they are allowed to consume, and the deep-fried foods that are metabolic poison to anyone, let alone children. And if there is obesity, make no mistake that you are storing up all manner of complications with it.

This may not always result in food intolerance, though it usually does, but it most certainly is ecological illness and it is a totally avoidable national epidemic.

Sugar is so frequently a cause of disturbed behaviour in children (and of course in adults) that many parents have found that the simply exclusion of sugar and sugar-containing foods is enough to bring about a marked improvement in the behaviour of children who before were highly antisocial. Glenn was one of my patients whose antisocial behaviour was due to malnourishment.

Controlled studies in other countries, particularly America, confirm that Glenn's case was no fluke result. In one of the most remarkable experiments 800,000 children in New York State schools, who were below average academically, were put on a 90 per cent sugar-free diet and, at the same time, were given only food without additives or preservatives. Sweet dispensers were removed and parents were educated to cooperate. The children

GLENN'S ANTISOCIAL BEHAVIOUR

Glenn was 13 when he was referred to me. He came into my rooms looking round-faced, red-haired, morose and depressed. He had been sent along primarily because of his extreme antisocial behaviour and he was on the point of being expelled from his boarding school. He broke every rule in the book and among his recent exploits were ringing the police and telling them there was a bomb in the police station timed to go off at midnight, and calling the fire brigade to inform them that the school was on fire.

He bordered on being hyperactive, without displaying all the symptoms normally necessary for a formal diagnosis of hyperactivity: in particular, he had no sleep disturbances. His history showed that he had suffered from a behaviour problem virtually all his life.

His diet was filled with refined carbohydrates and in fact the whole school diet was most unsatisfactory. The boys seemed to survice on deep-fried potatoes, a few vegetables and almost no fresh fruit. They drank cordial laced with sugar, had desserts that were invariably something sweet with ice-cream, and were clearly malnourished.

To his credit the head-master, who knew nothing before then about ecological illness, was impressed enough by what I told him of the dangers of refined carbohydrates to order a complete overhaul of the school's diet. Without doing any further tests, I recommended that Glenn's diet should in future omit refined car-bohydrates plus all fatty foods, and this led to an almost complete turnabout in his behaviour. Two years later, his examination results and his general conduct in the school confirmed that he was once again an entirely normal, well-behaved and well-adjusted boy.

The effect of the new diet on the other boys was so striking that teachers and parents alike commented on the improvement in every department. Conduct improved, academically and at sports the boys thrived as never before.

were carefully monitored for four years. Overall, they went from being below-average achievers to 11 per cent *above* the national average — and they preferred their new diet!

A seminar held recently at the John Radcliffe Hospital in Oxford, UK, was told that antisocial behaviour among adolescent delinquents in fourteen British institutions, such as fighting, lying and stealing, was reduced by more than 40 per cent when refined carbohydrates (sugar and white flour), desserts high in sugar, soft drinks and cereals were removed from their diet. In one institution the suicide rate fell from a steady five a year to none at all.

Another very rebellious boy, an 11-year-old patient of mine whom we shall call Tom, was just as destructive as Glenn. In fact his school had gone a stage further and expelled him for his aggressive and destructive behaviour. He had been seen by many experts, including a psychologist and a psychiatrist, none of whom had achieved anything for him. His mother had tried him on a Feingold diet without worthwhile improvement, and all in all the prognosis was pretty bleak.

Tom's glucose tolerance test was revealing, climbing quickly to a high peak and then plummeting to hypoglycaemic levels, by which point he was hyperactive and almost uncontrollable.

I put him on a mono-exclusion diet of brown rice for five days and by the end of that time he was socialising normally and relating extremely well to the staff and the other patients. There was no sign of his old antisocial behaviour.

Food testing showed that he was reacting to a number of foods including wheat, animal fats, green beans, tomatoes and cow's milk, as well as to the sugar that was responsible for his hypoglycaemia. Some of these are difficult foods to exclude completely from a diet, but his parents applied themselves diligently and were rewarded by having their formerly rebellious son reinstated at school, where he went on to achieve excellent results in his examinations.

Just occasionally, he slipped from his diet, either by mistake or when the temptation of a sugary drink on a hot day was too much. Each time, the old symptoms returned, not as severely as before, but enough to make him draw in his horns very sharply and return strictly to his diet. At the time of writing, he has been on it for four years and continues to do as well as ever. In his case, the exclusion diet that we worked out will probably be a necessity for life if he wants to remain symptom-free. Tom would be the first to agree that it is a bargain price to pay for his new life.

PART THREE

The Chemical Burden

19 The Poisoning
of the Planet

A hundred years from now, the last half of the twentieth century will probably be remembered, with a good deal of irony, as the Age of the Environment: the time when the human race, having polluted its environment to the point of endangering its own survival, sometimes in ignorance, often wilfully, at last began to understand the awful truth of what it was doing. It was the time when it first dawned on people that their health could only be safeguarded if their immediate environment was also safe, meaning also the environment in which their food was produced and processed.

I hope that it will also be remembered as the time when a growing number of doctors and other health-care professionals, weary of not being able to treat so many patients by conventional medicine, turned to the environment and there found many of the answers that had eluded them.

We have seen how many ordinary foods, as well as the chemicals in those foods, can create intolerance, which manifests itself as many of the disorders and symptoms that plague modern Western Society. Now we must look at the second major cause of these same ecological illnesses, the chemicals that are all around us in our environment.

It used to be thought — and it still is thought by many doctors and lay people — that, although some things cannot be inhaled or eaten without causing injury, most of the chemical substances that get into our body one way or another go in at one end, as it were, and come out at the other without any ill effects.

Once a substance was declared by the toxicologists either to be safe at any dosage, or to be harmful only above a certain level of exposure, anything less than this was automatically assumed to be safe. We know now that this is absolutely wrong.

It was Dr Theron Randolph in the United States who put a spanner in the works of this comfortable theory in 1951, by showing from his own clinical experience over many years that chemicals, even in minute traces of substances that had previ-

ously been declared safe, cause illnesses and symptoms in susceptible people.

My own experience after many years is that probably everyone is sensitive in some degree to one or more substances in their
environment, even if the only reaction is that they are not achieving their full potential.

Not all chemicals are dangerous; some present no danger
when they are inert, but are an extreme environmental hazard
when that stability is disturbed. The chemical toluene di-
isocyanate (TDI), for example, which is a commonly used component in paints, lacquers, plastics and polyurethanes, turns to
acid when it comes in contact with moisture. The victims not infrequently are firemen battling chemical fires in factories or ware-
houses where any of these products are manufactured or stored.

In a typical case, a fireman was exposed to TDI when his
mask was accidentally knocked off when he was fighting a chemical fire. The brief exposure so affected his immune system — the
most common target — that he was unable to drink normal tap
water, he couldn't walk down the street or even eat food kept in
plastic containers or wrapped in plastic film. This heightened
sensitivity included such intolerance of any perfume or deodorant, that the merest whiff of it sent him into a towering rage (he
had always been a mild, placid man), or forced him to bed for
days.

Not all chemicals adversely affect all people; but probably
all of them can adversely affect some people some of the time.
The vital point that we need to understand is that chemicals can
do this regardless of the extent of exposure — even when it is so
small that toxicologists have always insisted that it poses no
threat at all.

HOW SAFE IS OUR ENVIRONMENT? ■

How safe, then, is our chemically saturated environment? The
truth is that nobody knows. The nuclear disasters at Three Mile
Island in New York and at Chernobyl in the Soviet Union are
constant reminders that nothing that is potentially dangerous can
ever be said to be totally safe.

Almost everyone in Western society today is aware that
some chemicals can be extremely dangerous. We are forcefully
reminded of this whenever we read of industrial disasters like
those at Seveso in Italy in 1976, when a factory spewed deadly

dioxin over a wide area; or at Bhopal in India eight years later, when a Union Carbide factory leaked methyl isocyanate which killed 1700 people and injured 200,000 others, leaving many of them blind.

Only eight months after Bhopal, in August 1985, Union Carbide accepted responsibility for leaking the same gas from another of its plants, this time in West Virginia, USA. More by luck than by good management, no deaths have so far been reported from this incident, although 135 people were injured.

A year after Chernobyl, the number of mongoloid babies born in Berlin rose to five times the normal level and an immediate study which followed throughout West Germany revealed an alarming increase in deformities. These were babies conceived in the weeks immediately after the disaster. The head of the Genetic Institute in West Berlin, Professor Karl Sperling, remarked cautiously, "From the data it is clear there could be a connection between Chernobyl and the deformities . . . the statistics indicate there must be a connection."

Most people can easily make the association between this high level of exposure to chemicals, and disease and death. It requires a considerable leap of the imagination, however, to accept the reality of ecological disease, in which chemicals — even in minuscule doses — are affecting us to the point of serious illness.

How do we know that this is happening? Very simply! We separate affected patients from the offending chemicals and they get better. We do it thousands of times every year, in the surgeries and consulting rooms of doctors taking a clinical ecology approach to their practice of medicine, and we still get the same results. We do it single-blind or double-blind in patients of all ages, all sexes and with almost every imaginable illness and symptom, and still it works. Then we introduce them to the same substances, if they are willing or we wish to satisfy ourselves, and their illnesses and symptoms come flooding back.

Nor should it be surprising that this happens. Commonsense alone should tell us that chemicals that can be lethal or harmful at a given dose do not suddenly become totally safe, as most toxicologists imply, because they are being ingested or inhaled at a slightly smaller dose. The only surprise is the quite devastating extent to which low levels of chemicals are affecting the health of practically all of us, and that when medicine does find an explanation and a solution for the majority of these cases, many doctors bury their heads in the sand and refuse to consider it because it was something they were not taught at medical school.

UNCONTROLLED POLLUTION ▌

In this century, indeed in the last half-century, we have done more to upset our environment than in the previous millennia. We have poured chemicals into the air, water and food, contaminating the very earth upon which we depend for our survival. We have done this on such a massive, largely uncontrolled scale, polluting almost everything we have touched, that there is scarcely a corner of the planet that has not been defiled in some way.

By 1980, 400 synthetic chemicals had been identified in human tissue, mainly in blood, breast milk, liver and nervous tissue. By 1986, there was not a single known animal species on earth, humans included, from Antarctica to the most frozen north, that was free of traces of DDT, a chemical manufactured specifically to kill.

In the United States alone, 227 thousand million kilograms (500 thousand million pounds) of chemicals are manufactured each year, 45 kilograms (100 pounds) for every man, woman and child on earth! More than 63,000 chemicals are in common, everyday use in the world, 3500 of them, as we have seen, in food processing and production. Even this is the merest drop in the ocean compared with the 350 *million* separate synthetic chemicals listed on the American Register of Chemicals. Many of the chemicals used specifically for foods are direct-line derivatives of chemicals that were designed for one purpose only: to kill people in war.

It is incredible that anyone should seriously doubt that this immense chemical contamination of the world — which is known to take the lives of thousands each year from acute poisoning, and to which we are totally ill-adapted as a species — is also having a deleterious effect at levels lower than those that result in gross poisoning.

The dangers ought to be sounding warning bells around the globe: instead, all that we hear is the feeblest tinkling. In an era of unprecedented scientific knowledge, we learned too much too quickly. We invented an excellent drug for controlling morning sickness in pregnant women, for example, but were not clever enough or careful enough to understand that it came at a price that would leave a legacy of deformity in its wake.

Then greed came to the fore, and even when we *did* know of the dangers of thalidomide, for that was the drug in question, the manufacturer continued to make it and sell it until dragged, complaining bitterly, from the marketplace. It relied on the naïve trust of ordinary people that no manufacturer of pharmaceuticals, the industry above all others with a special responsibility to its customers, would ever knowingly allow people to be hurt by its products. How tragically wrong they were!

Thalidomide is still, at the time of writing in 1988, being distributed and sold in many Third World countries, often without any warning of its potential to cause birth defects. In these countries consumer organisations and governments interfere less in the way foreign companies choose to conduct their business.

"DON'T WORRY — YOU'RE BLACK" ■

Industrial deception occurs at every level, often condoned by governments in those countries that most pride themselves on their morality and ethics. When we look at pesticides shortly, we will see that some of the research data was falsified. We need to be aware of this deception, for it has a marked effect on the general attitude to chemicals at any dosage. If the chemical industry, which is immensely powerful, successfully manipulates the truth to allay fears about heavy pollution, it inevitably reduces people's concern about the dangers of low levels of those and other chemicals.

The manufacturers of vinyl chloride, first in Italy and then later in the United States and the rest of the world, including Australia, knew that it was causing cancer of the liver in their workers, largely because of inadequate safety measures in their plants. Yet they suppressed this information for years.

One study, sponsored by the industry itself, confirmed that vinyl chloride was carcinogenic and a major hazard to workers, yet because of a secrecy undertaking, the members of the study group felt obliged to withhold the information until management, much later, was compelled to release it. Among these were doctors of medicine. Thousands of workers worldwide were needlessly exposed to the dangers of vinyl chloride, for years in some cases.

The asbestos industry, which hovers at the edge of the

chemical industry, perpetrated an even more blatant deception on its workers. It knew for sixty years that its products caused cancer and other fatal and crippling diseases, yet it conspired for all of that time to deceive not only its own workforce, but untold thousands of unsuspecting people in the community who were contaminated by its products or its manufacturing processes.

"Don't worry", management told the Aboriginal workers at one New South Wales asbestos mine. "Asbestos dust might affect whites, but not Aborigines."

Now asbestos is the pariah of the 1980s, and the two or three companies in Australia who made their fortunes from it are engaged in an unedifying scramble to put as much distance as possible between themselves and the substance which in 1979 the US Department of Health, Education and Welfare predicted was responsible for 17 per cent of all cancer cases in the United States.

In spite of the enormity of what they have done, it seems most unlikely (in Australia at any rate) that those responsible for conspiring to perpetrate this dreadful crime will ever languish in prison as would be their fate in many other countries, or will even incur much opprobrium. Such are our values.

This kind of behaviour and this attitude to it, repeated countless times in countless countries (in many Third World countries nobody even bothers to go through the charade of covering anything up), has a very profound bearing on popular attitudes to the role of chemical contamination in ecological illness. If you don't care very much when industry claims the lives of its own employees for profit, you aren't likely to worry unduly about the migraines, anxieties, depressions, arthritis and aches and pains induced by low levels of chemical exposure. Unless, of course, it is you who happens to be the victim.

It is easy enough to see how this manipulation and deception have succeeded. Half the world's population had no knowledge or understanding that these chemicals were even dangerous, if they knew they existed at all. The other half, which did have the education and sometimes the knowledge, were persuaded that they must be safe or "they" — that comforting, amorphous Big Brother, constantly safeguarding our health and welfare — would never allow them to be sold. Those who did know, and were not convinced that all was rosy, were either too few in most countries to make any impression, or had some vested interest (not least their jobs) that secured their silence or perpetuated the lies.

Among the victims of this whitewashing were the victims of chemical intolerance.

WHAT CHEMICALS DO TO US ■

All chemical intolerance involves a poisoning of our systems, but it is a poisoning with a difference. If you expose a hundred people to arsenic, for instance, in sufficient quantities, you will eventually have a hundred people affected by arsenic poisoning. The only question in doubt is whether the reaction will be acute and very rapid if the dose is large enough, or chronic and cumulative over a much longer period if exposure was to small doses over a longer period of time.

If you expose a hundred people to formaldehyde in the atmosphere, on the other hand, at concentrations of one part per million (which is normally considered to be an acceptable and safe level), only one or two of them will develop any kind of intolerance response. (At very high doses, of course, the acute reaction may be almost as swift and dangerous as to arsenic.) The reason is that individual susceptibility determines not only what symptoms will appear, but whether they will appear at all.

The course of chemical intolerance is very similar to that of food addiction. Once it has developed, there may be a stage of preadaptation when unpleasant symptoms occur as soon as we are exposed to the chemical molecules. Usually the victim ignores the warning and the intolerance inexorably gets worse.

The next stage sees a gradual improvement in the symptoms, not because the outgassing has disappeared, but as the body adapts to living with this unwelcome intruder. Masking develops, removing any recognisable link between the exposure and the symptoms.

If a girl removes her nail polish on Wednesday and has a low-grade migraine on Friday, why should anyone associate the two unless they know what to look for? There have probably been dozens of other stressors in between the two events, each of them capable of producing a mild headache.

More often than in food intolerance, blind adaptation occurs in which the first preadaptation stage is bypassed altogether and the patient goes directly into a state of masked adaptation. It makes it even more improbable that the cause and the effect will be linked.

Finally, and inevitably as in all intolerance, the time comes when the level of exposure — the "dose" — to the unsafe chemical, which has probably been sufficient to maintain a measure of normality at about the +1 level, is no longer enough. Ever increasing doses are necessary which often take the form of new intolerances to other chemicals developing and eventually the immune system breaks down altogether, masking disappears and the reaction to exposure is immediate and unpleasant.

EXPLAINING CHEMICAL INTOLERANCE ▌

The exact progress of chemical intolerance, from first exposure to final illness, is still not fully understood, but what probably happens, depending on whether we ingest or inhale the molecules, is as follows.

In food intolerance we have seen how a protein, or protein fraction, gets through the wall of the gut and into the bloodstream. Then it travels to the organs and tissues and eventually may provoke an entirely inappropriate reaction as the immune system tries to get rid of it.

When chemicals are involved, it is not a protein but a molecule that is responsible. If it has been ingested through the mouth, it either follows the route taken by the food protein, forcing its way through the gut wall and into the bloodstream; or it passes along the gut and is harmlessly evacuated. Once through the gut wall, similar molecules will follow it, like sheep through a hole in a fence.

Eventually, if there has been regular and frequent exposure, and there is individual susceptibility, these molecules will upset the nerves in one of the organs that they visit and there will be a reaction as the immune system tries to get rid of them. There may also be interference with the neuropeptide transmitters, the hormone messengers in the brain, which will cause further inappropriate reactions.

When we inhale the molecules, which apart from food chemicals is the most likely way that chemicals get into our bodies, the process is initially more involved until they reach the bloodstream. Absorption through the skin is yet another way of entry.

Chemical molecules tend to get to their target area more quickly than food proteins and, perhaps because of this, they usually produce a faster reaction. The victim also recovers more quickly.

THE WAY WE SMELL ▪

Understanding how we smell things is a good guide to the journey that awaits inhaled molecules. When we smell something, molecules from that substance rush through our nostrils (in fact we can smell either through the nose, or through a passage at the back of the mouth joining the mouth and the nasal passages when we are eating); then they proceed up two narrow chambers to a pair of mucus-covered patches, each the size of a one cent coin, just below the brain and behind the bridge of the nose. Here, by some means that we still do not understand, the molecules bind to receptors on tiny, hair-like processes called cilia on the end of the olfactory nerves, which are the nerves concerned with our sense of smell. The olfactory nerves send the message to the brain and this makes us aware of the smell.

The message goes more directly and faster to the brain than with any of the other senses. The part of the brain that receives it is the limbic lobe, the oldest part of the brain and the part that is involved with emotions and memories as well as with our autonomic functions (such as heartbeat and hormone release over which we have little or no direct control). Once the message has reached the limbic lobe, the smell can stimulate associations, evoke memories, arouse us, frighten us, or trigger our appetites, for example.

The brains of primitive humans, and all other mammals, were mostly limbic lobes, or "small brains", and only much later in our evolution were the limbic lobes gradually covered with neocortex (cerebral cortex), the grey thinking matter that controls our reasoning and much of our conscious behaviour.

Our sense of smell is a marvellous piece of machinery, so acute that it is probably 10,000 times more sensitive than our sense of taste, which can detect only salt, sweet, bitter and sour. Pinch your nose and see how difficult it is to know whether you are eating a slice of potato or a slice of apple!

Although smell has become much less important to the human race today, because of the development of the other senses, the amount of our brain tissue that is devoted to smell is very large, a reminder of how important the sense of smell must once have been. Another reminder is that, unlike other vital nerve cells, the olfactory neurons constantly replace themselves. It is an attribute that neither the eye nor the ear, nor even the spinal cord and the brain, share.

Smell allowed us to find food, to determine whether that food was good or bad for us, to mate and to be warned of approaching danger. A blind rat can live perfectly well, but take away its sense of smell, and it cannot mate, eat or sense approaching danger.

To a much less important degree, our sense of smell still warns us. We smell rotten meat or sour milk and know that we mustn't consume it: if we are offered something to drink and don't recognise it as being safe or agreeable, we still instinctively sniff it.

There is no such thing, from our body's point of view, as a pleasant or an unpleasant smell. Anything that deviates from 78 per cent nitrogen, 21 per cent oxygen and the eight other gases in unpolluted air is perceived as being different and therefore potentially threatening. It was logical that some smells should be repugnant, simply to protect us: rotting animals and sulphur dioxide are potentially dangerous. What is not so clear is why other smells, such as newly mown hay or baking bread, should be so universally enjoyed.

HOW PARTICLES ENTER THE BODY ■

A factor that seems to be important in determining whether intolerance will develop from the chemicals that we inhale is the size of the molecules, for they are not all the same size. The largest are called particles, which are actually large clusters of molecules as well as large, complex individual molecules. Vapours, on the other hand, are single molecules floating free in the atmosphere. The main distinction between vapours and gases is that vapours, as the word implies, usually come from evaporation of solvents, chemicals or any other substance that is normally liquid at room temperature; while gas is generally not found in a liquid state at room temperature.

Particles are usually trapped by the cilia, which are also moving in unison to propel the mucus, with the particles stuck to them, into the throat, from which they are expelled. Anything smaller than a particle, however, gets past the filtering system — through the hairs in the nose, over the sticky bronchial substances, across the tracheal and then the bronchial cilia. As the inhaled particles brush past the olfactory nerves, they leave a sense of smell, but are not trapped. Instead, they can penetrate right into the alveoli, the minute sacs deep in the lungs where the exchange of carbon dioxide and oxygen from and into the blood takes place. Here they can easily pass through the permeable membranes and into the bloodstream, where they set off on their journey to the organs and tissues. Once the molecules, whatever their size, are in the bloodstream, the steps that lead to eventual intolerance are identical.

It is not always necessary for them to get even as far as the alveoli. Chemical molecules can also be absorbed anywhere along the full length of the bronchial tree. Medically, drugs (chemicals in solution) are sprayed into the nose for a number of purposes and they quickly enter the body and rapidly take effect, without having to go near the alveoli. The same happens with other non-medicinal drugs such as snuff, which is powdered tobacco.

Most of the common allergens, such as pollens, grasses and danders, enter the body as particles. Trapped by the cilia or on the sticky bronchial substances, they provoke a classic antibody response, which is why so many truly allergic reactions involve the eyes and the nose. As a general, though far from invariable rule, patients who are bothered by particles in the air tend to be more troubled by conventional allergy; the smaller molecules result in all the symptoms of intolerance and ecological illness.

Usually, the extent of the exposure is directly related to the severity of the symptoms once intolerance has developed: the bigger the dose, the worse the reaction is likely to be. Very often, sensitivity to chemicals is closely associated with intolerance to food and sometimes also with true allergy — to give an overall picture of environmental illness.

Sometimes more than one substance must be involved, to provide a reaction, like the man who was highly intolerant of white wine only when he sat down to dinner with his friend's dog beside the table. He was slightly intolerant of wine and slightly intolerant of dog dander, but neither on their own presented any problems for him.

When symptoms are severe, it is an indication that more than one source is involved. In my experience, it is comparatively rare for anyone to be intolerant of only a single chemical and nothing else, whether food or chemical.

There is rarely any warning that an intolerance is about to develop. Hypersensitivities come when they come — you either have them or you don't — so that there is very little that can be done to avoid them, apart from trying to ensure that your overall stress load remains as low as possible so that they never develop in the first place.

SUSPECT THE THINGS THAT ARE CLOSEST ■

In any kind of ecological illness, there must be two factors present: individual susceptibility and either a single heavy exposure to the substance, or frequent and regular low-level exposure. It is inevitable, therefore, that most people are likely to become intolerant of those things with which they come in closest contact.

If you are allergic to cats, for instance, meaning cat dander, the chances are that you are either a cat lover, a cat hater, or at least have spent much of your life at some time with cats. (Laboratory assistants working with small research animals can become allergic to research guineapigs for the same reason.) It isn't a random quirk of fate that makes us react to the very things we love most, but the inevitable outcome of the fact that constant and repetitive exposure to any substance greatly increases the risk of becoming intolerant of it.

As in all ecological illness, stress is a key factor. We are always concerned with the total stress load to which patients are exposed. Chemicals that may produce only a mild reaction on their own (or no reaction at all) can have a far more serious effect when they coincide with other stressors, which may be different chemicals, food, infection, or some stress in our lives. When our individual stress bucket overflows, taking us past our threshold of tolerance, any kind of intolerance can follow, whether to food or chemicals.

20 *Outgassing* |

In food intolerance we saw how hypersensitivity or intolerance often develop to staple items in our diet, such as wheat, potatoes, eggs or cow's milk. In chemical intolerance it is the constant low-level exposure to numerous molecule-discharging chemicals that causes the trouble, in our homes and workplaces, and in the atmosphere outdoors.

Most people think of their immediate environment as consisting of a number of solid objects, like furniture, trees and people, with nothing in between them except empty space. In fact this "air space" is very far from being empty. It is made up of the air — consisting of 99 per cent nitrogen and oxygen, the other 1 per cent being made up of water vapour, carbon dioxide and traces of eight other gases — and a usually invisible mass of millions of minute particles of matter from innumerable different substances. They include dust, pollens, organic debris, and also the molecules of everything that is "outgassing" into the environment.

Outgassing is the rather ugly jargon for the emission of molecules by any substance and it is the most important cause of chemical intolerance. Vapours are molecules that are the result of evaporation, so that when we smell petrol, paint, or perfume, for example, we are inhaling the outgassed molecules that come from that evaporation.

It is not only the obviously smelly things that are outgassing. Many substances that appear to be entirely inert, like plastic, wood and even stone, may outgas their molecules for months and often years. Certainly not all of them are dangerous. Not all those that are potentially harmful affect all people, but some of them are capable of affecting some people most of the time. The trick lies in establishing who is being affected by what.

The amount being outgassed is minute, but the effect is often continuous. As we have seen repeatedly, low-level, regular and frequent exposure to substances does just as much harm in ecological illness as the sudden high-level exposure that follows an accidental discharge of chemicals or a food binge. As almost nothing in the home is inert, at least in the months and years following its manufacture, the opportunity for low-level exposure that meets all the other requirements for triggering ecological illness is obviously often greatest behind our own front doors.

In an attempt to find the substances that would outgas the least in American spacecraft, where there is almost total recirculation of air for long periods, Nasa conducted a study that graded substances according to the level of their outgassing. Topping the list as the worst offender were the polyesters, and the safest, though not very practical in a spacecraft, was stone. The list was as follows:

Polyesters	Aluminium
Polyethylenes	Copper
Polyvinyls	Hardwood
Silicones	Iron
Epoxy resins	Steel
Polyurethanes	Ceramics
Fluorocarbons	Stone

It will probably come as a surprise to many people to realise that some of these substances are even capable of outgassing. What it means is that unless we go through life wearing a gas mask, or cocooned in a sterile environment, a little bit of all these things is being constantly inhaled and entering our bodies.

If we are exposed to any of this outgassing for long enough, and if genetics, fate, and all the other factors that added together make up our individual susceptibility, determine it, we are likely to become intolerant to one or more of these substances. (Only very rarely, mercifully, does a person become intolerant of all of them.) With this intolerance comes any or all of the familiar symptoms of ecological illness.

TRACKING DOWN OFFENDING CHEMICALS ■

Once chemical intolerance has been implicated, nothing in the home or at work is beyond suspicion, as we try to track down the offending molecules. Luckily, as we shall see, most of the common causes of chemical intolerance fall into a relatively very small number of chemical families so that we can at least whittle down what is likely to be responsible, although it can still be a long job. Patients come to look at the most familiar objects with a jaundiced eye until they have been proved innocent.

Mr Sheen-induced depression, Dynamo-activated migraine and Gladwrap-provoked anxiety or arthritis are all possible household reactions. Look at the furniture in your lounge room, at the curtains and the television set. Open the cupboard under the sink and look at the accumulation of cleaners, bleaches, sprays, polishes and disinfectants; then turn to the proliferation of smelly things in your bathroom cabinet. All these things regularly cause chemical intolerance.

I have had women patients who swore that they were allergic to their husbands: they couldn't go near them without feeling sick or coming out in a rash. They weren't exaggerating — except that (presumably) it wasn't the unfortunate husbands who were responsible. What made them unbearable to be near was their aftershave or deodorant, to which the wives were intolerant. Even the most expensive perfumes can have the same effect, and most women know at least one scent that, however expensive, they cannot wear because it gives them a headache.

Look suspiciously at the vinyl tiles on the kitchen floor, at the carpets and rugs in the rest of the house and especially at the sheets, pillows and blankets in the bedroom. The bedroom is a trap for the unwary, because we spend about a third of our lives there, exposed to anything that is outgassing. Even the clothes we wear cause endless trouble, ruining some people's lives with symptoms that nobody should have to put up with. A lot of clothing is made from polyester, the arch-villain on Nasa's outgassing list, and almost all clothing has chemicals added to it during manufacture, often to make it crease-resistant or drip-dry.

View with the greatest suspicion the gas cooker in the kitchen. Gas and formaldehyde, as we shall see, are the two most common offenders in the home. Try to isolate the garage from the rest of the house, a difficult task if they are both under the same roof.

Most garages are used as storehouses for everything from swimming pool chemicals, weed and pest killer, to fuel for the lawn-mower, let alone for the car itself, which is outgassing continuously even when the engine isn't running. On a hot day, you can see the fumes rising from the bonnet. One American study showed that the fumes from the cars in an underground garage found their way up ten stories of a high-rise building and were adversely affecting people living there. How things have changed! In the days when he had horses instead of cars, not many people would have put up with the pollution of stabling the horses in the house.

THE HAZARDS THAT NO-ONE SUSPECTS ∎

Because many of the most troublesome chemicals are so common, and unlike food may be invisible, they are usually unsuspected, so that no attempt is made to avoid coming in contact with them. Indeed, if it is true, as appears to be the case, that there is an addiction component in chemical intolerance, as in food intolerance, it is possible that we subconsciously actually seek out the smells and so the molecules of the very substances that are hurting us.

Even when the problem is staring us in the face we often still do not make the association. Something as simple as a thick rubber band on an office desk (which is usually not rubber at all, but made from a petrochemical derivative) can cause nausea and instant headache in many people if it is held close to the nose and inhaled.

Sitting on a desk 2 metres away from the face, the same rubber bands may not produce such an instantly unpleasant reaction, but they are outgassing all the time, exposing the secretary to much smaller doses over a much longer period. In the end, the reactions are likely to be the same as the acute reaction that followed when the molecules were inhaled deeply at close range.

In an odd case, a man decided to economise by dying a pair of white shoes black. The first time he went out in the rain, the shoes got soaked and an hour later he collapsed and appeared to be dead. Oxygen and adrenalin brought him round and the treatment he might then have received hardly bears thinking about. Fortunately for him, he was already being treated by a clinical ecologist for other symptoms.

This doctor suspected the problem immediately when he saw the dye running out of the shoes. It was not the man's heart at all that had caused his blackout, but the colouring agent he had used on his shoes. This agent, paraphenylenediamine, incidentally, was also used in hair dyes in Australia until comparatively recently, when it was found to be causing a battery of side effects, from hair falling out to vomiting and diarrhoea.

Although it is no longer used in hair dyes, paraphenylenediamine should still be suspected by anyone who has otherwise inexplicable symptoms that occur only when they are wearing dark clothing or furs, where it is still used as a dye.

Some people cannot tolerate acetone, which is the active ingredient in nail polish remover (among numerous other products), even though they use it regularly and may even like the smell. Every few days, they breathe in the acetone molecules and because of masked adaptation, they develop a mild headache two days later, but no symptoms at all at the time of using the acetone. Inevitably the two are not remotely linked.

ONE SMELL AT A TIME ■

There is a very common form of adaptation that is closely linked to our sense of smell. We have seen that our ability to smell is above all a defensive mechanism, designed to warn us when there is any change in our immediate environment. Change for primitive humans spelt danger.

One of the limitations of smell, however, is that it is very difficult to smell more than one thing at the same time and to differentiate between the smells. Like colours on a palette, smells tend to merge together when they are mixed. To cope with this, we adapt with remarkable speed to any smell, even to the foulest smell as when we are cooped up with a rotting animal. Often after as little as ten minutes, we begin not to notice the smell and the easy assumption is that it has gone away. In fact it has done nothing of the sort.

What has happened is that our sense of smell has done its job. It has warned us that something new is in the environment; our subconscious mind has evaluated that warning; and if we choose to ignore that warning, that is entirely our problem. The olfactory nerves must quickly prepare themselves to be ready to smell the next intruding molecules and, because we cannot accurately smell more than one thing at the same time, they achieve this by very rapidly adapting to the new smell and, as it were, clearing the slate.

We see this at work in the city. People who move there from the much cleaner air of the country, or even from other cities where different smells predominate, first notice the smell of the place, but then quite quickly adapt and find that they are not aware of the smell at all. If they were born in the city, they probably adapted when they were children.

These people are likely to have a bad reaction only when they move into the clean air of the country! They are like the coffee addicts who get their headaches only at the weekend because their regular dose of coffee doesn't arrive on time.

In the city, with thousands of cars pouring their exhaust fumes into the atmosphere, we are often not aware of the smell at all; in the fresh air of the country, not only do we smell the occasional car that drives by, but we can usually tell whether it is running on petrol or LPG!

There is another more worrying side to this, however. Not only do people living in the city stop noticing the smell of the ozone and the other hazardous substances in their polluted air, but they no longer react to them. Where once they suffered from wheeziness and breathing problems, adaptation and masking have removed these preadaptive symptoms and replaced them with perhaps a constant feeling of lethargy and tiredness. From now on, those who are susceptible will have no warning as the effects of the pollution gradually take their toll.

THE SMELLS WE REMEMBER ■

Not all bad reactions to smelly substances or to things that we inhale can be attributed to intolerance. Some smells are so evocative that they can trigger a reaction without any assistance from maladaptation. I had a patient who was forced to eat cold, greasy bacon as a child until she vomited across the table. For years afterwards, until hypnotherapy came to her aid, the smell of bacon made her vomit immediately.

We also know that red wine, among other things, often triggers migraine, not necessarily because of intolerance to any of the chemicals in the wine, but as a direct reaction to the aldehydes and various other components in the wine that are vasoactive, meaning that they can alter the blood vessels. This in turn causes the headache in people predisposed to having migraine.

This may also be what happens when you go into a room where the air is thick with tobacco smoke, or a particularly cloying perfume. You immediately feel a tightening of the head that you know is the forerunner of a wicked headache an hour later. Many non-smokers can detect the presence of a smoker hours after he has left a room, and the smell of cigarettes hangs around in clothes and curtains sometimes for days. Reacting to this smell of smoke certainly may be the result of intolerance, but it can equally well be the unconscious mind responding to something profoundly unpleasant, just as the woman reacted to the bacon.

Nathan Pritikin gave a remarkable example of how even normally harmless, indeed essential substances can become harmful.

Among some of the Bantu people of Africa, he reported, iron pots have been used for cooking for generations. Iron is a substance that is normally considered unthreatening and that we must have for survival. If we are short of iron, we are anaemic; and if we have none at all, we are very soon dead. The red blood cells contain iron, which accounts for about 5 per cent of a healthy cell's weight.

Over the years, the Bantu cooking pots rusted and traces of this rust went into their food until, over a period of years, it so overloaded their livers that they became cirrhotic. The normal tissue was replaced by scar tissue, and this became the principal cause of death among the adults of these tribes. As Pritikin put it, "The iron fills the liver to such an extent that it is just like an alcoholic with cirrhosis of the liver who dies from that cause".

That too much of anything has the potential to cause harm is one of the fundamental lessons of clinical ecology!

THE INESCAPABLE HYDROCARBONS ■

The great majority of chemicals in use today, and particularly the petrochemical derivatives which include plastics (see p. 268), were discovered only after the Second World War. Obviously our systems have had no time to adapt to them (and probably won't adapt for at least another 10,000 years).

Many people still think that our only exposure to petrochemicals, which are hydrocarbons, is from the fuel used in transport. In reality the petrochemical derivatives include everything from furniture to toothpaste, pharmaceutical drugs to carpets, and paints to beds and mattresses.

Not only garage mechanics, but beauticians, painters, actors (because of their make-up and the paint on the sets), process workers and undertakers are just as likely to become victims of petrochemical fumes because of the products and substances they work with.

The petrochemical, or hydrocarbon, problem can be seen in better perspective if we look first at just one group within the hydrocarbon family, the phenols. This example also vividly highlights the difficulties in pinpointing a specific item that is causing intolerance.

Phenol (which is also known as carbolic acid or hydroxybenzene) is very remarkable for its versatility. It is the starting point for production of epoxy and phenolic resins, as well as for aspirin and other drugs. It is commonly found in nasal sprays such as Afrin and Neo-Synephrine that relieve congestion, bronchial mists and numerous over-the-counter drugs including cough syrups, eye drops, antihistamines, cold capsules and decongestants.

It is in cosmetics, particularly Revlon products, where it is found in mascara, liquid eyeliner, creme rouges and eye-shadows. It is also an ingredient in ointments and first-aid creams and in hair products, including lotions, hair sprays, dyes and shampoos. It is in virtually all perfumes, aftershave lotions and scented deodorants. Almost the only way of establishing whether any of these products are free of phenol is to ask the pharmacist or doctor, and if this fails, write to the manufacturer.

Phenols are also used in the manufacture of explosives; as constituents of herbicides and pesticides; in the manufacture of nylon, synthetic detergents, polyurethane, petrol additives, dyes, photographic solutions; and as a preservative for the antigens in allergy shots. They are in bakelite and many moulded products such as telephones, thermal insulation panels, laminated boards, children's toys and refrigerator storage dishes.

Phenols are in creosols, as in Lysol disinfectant; and in menthol and camphor, as in Vicks Vaporub and cough medications. Almost inconsequentially compared to their uses when artificially made, they occur naturally in thyme oil, clove oil and menthol, in some spring water and as the toxic agent in poison ivy and poison oak!

Anyone intolerant of phenol can react to any one of these items or substances!

PLASTICS ▮

Plastics is a generic word for a series of materials which are composed of polymers and synthetic chemicals. Among them are polyvinyls, polyethylenes, polyesters and polyurethanes. The prefix "poly" means "many" and signifies that there are many molecules in long chains, called polymers.

Plastics also include some of the worst offenders in any blacklist of items that heavily outgas. However inert most plastics look, particularly the harder forms of plastic, most of them are capable of outgassing for years, constantly emitting molecules of hydrocarbons which float around in the atmosphere waiting to be inhaled. The softer, more pliable and more smelly plastics are, the more they are outgassing and so the more they are likely to result in chemical intolerance.

The special hazards in soft plastics are the plasticisers, which make them soft and flexible. These plasticisers work by facilitating the internal movement of polymer chains, which in turn makes the whole product tougher as well as flexible. The most commonly used plasticisers are chemicals that are called esters, and the two most frequently used of these in soft plastics are dioctyl phthalate (DOP) and di-octyl adipate (DOA), both of which are suspected carcinogens (that is, they may cause cancer) in rats and mice, in addition to being powerful and common triggers of intolerance and ecological illness.

Once a substance has been shown to cause cancer in laboratory animals, there is at least a prima facie case for suspecting that it *may* do the same in humans.

Beware of Plastic Wrapping   Plasticisers can constitute 50 per cent or even more of the total weight of many plastics. They can outgas their molecules into the atmosphere, or leach them into any food they may be touching. Probably the most alarming of all plastics, because it is so abused and leads so often to intolerance reactions, is plastic wrapping. Epitomised by Gladwrap, but with many near-identical clones, it has been on the market in Australia for twenty years. It was originally used almost exclusively for wrapping food, and that is still probably its main use, although the possible applications are limited only by people's imaginations.

In fact, because of its tendency to leach molecules into any food wrapped up in it, this use is the worst imaginable application for it. There is no Australian standard limiting the amount of plasticiser that can safely be allowed to leach. The leaching is greatest with high-fat foods such as cheese.

Nearly all plastic wrapping (at least in Australia) is made from either polyethylene or polyvinyl chloride (PVC), which are chemically very similar. There is, however, one very important distinction in that polyethylene is naturally flexible, while PVC is more brittle and has to have plasticisers added to make it flexible enough to use as a wrap. Although both forms should be avoided like the plague by anyone who even remotely suspects that they might have any chemical intolerance, PVC is probably marginally the worse of the two because of the added plasticisers. You can tell the difference between them by their appearance (except when the manufacturer has added colour). When polyethylene is on the roll, it has an opaque, white colour, while PVC has a clear, shiny look.

Plasticisers are not the only additives used in plastics. Sometimes, for example, plastics (particularly polypropylene, polyethylene and polystyrene) are prone to oxidation that leads to breakage in the polymer chain. When this happens, there is a loss of toughness and the manufacturers use anti-oxidants, particularly butyl hydroxytoluene (BHT) and butyl hydroxyanisole (BHA). These are both notorious health hazards, as we have seen when they are used in foods for the same purpose (see Chapter 10, p. 130).

Stabilisers are also sometimes added to plastics, to prevent discolouration at processing temperatures, particularly with PVC. Lead compounds are still the most important group of plastic stabilisers.

Christmas Trees and Car Seats Of Nasa's top three outgassing substances (listed on p. 262), polyesters are most often found as soft plastics in clothing (see p. 293), upholstery and curtains; and as stuffing for quilts, pillows, furniture and winter clothing. Polyethylenes are hard plastics used predominantly for food and milk containers, for instance.

Polyvinyls can be either soft or hard. In their soft form, they include such household items as shower curtains, artificial leather upholstery, electrical insulation and even artificial flowers and Christmas trees. Hard polyvinyl chloride (PVC) includes gas pipes, polyvinyl water pipes and conduits, and numerous moulded products, from toys to tables.

Of all the plastics vinyl is the main source of trouble in furniture partly because it is so difficult to prevent it from outgassing. In the car, a covering of sheepskin or some thick material such as denim, provides an effective barrier against the outgassing vinyl molecules. About the only way to cope with the problem in furniture at home or in the office, however, is to remove it altogether because it can go on outgassing for much longer than its normal useful life.

Vinyl wallpaper can be a problem, particularly in rooms that are always heated, because warmth increases the rate of outgassing. In extreme cases, it is sometimes necessary to strip the walls entirely of vinyl wallpaper.

Polyurethane is extensively used in furniture and furnishings, including chairs and lounge suites. Polyesters are also used in furniture and curtains, but very extensively in clothing. A troublesome use of polyurethane is that it is nearly always present in modern mattresses, as a thick outer layer. Wrapping the mattress completely in several layers of blankets is usually effective in reducing the risk from the outgassing — a significant risk, because you lie awash in the molecules for eight hours every night.

A Valuable Check List Drawing up a check list of the most common uses of plastics in the last quarter of the twentieth century is a forlorn exercise, because there can hardly be a home in the Western world that is without them. Any such list, however, would have to start with the most common soft plastics because they do by far the most harm in ecological illness.

Gladwrap and other plastic wrappings would head the list, no mean feat when you consider that about 99 per cent of all plastics will appear on it. It qualifies doubly for this unenviable position because it is probably also a carcinogen. Tablecloths, plastic curtains, garbage bags, vinyl cushions, handbags, soft briefcases, curtains and mattress covers would all be included near the top of the list.

After that it is really a case of following the guidelines of Nasa's list. To give some idea of how broad the canvas is, the following items would barely make an impression in any definitive list.

Plastic brushes, spectacle frames, toys, combs, dolls and false teeth (which cause chronic ulcers in plastic-intolerant patients) have all been implicated in plastic reactions. Even telephones have affected people's health because of their outgassing.

One young housewife suffered a severe headache almost every day of her life, but could find no reason for it until a clinical ecologist tracked down the cause to her telephone. With help from the telephone company, she found an old bakelite telephone to replace her modern plastic instrument (hard plastics such as bakelite and formica are rarely incriminated in chronic illness resulting from intolerance), and the problem disappeared. She remained symptom-free — until she took a job in an office which required her to use ordinary telephones again. Within three weeks, the headaches had returned, even more painful than before.

Some people are so sensitive to plastics that even the out-gassing of plastics in the television set, particularly colour television where the temperatures in the set are much higher than black and white, is enough to leave them with unpleasant symptoms that persist for hours. If the patient baulks at the idea of getting rid of the television, I usually recommend that it be built into the wall so that the fumes are kept out of the immediate environment.

Far more people than most doctors can imagine are adversely affected by food that has been stored in plastic containers. A few people even react to food that has been kept in open glass containers in a plastic-lined fridge, because of plastic outgassing into the food.

Put a glass of fresh water into the fridge without covering it and within twenty-four hours it will have a most unpleasant taste that makes it almost undrinkable. Any food left uncovered in the fridge, or stored in plastic, will acquire this unpleasant taste. The answer is simple — use glass for storing any food and make sure the container is covered, but not with Gladwrap!

The bad taste means that the plastic molecules have found their way into the food or drink and from then, every time you eat it or drink it, those molecules will be taken into the body. Once there, they have the potential to cause harm and they not infrequently do.

The longer any food is stored in a plastic container and the more liquid a food is, the more likely it is that chemical contamination will occur. No plastics of any kind can be totally relied on. Even Tupperware has been known to cause skin eruptions in the children of mothers who frequently hold Tupperware parties and so have large stocks around the house.

Because glass cannot be put into the freezer, it is often difficult to get over the problem of finding an alternative to plastic. There are now wood cellophane freezer bags (available from allergy associations) which fill this gap very effectively.

Plastics in the Car   In addition to the glass-of-water test, another effective proof of the existence of outgassing is the coating that appears on the inside of the windscreen of almost any mass-produced car (that is cars with seats of plastic, not leather) less than two years old. This smeary coating is the accumulation of the outgassing molecules from the plastic interior. It is especially noticeable in new cars and in cars where the interior has grown hot when the car has been left in the sun.

Plasticisers have a special purpose in vinyl car seats, where the plasticiser migrates to the surface and gives the seats an oily, supple feeling. In time, this is lost and the plastic gradually becomes more brittle and eventually cracks, a process that is greatly accelerated if the car is left out in the heat and the sun. This same breakdown occurs with plastic curtains and garden hosepipes.

Washing vinyl seats with a strong solution of cider vinegar and then rinsing and drying it well before repeating the procedure again, substantially cuts down the amount of molecules that are released by the plasticisers, which cause most of the trouble. Because heat always increases the release of molecules, try to park in a shady place and cover the dashboard and the seats with flannel towelling — not with the plastic sunshields that are widely marketed. Finally, always air the car well before driving off to get rid of any accumulated molecules.

PAINTS AND VARNISHES ▮

Paint and varnish may appear to dry within a few hours, but the outgassing of their molecules in reality goes on for months after the paint has been applied. The molecules continue to float around the house or whatever room has been painted, and, despite appearances, varnishes take even longer to dry completely (that is to reach a stage when they are no longer outgassing) than paint. Don't fall into the trap of thinking that the drying time claimed by the manufacturer has any relationship with the time that it takes for the paint to stop outgassing.

The paint industry uses more than 600 ingredients and it is often extremely difficult for patients or doctors to find out what particular chemicals are in a product. The manufacturers insist that their ingredients are a trade secret, even when we know that the product contains something that is causing serious reactions. Even without intolerance, painting has long been recognised by industrial health experts as a dangerous occupation.

As in all ecological illness, there is no need to list the

symptoms that intolerance to paint and varnish can cause: the molecules get to every organ and can result in every illness and disorder that each organ is capable of producing. Headaches and nausea, though, seem to be particularly common and I have noticed that almost any symptoms that are already being suffered by patients are made worse when they come in contact with out-gassing paint, even when there is no specific intolerance to paint. Low-grade chronic headache turns into full-blown migraine and low-level aches and pains may take on all the appearance of arthritis.

Purple Frogs, a Lion and a Gorilla Generally the solvents in paint cause the most trouble, and it makes no difference whether they are water- or oil- (meaning petrochemical) based. They seem to have a special affinity for the central nervous system and I have had a patient who went into an epilepsy-type seizure as soon as he went into a newly painted room.

Sometimes reactions to paint can be quite bizarre, as in this case reported by a colleague. When a patient of his slept in a recently painted room she saw purple frogs hopping about the room while a lion sat at the foot of the bed and scared her out of her wits. She was so upset that she decided to go home — then found that in the sleeping berth on the train, she was sharing her bed with a gorilla!

Water-based paints are also called plastic and latex paints, latex because the ingredients are held in water as an emulsion and latex rubber is a naturally occurring emulsion of polyisoprene. The emulsion can be vinyl chlorine and vinyl acetate. Plasticisers are also added and these tend to migrate to the surface where they outgas throughout the drying process. Finally, there are other additives that are stabilisers, thickeners or aids in the dispersion of the colouring agent. Any or all of these can affect the sensitive.

Water-based paints usually dry more quickly than oil paints (though not necessarily in damp or humid conditions), and they contain fewer petroleum derivatives, but they still cause many problems for many people.

Oil-based paints, on the other hand, contain a higher proportion of volatile hydrocarbons, with the result that exposure to potentially poisonous compounds, including toluene, xylene and benzene, is greater. There are also known as alkyl paints. They contain oils or alkyl resins in solvents such as turpentine, white spirit or kerosene. The oils themselves are usually natural, often linseed, castor or soya.

Epoxy paints have excellent durability, but take an exceptionally long time to dry. They are better avoided altogether if anyone sensitive to them lives in the house, unless the paints can be aged for at least three months, and preferably six, before bringing them into the house. This virtually eliminates their use on the walls.

Timber Coating Polyurethane paints, such as Estapol, are widely used as a surface coating on timber. Polyurethane is a polymer of an alcohol and toluene di-isocyanate, which is highly reactive and often causes acute illness among workers making the polymer, as well as chronic illness among those who are intolerant of it. These paints take twelve hours to cure (usually stated as the drying time by manufacturers), but it is at least a month before they stop outgassing.

Creosote is distilled from coal tar, which in turn is extracted from bituminous coal, which is also the source of paraffin, naphtha, benzene, and aniline dyes. The main use of creosote has traditionally been as a wood-preservative.

Rarely used indoors today, it is still popular for treating timber fences and posts. It has made the lives of many people very miserable when they have developed hypersensitivity to it, even to the point of having to walk away permanently from their homes when it has been used on exposed timbers in the house. Anyone using creosote should watch carefully for symptoms, including masked symptoms which may appear as a low-grade headache, for instance, two or three days after the creosote was used. If there is any suspicion that the creosote is causing intolerance, find a substitute, for the symptoms can be very distressing once they take hold.

Strippers Paint and varnish removers often contain benzene. Researchers from the US National Institute for Occupational Safety and Health bought a standard paint remover that contained 52 per cent benzene and used it in an ordinary two-car garage to strip the paint from a table. At the same time they measured the fumes.

They found that a person exposed to it for five minutes would inhale more than forty-three times the maximum amount permitted by occupational health standards. The dose was so high that there was an even greater risk of outright poisoning occurring than of intolerance developing.

Most paint strippers contain other chemicals as well as benzene, but there are many good reasons for avoiding benzene (it has been linked with leukaemia since 1928). A colleague has provided the following cautionary tale of an executive who stripped a wooden chest of drawers with a common paint stripping agent containing methylene chloride. He then worked for three hours, indoors, relaxed for an hour and suffered a heart attack.

He survived and, after relaxing for a while, he again went back to work on the chest when he got home. This time he had been working for three hours when he collapsed and had a second heart attack. He was rushed to hospital, and six months passed before he went back to work on the still not finished chest of drawers. The inevitable third heart attack was the last: he was dead before he reached the hospital.

The moral of this salutary story is that if you must use paint stripper, do it outside, stand upwind and at the first sign of any reaction — which may be no more than a slight tightening of the neck muscles, or mild nausea — abandon the job. If possible, also use a charcoal filter mask, which traps the airborne molecules, and protective gloves.

Drying always occurs faster in warm, well-ventilated conditions, so try to put off any painting jobs until you can open up the house on a warm day and let the vapours escape. Adding baking soda to water-based paint is an old trick that speeds up evaporation and so reduces the time of outgassing.

GLUE AND ADHESIVES ■

The adhesives that seem to give the most trouble are those used for floor and wall tiles; for joining carpet; and for sticking large fittings such as kitchen units. Like paint, they can be either water- or oil-based, or 100 per cent epoxy resins; and most of the points that apply with paint hold good for adhesives.

It is impossible to avoid mentioning the pernicious and increasingly common habit of glue sniffing, which some see as a cheap way of getting a high. Unfortunately, it can also be very dangerous and every year a disturbing number of deaths are reported. Its discovery by Aboriginal children has been particularly tragic.

It got its name because the first substance that was sniffed was mainly the glue sold with model kits. The habit spread quickly and soon other things were being sniffed, including anti-freeze, cold-start, paint thinner, lighter fuel, dry-cleaning fluids, hair lacquer, a number of aerosol sprays and particularly, petrol. The activity could more accurately be called hydrocarbon sniffing, because hydrocarbons are the main constituent of almost all the substances that are regularly sniffed.

When a 15-year-old boy was found dead recently after sniffing glue in his school's playing fields, the coroner warned that the practice was "as infectious as measles", and this was no exaggeration. A bottle found near the boy showed how complex the problem is: it contained sixteen different compounds, including paraffins and other hydrocarbons, which he must have mixed, and fifteen of them were found in his blood at autopsy.

It quickly becomes an addiction, following the pattern of all addictions and producing both acute and chronic symptoms. The physical effects of long-term hydrocarbon inhalation (and because it is an addictant, it quickly becomes a long-term problem) include severe kidney damage, liver poisoning and brain damage; abnormal behaviour, even mental illness; and sometimes death. We do not seem to be getting the message across to those who see it only as an easy release from boredom and worry that it is a very dangerous game to play.

What is more, as hydrocarbons increasingly contaminate our environment, glue sniffing can be seen as an extreme form of an increasingly prevalent type of illness and intolerance that is developing.

PRINT AND PAPER ■

Print on paper is such a problem for some people affected by the outgassing of fresh print (and sometimes of the paper as well), that they have to wear a charcoal respirator before they can read it. Some of my patients actually have to peg the newspapers on the washing line or bake them in the oven before they can risk handling them. One man became so weak that he collapsed on the floor if he inhaled deeply with a newspaper close to his nose. Telephone directories are a special source of agony for these people, because the print is so small that they often have to put their faces quite close to the page to read it.

Drying the ink was the main reason that the butler used to iron the newspaper before bringing it in to the master, not as legend has it, so that he wouldn't have to put up with creased pages. If you don't want to put a favourite book in the oven or the microwave, then stand it on its edge in the sun and let it air for a while.

The easiest way of proving the instability of printer's ink is to look at your hands after reading most newspapers. They will be black. The ink smells strongly as well, which is a sure indication that it is outgassing molecules into the atmosphere. Again, the problem is the hydrocarbons in the ink. When web offset presses are used, which are fitted with ink dryers, there is rarely any intolerance.

Most modern photocopying machines are dry-process and present no threat, but glossy magazines are notorious for the intolerance reactions they can cause. Trying to read a magazine like *National Geographic* or many of the more expensive women's journals is an impossibility for some people. Even the *Journal of Clinical Ecology* in the United States outgassed more than a few doctors could tolerate. (The problem was overcome by sending dry-process photocopies of the entire journal instead.)

PINE ■

There is one natural product that causes special intolerance problems for many people and that is pine, either as wood or as the perfume in innumerable household products.

It is perhaps not surprising that pine, more than any other wood, is so often incriminated in chemical intolerance — chemical because it is the pine molecules that do the damage. The hydrocarbon fuels, coal, oil and natural gas, are believed to be derived from huge prehistoric pine forests which millions of years ago were crushed beneath the earth in some cataclysmic geological upheaval.

Hardwoods rarely give any problems to the chemically sensitive, but pine and its relations, cedar, spruce and other conifers, can outgas for many years as their resins evaporate.

A young apprentice carpenter, a most talented boy, was once one of my patients. In spite of all the treatment that I could offer him, he was eventually forced to give away his apprenticeship. He was so intolerant of western red cedar, a commonly used timber in Australia, that it left him helpless and so weakened that he could hardly stand up, let alone work.

This intolerance (sometimes true allergy) to western red

cedar is quite common, and anyone contemplating using it in a new home, or taking up carpentry, should take every opportunity for a couple of weeks to smell it and sleep with it close to the bed as often as possible. Make sure that every member of the family comes in contact with it as well. It will outgas for at least five years and often for much longer once it is in position. A good many people have been forced to move house because the pine outgassing has become so intolerable.

Pine sensitive people often go through agonies at Christmas time when the Christmas tree is brought into the house. Burning pine logs in an open fireplace leaves them gasping for breath; and the pine-scented products, from toilet disinfectant to floor cleaners, bath oils, shampoos and deodorisers, bring an array of unpleasant reactions in their wake. Typical was one patient who felt dizzy, excessively irritable and tense whenever she smelt pine, and one of whose children rapidly developed asthmatic symptoms from it.

It is impossible to escape deodorants and disinfectants in public places, particularly public toilets, which for some reason always smell as though they have been drenched either in pine or artificial fruit.

Turpentine is obtained by distillation from oleo-resins in pine trees and so can produce the same reactions as any other part of the tree.

THE MATTER OF CREDIBILITY ■

Just as with food intolerance, there is a credibility gap when patients who are aware of ecological illness try to persuade doctors who know nothing of it that they should at least try this approach. The doctors, by this time, have usually failed to come up with any treatment that has achieved any good, but that is no guarantee that they will consider chemical intolerance.

Yet whatever the dispute over the relevance of clinical ecology in modern medical practice, it must be beyond argument that there is no conceivable way in which any of these outgassing chemicals can *benefit* the body. That alone should make it worth trying to get rid of them from our environment.

The only sound advice that any doctor can give when asked about the possible hazards of, say, aerosol sprays or any other chemicals, is "If you wouldn't eat it or drink it, then don't breathe it!" If you wouldn't take a swig of fly spray, fearing that it may harm you, then don't spray it in such a way that you, or anyone else, will inhale it. Either way, it will be in the bloodstream within seconds. And if the directions on the can or pack say "Don't spray near pets or fish", then read that as meaning "Don't spray near anything that is alive", which includes people and most especially, children.

It is a difficult concept for many people to come to terms with, but air pollution in their own homes often poses a greater threat to their health than the pollution outside their front doors, serious enough as that is.

Theron Randolph maintained that indoor pollution is between eight and ten times as great a threat as outdoor hazards, and I suspect that even this understates the real extent of the problem. A house may shelter us from the wind, the rain and the sun, but it can still be a very hostile environment.

Indoor air pollution is particularly troubling because there are so many substances outgassing and because exposure to them is constant. Outdoor pollution comes and goes, depending on the weather and many other factors, or else our contact with it varies as we move around; but the pollution in the house, office, supermarket and school is always there.

Far more harmful molecules are inhaled in the average kitchen by cooking dinner on a gas stove than in the typical workplace, or driving home through heavy peak-hour traffic.

We spend a third of our lives in the bedroom, which often has more things outgassing in it per cubic metre than a lot of factories. Many of us spend about 2000 hours a year in an office that more often than not doesn't even have windows that can be opened; yet it is awash with the molecules being outgassed from all the stationery, spirits, equipment and furniture. Office workers habitually go home nursing a headache or feeling far more exhausted than the work they have done warrants. They blame the job, the boss or the journey to work (all of which may certainly contribute to their gloom), but very rarely the ultra-modern office with its state-of-the-art equipment and expensive, comfortable furniture.

The way we build our houses today doesn't help, either. Old homes may have been draughty, but at least the air was being constantly changed in them. Now that more houses are better sealed to conserve energy, especially in winter, the all-important air exchange rate has gone down from about once every two hours at worst in older homes, to once every four hours in recently built houses.

At this rate it is estimated that the level of carbon monoxide could rise to three times that in heavily polluted outdoor areas; nitric acid to five times peak outdoor levels; and nitrogen dioxide to ten times the level in the middle of a busy city street.

A relatively new threat — new only in our understanding of it — comes from a naturally occurring gas called radon. It is produced when uranium decays and it is odourless and invisible. It is found in many parts of the world and it has been discovered under many homes, where it has been accumulating for years. Radon has become a cause for great concern in the United States, where one study put the likely incidence in several parts of the country at one home in eight. It can cause lung cancer and cancer of the nose, vivid testimony to the route that it takes into the body.

Tests conducted so far in Australia suggest that it will not be such a serious problem as in America, but traces of uranium are found in soil and rocks in many places. Local health authorities can check.

There are so many sources of potential trouble in the home that a comprehensive check list is almost out of the question. There are, however, three areas that are continually implicated — gas, formaldehyde and plastics. Gas and formaldehyde have no challengers at the top of the Most Unwanted list.

GAS ■

Gas in the home is a notorious troublemaker and it makes no difference whether it is natural gas or the increasingly obsolete coal gas. The only sense in which natural gas can truthfully be described as a "clean" fuel is that, unlike coal gas, it does not produce the highly visible smog-producing residues. For those who, ecologically speaking, cannot tolerate it, natural gas is among the worst of all pollutants and it causes an enormous amount of illness.

Gas is particularly troubling in older homes and buildings where the pipes and fittings frequently leak. Leakage became especially widespread when the old coal gas pipes were used unaltered for natural gas, which is reticulated at a different pressure. As gas is lighter than air, it tends to rise into the rest of the house from under the floor if there is the slightest risk.

The fact that it is leaking in quantities that the gas utility insists pose no threat of explosion (which is true) does not for a moment mean that it is safe from an ecological point of view. It is highly pervasive, with some unfortunate people sensitive to parts per billion in the atmosphere. One woman reacted with uncontrollable weeping in a house that hadn't been connected to the gas mains for ten years. The old gas meter had been thrown under the house and had continued to outgas for all that time. The woman was not even aware that it was there.

Cooking in Heavy Smog Of all the sources of gas contamination in the home, the gas cooker is by far the worst offender, and not only because it is also by far the most common gas appliance. A gas oven, for example, operating at 200°C for an hour can cause air pollution in the kitchen, even with the exhaust fan working, comparable to a heavy city smog. Combustion of the gas molecules is never complete and without a fan, the levels of carbon monoxide and nitrogen dioxide quickly leap to three or four times even that level.

Women, because they tend to do most of the cooking, but frequently other members of the family tend to be the victims who suffer most. If their headaches, aching legs, nausea and constant fatigue miraculously get better when they go away on holiday, they probably put it down to a change of air, little knowing how accurate they are!

Take the example of Doreen, a middle-aged secretary who lived alone in a three-room flat with a gas cooker in the kitchen. For years, and for no reason that she could understand because it seemed to happen whether she was feeling low or cheerful, Doreen became weepy and tearful when she was at home. Sometimes it got so bad that she became profoundly depressed and indeed she was recommended for electric shock therapy by a psychiatrist. Only a call from a friend who had heard a broadcast I was giving encouraged her to put off this treatment and get a referral to come to my rooms instead.

It needed only a glance at her history to realise that gas, in a small flat in a high-rise block of units, was at least a possible explanation. It was clear that in every other way, Doreen appeared to be well-adjusted socially and at work. (Whenever I see a child with asthmatic symptoms, one of the first questions that I ask is about the presence of natural gas at home: my frequent experience is that the incidence of asthmatic problems and upper respiratory difficulties in children is significantly higher in homes where natural gas is used.)

Doreen's treatment was initially very simple: I sent her to stay with a friend who had an all-electric home for a few weeks and miraculously all the symptoms disappeared. Then she went home and within hours she had dissolved in tears and was so depressed that she rang me in alarm.

Removing the gas from her unit turned out to be impossible and, while she was looking for a new, all-electric unit, she avoided the gas cooker and kept the exhaust fan in the kitchen running whenever she was in the flat. She needed to do this because in severe cases of gas intolerance, it is rarely sufficient just to stop using the appliances. Even turning the supply off at the street is unlikely to be enough because of the ability of even the empty pipes and fittings to go on outgassing for years.

Other patients have reported dropping things and becoming very clumsy whenever they are near gas, something that is normally quite alien to them, as well as the common symptom of just bursting into tears when they come within range of the cooker.

Changing to electricity, incidentally, is usually very expensive. If you suspect that gas is the villain, try to go to a completely gas-free environment for a few weeks to see if, as in Doreen's case, the symptoms really do disappear. Going through the trauma and expense of converting your home to electricity, only to find that it was formaldehyde in the curtains and lounge suite and not gas that was the cause of the trouble will be no aid to getting over depression!

Gas space-heaters can cause even more trouble than cookers and their only saving grace is that they are not nearly so common. Natural gas is also used for central heating, with the furnace often located right in the house or just outside in the garage, from where the fumes effortlessly leak into the house. The gas is so insidious that it can find its way through hairline cracks in a brick wall so small that they are invisible to the naked eye.

The best substitutes for gas space-heaters are the oil-filled electric column heaters, such as Dimplex, but they are expensive to buy and can be exorbitant to run. Even these have problems for the intolerant. I know of patients so sensitive that they react to the chemicals given off at the site of the switch and the thermostat, and to the heated paint. Sufficient people are seriously

affected by this problem for a firm in the United States to be producing oil-filled column heaters free of paint and with special
electrical fittings.

Fluorocarbon There is another rarer gas that can also
cause unpleasant symptoms in the home, and that is the fluorocarbon used as the refrigerant in fridges, freezers and air-
conditioners. It is the same gas that is often used, because of its
stability, as a propellant in hair sprays, whipped cream and
toppings, fly killer and some drugs, mainly the inhaled nasal
aerosols.

The gas itself provokes intolerance and because many of the
substances being propelled can themselves cause intolerance reactions, the victims risk being hit simultaneously with both
barrels, as it were. There is yet another danger from these sprays
that has nothing to do with intolerance and that is the damage to
the sensitive cornea of the eye that they can cause. This "spray
kerotitis" is a good reason for being very light-handed with
aerosol sprays.

OIL AND KEROSENE HEATERS ■

The unhealthiest alternatives to gas or electric heating are open-
flame oil and kerosene heaters, particularly kerosene, which is a
very bad source of chemical intolerance especially when the heater
is free-standing in a room.

This kind of space-heater produces fumes primarily as a
result of the incomplete burning of fuel, but the problem is more
complex than that. The air that fuels the flame of the heater contains suspended dust and other chemical molecules that have been
outgassed and this chemical-containing dust can break down into
a complex mixture of gases when it is burned, or even heated to
high temperatures.

These gases may only remotely resemble the molecule
clusters that went into the heater and what would normally be
relatively harmless particles from a synthetic carpet, for example,
can be changed into potentially very harmful vapours simply by
virtue of going through the heating system. It makes these
heaters very bad news.

They are, of course, relatively cheap, so they tend to be
favoured when economy is necessary by people who frequently do
not understand the dangers of chemicals, even when they are
explained to them. To conserve fuel, they are likely to keep the

room tightly sealed for maximum heating. This in turn means that the room, probably already small, becomes a trap for the recycling of the products of combustion and the other burned substances. These burned synthetic substances can be extremely toxic, even carcinogenic, quite apart from their ability to trigger intolerance reactions. The last straw is that some of the free-standing kerosene heaters are poorly ventilated and poorly designed. It is a very unhealthy combination.

If you must have an oil or kerosene heater, at the very least make sure that there is some way for the fumes to escape. If the heater is free-standing, there is little alternative but to leave a window open, though a better solution is to have a proper flue installed carrying the fumes outside.

FORMALDEHYDE ■

Formaldehyde is a simple organic chemical, manufactured from low molecular weight petroleum products. With the possible exception of natural and coal gas, it is the most troublesome of all the chemicals to which we are regularly exposed.

Exposure to formaldehyde can bring on the whole spectrum of symptoms and disorders that can be caused by chemical intolerance, meaning that it can affect every organ in the body. In West Germany formaldehyde has been seriously equated with dioxin as a health hazard: some nursery schools were closed when the glue in wood panelling was found to be outgassing formaldehyde.

Respiratory, skin and gastric ailments, as well as fatigue, headache and migraine, muscle and joint aches and pains are all commonly encountered as symptoms of formaldehyde intolerance. There cannot be a doctor with a bias towards clinical ecology who has not encountered memory loss, depression, insomnia, apathy, contact dermatitis and vasculitis as reactions to formaldehyde hypersensitivity — and all this in addition to the acute effects that formaldehyde provokes.

Russian studies suggest that formaldehyde exposure may also lead to menstrual disorders and complications in pregnancy. The possibility that it also may cause cancer is causing increasing concern, because formaldehyde is so widely used.

In March 1980, the American National Academy of Sciences added its formidable weight to the controversy when it concluded that formaldehyde, even at low levels, posed a serious health threat. A concentration of five parts per million in the atmosphere is normally considered safe, but there are many people who cannot tolerate exposure to formaldehyde at levels as low as one hundredth part of this.

Another American survey estimated that one-fifth of the entire American population is affected to some degree by the presence of formaldehyde, often at levels far below those traditionally considered to carry any risk. Even if the figure were significantly less than this, it would mean a very big problem.

You Can't Escape Formaldehyde! Formaldehyde is almost unavoidable and it is used in a dizzying array of products and processes, many of them in everyday use. During chemical testing I ask patients to read an abridged list of the common uses of the chemical and most of them, as well as being astonished at the variety of it, immediately recognise familiar items in their own homes.

The major source of formaldehyde pollution is the incomplete combustion of hydrocarbons in petrol and diesel engines, as well as the burning fumes and incineration of waste. Backyard incinerators are a serious source of formaldehyde pollution, emitting up to eight times the amount of formaldehyde of a malfunctioning, dirty petrol engine. It is believed to be the principal agent responsible for the unpleasant eye-burning sensation in smog.

It is a cheap and effective form of insulation and millions of homes and caravans have had urea formaldehyde pumped into the cavities of the walls and ceiling for this purpose. In America the reactions to urea formaldehyde exposure, particularly in the confined area of caravans, have led to the disorder known as mobile home syndrome, which is taken so seriously that, at the time of writing, urea formaldehyde is about to be totally banned as an insulating material in caravans. The outgassing is exacerbated because caravans are often heated, with the doors and windows closed against the outside elements.

Formaldehyde is used as a rat poison and an insecticide for killing flies, mosquitoes and moths. It disinfects equipment in the fermentation industry and in the manufacture of antibiotics, destroying bacteria, fungi, moulds and yeasts. It deodorises public places, and it is a commonly used intermediary in the synthesis of explosives.

It is in toothpastes, air-fresheners, shampoos, cosmetics and perfumes; hair-setting lotion and mouthwash; in plywood and particle boards (a particularly troublesome application because it is so widespread), which consist of woodchips bonded together by a resin that contains the formaldehyde.

It can be found in every hospital and biology laboratory as formalin (a 40 per cent solution in water), where it is used as a disinfectant and preservative. It is used in the fur and leather processing industries (so that it may always be present and out-gassing in furs and leather goods), in newsprint, industrial filters and photographic paper; and — in high concentrations — in cigarette smoke. It is a component of latex paint and many glues.

It is used as an agent to make concrete and plaster impermeable to liquids, and, with other chemicals, in preparing fireproofing substances to put in fabrics. It is even used in the preparation of vitamin A and for improving the activity of vitamin E. It turns up as a resin in nail polish and improves the wet strength of paper products.

It is widely used in fabrics of all kinds and for all purposes, making wool moth-proof and more elastic, and almost all natural and synthetic fibres water- and flame-resistant and crease-resistant; and it improves the colour stability of dyed fabrics. Although there is no mention of it on the tin, you are getting a blast of formaldehyde every time you spray Fabulon on your ironing.

The best test for determining whether clothes or fabrics contain formaldehyde, incidentally, is to crumple them up and put a few drops of water on them. If the material doesn't crease easily and if the water sits on the surface rather than being absorbed, then it is odds on that it contains formaldehyde. Always wash any new washable clothes or bed linen in borax or rinse them in vinegar, both of which are effective removers of formaldehyde; and several washings in soapy water will usually have the same effect. Simply because of the cost, fabrics are rarely washed before they leave the factory after being pre-treated.

There is an argument that any concentration of less than two parts per million (the level normally allowed in the atmosphere in factories) can be safely tolerated by humans. This was claimed to be reinforced by the apparent discovery that formaldehyde occurs naturally in the human body as a metabolite at a concentration in normal tissue of between three and twelve parts per million.

But it is a specious argument because, even if it is true that

in the average person levels lower than this are successfully repelled by the immune system, it takes no account of those whose
susceptibility is less than average (and we have seen that such
factors as sickness, malnutrition and age play a big role); and it
takes no account at all of the untold thousands who are affected to
the point of developing all the illnesses and symptoms of intolerance at levels of exposure that are only a tiny fraction of this.

As usual in the chemical debate, the stakes are very high.
There is a huge investment involved in what is one of the most
profitable of all mass-produced chemicals. In the United States
alone, about fifty chemical works make more than 3 million
tonnes of formaldehyde a year. The West German chemical
giant, BASF, the world's largest producer, manufacturers
400,000 tonnes a year, worth almost $A1 billion. When the
stakes are that high, such concerns as being made ill and possibly
dying because of the effects of a product all to easily take a back
seat.

INSULATION ■

While urea formaldehyde is particularly favoured as insulation for
cavities, the space under ceilings and other hard-to-reach places,
the ubiquitous pink and yellow batts are another popular form of
insulation.

Urea formaldehyde outgasses its chemical molecules for
years, particularly when the weather is hot and the house heats
up. The problems associated with batts, however, are likely to
be the result of outgassing by the plastic resin holding the fibreglass particles together, rather than the glass fibres themselves.
Although the fibres are very unpleasant to work with, they have
never been proved to cause any lasting harm.

Once batts have been laid in a well-ventilated roof space,
preferably backed with an aluminium foil (which is rarely done),
they seldom cause any problems of intolerance or sickness. About
the most serious side effect of fibreglass is that occasionally tiny
specks of glass may break off and embed themselves in clothing.
If they then get into the skin, an extremely irritating dermatitis
can result.

HOUSE DUST ■

We need to say a special word about house dust. This is not entirely chemical, but it poses a serious problem for many people
and has implications that extend to ecological illness even though

it is normally associated with true allergy. It is often accompanied by chemical outgassing in the home, and because it imposes considerable strain on its victims, there is an additional tendency for it to be linked with intolerance reactions.

House dust is a very complex mixture of human hair and skin; animal danders, which are the scales of hairy skin particularly of dogs, cats and horses, simply because these are the animals most often in contact with people (small-animal keepers in laboratories quite often develop the same sensitivity to guinea-pigs); food particles; fragments of insects and other creatures, and their faeces; wool and cotton; and a great many other substances that float or are carried into the house, including the molecules of outgassing chemicals.

No matter how good a housekeeper a person is, there will always be dust. The average six-room house in the city accumulates about 18 kilograms (about 40 pounds) of dust a year, yet most of the time we don't see it, unless it collects on the surface of furniture or in forgotten corners. Only when a ray of sunshine streams through a window can we see it suspended in the air and get some idea of what we are constantly inhaling.

Even though we may say that we are allergic to house dust, the allergy is usually to a creature that lives in the dust called the dust mite. More precisely, it is generally not the mite itself that causes the trouble, but the mite's faeces, which are about the same size as particles of pollen. Each mite produces up to fifty tiny faeces each day.

There are several types of dust mite, each preferring a slightly different environment. One may select the mattresses, another goes for the kapok in old stuffed furniture, while yet another lives in the carpet.

Magnified 300 times, dust mites are fearful-looking creatures, and the very idea that we are breathing them in or eating them (let alone their faeces), still alive, is unsettling for some people. In fact, apart from the allergy and intolerance they provoke, the dust mites (faeces and all), and indeed all dust, appear to be harmless, which is just as well. Like them or not, they are here to stay in everyone's home.

The symptoms of house dust intolerance and allergy are familiar to many people. They often resemble those of the common cold, with sneezing and wheezing, a runny nose and itchy eyes. Unlike a cold, however, they disappear quickly when the victim gets out of the house. That is why many husbands find that their symptoms disappear when they go to work, while the rest of the family, left at home, goes on snuffling and sneezing all day.

Just as the large particles of other allergens, such as pollens and grasses, get caught in the cilia and the sticky substances after being inhaled, so do the dust mites faeces get trapped. The immune system immediately recognises them as foreign and tries to get rid of them faster than the cilia can move them into the throat. As a result, this struggle, the antigen-antibody reaction, produces the familiar symptoms of dust allergy.

For obvious reasons, the symptoms are likely to be worse at times like bed-making, dusting and carpet- and furniture-beating, but sensitive people find their symptoms being triggered even after someone has unsettled the dust by walking across a rug or carpet. Send sensitive children out of the house while these chores are being done and keep the windows open if that is possible. In many high-rise buildings and hotels, you tend to be looked at as though you are a would-be suicide if you have the audacity to ask for fresh air to be allowed into the room, but it is worth persevering.

Vacuum cleaners are by far the most effective way of picking up dust, but most of them pollute nearly as much as they clean, in spite of all that accumulates in the bag. They suck in the dust at one end, but then blow out the smaller particles — the ones that are most likely to cause an intolerance reaction because of their size — through the filter or bag at the other end. They go straight back into the room where, instead of being confined to some part of the furniture or the carpet, they then swirl around in the air.

The most efficient vacuum cleaning systems are those that are built into the house and take the dust to a central unit from where it is blown directly outside. For the very sensitive, there are now vacuum cleaners on the market that use water as a filter instead of bags.

CURTAINS AND WALLPAPER ■

Curtains are likely to have been subjected to several chemical processes, even if they are not actually made of heavily outgassing polyesters. Rubber-backed curtains are an additional hazard for the intolerant, as are curtains coated with an emulsion of either acrylic resin or PVC: all are likely to have been treated with a fungicide as well.

Even wallpaper leads to reaction symptoms in some people. Fabric wallpapers can break down and produce a cellulose dust; and many conventional wallpapers are coated with plastic film to make them washable. Wallpaper paste (and even the paper itself sometimes) often contains insecticide and anti-mould chemicals. These may be necessary if the wallpaper is used in dark, damp places, but if there is intolerance, the price may not be worth the convenience.

Remember that as always in chemical intolerance, not everyone is hypersensitive to all these substances, or even most of them. The trick is to find out which ones are causing the problems, once chemical testing, with sublingual drops, has identified the group of chemicals responsible. It can be very tricky. Even if, by trial and error, the cause has finally been sheeted home to anti-oxidants, for instance, it can take a long time to realise that the anti-oxidants are in the adhesive used in the manufacture of shoes, and that the molecules outgassing from this, infinitesimally small as the exposure is, can cause as much trouble for someone very sensitive to anti-oxidants, as those in food.

CARPETS ■

Carpets, underfelts and underlays present a multitude of problems for anyone unfortunate enough to be sensitive to any of them. They outgas the chemicals that are put into them during manufacture, as well as the adhesives used when they are being laid, and they are the worst dust trap in any home. Clearly the newer the carpet, the greater the level of outgassing, but the outgassing can last for years, for much of the time without emitting any smell. If there is under-floor heating, or the carpet is in a home or office with a slow rate of air turnover, the problem will be greatly exacerbated.

The commonest fibres used in carpet pile are wool and nylon, frequently as a mix of 80 per cent wool to 20 per cent nylon. If the carpet has been woven, it will probably be by either the Axminster or the Wilton method (which are styles of manufacture, not trade names), where the backing, in which the pile is anchored, is formed from the weaving itself. From a tolerance point of view, this is the safest method of manufacture.

The usual alternative process (and it is not only used for cheap carpet) is tufted carpet, which is made by inserting the pile yarn into a separate backing material. An adhesive, usually a latex glue, has to be added to strengthen the anchorage. In addition, tufted carpet usually also needs a secondary backing to give extra strength and resilience, and this may be made from reclaimed rubber, or synthetic rubber, polyester, polypropylene or PVC. It needs no special expertise to realise that this process is likely to result in more intolerance than either Axminster or Wilton.

Underneath the carpet there may be an underlay, often made from rubber or synthetic rubber moulded into a hessian base. The carpet itself is often treated with chemicals such as Scotchgard or a moth-proofing chemical.

I have seen patients so affected by tufted carpet and the underlay that the only way they could go on living in their homes was to take it all up and revert to bare boards and rugs, which are much easier to keep relatively free of dust. If a sensitive person tries to sleep in such an environment, the inevitable result is sleeplessness, fatigue and constant irritability, producing more stress and so yet worse symptoms.

CLOTHES AND FABRICS ▮

Almost everything that people put next to their skin makes someone, somewhere, suffer. Even wool in its own right often causes dermatitis and extreme itching, and is a common allergen, but many of the intolerance problems associated with clothes are caused by the substances that are added to the fabric, rather than the fabrics themselves.

Nylon and rayon, for example, hardly ever cause reactions. One exception was the young teenage girl who began suffering from migraine when she turned 14, even though she had never before had a headache in her life. It took a lot of ground work to track down the culprit. On her fourteenth birthday, she was allowed to wear a brassiere for the first time, and the one she chose was made of nylon which, unknown to her, she couldn't tolerate. Outgassing all day only centimetres from her nose, the nylon provoked very painful preadaptive reactions. Fortunately we were able to pin the reactions down before adaptation and masking set in, which would have enormously complicated the search for whatever was responsible.

Orlon and dacron are unlikely to be involved in intolerance, even though dacron, in particular, is often blamed. Although cotton, on the other hand, is a natural fibre and probably fairly harmless to everybody, it has usually been exposed to a variety of chemicals before it appears in the shops in a made-up form. It has often been bleached with sodium chlorite or hypochlorite solution, and then mercerised or treated under tension with a caustic alkali such as caustic soda (sodium hydroxide) to make it stronger and more lustrous.

The cotton may then be coated with starches and gums to make it easier to weave; then a flame retardant and probably salicylanide, or copper sulphate, to protect it against microorganisms when it is stored and being transported. By the time the processors have finished, the harmless cotton is a very potent product, just waiting for anyone intolerant to any of those chemicals to come along and inhale them or put them next to their skin.

Wool usually suffers an even worse fate because it is so prone to attack by moths and beetle grubs. Many woollens are still moth-proofed with dieldrin, a very dangerous pesticide that is now banned in baby clothes and underwear. When dieldrin cannot be used, permethryn, a relative of the natural pesticide pyrethrin, is commonly used. The reason why it is not used all the time is because it is much more expensive. Wool is usually bleached with sulphur fumes or sodium hydrosulphite, which commonly provoke intolerance and whose molecules linger in the wool for months, even after repeated washing.

Chromium is sometimes used in the rapid tanning of leather and makes susceptible people ill. If it is in the leather band inside a hat or a cap, it can elude suspicion for a very long time. Another unsuspected irritant (which may be just that and not an intolerance-provoking substance) is the rubber in brassieres and elastic-topped underwear.

Virtually all wash-and-wear or crease-resistant clothing contains formaldehyde (and we discussed its dangers earlier in this chapter). In addition, any of the chemicals that are used for washing and treating clothes — detergents, fabric softeners, antistatic agents, water softeners, bleaches and so on, as well as the chemicals like chlorine and fluoride that are in the water itself — can trigger reactions in the hypersensitive.

I have treated frightened patients who without warning suddenly find themselves too weak even to stand up from a chair, or who break down in uncontrollable crying for no apparent reason. When they get undressed for bed, the symptoms pass just as quickly. The not uncommon reason is that they cannot tolerate polyesters and if their clothes are made from polyesters, even in the smallest proportion, they quickly develop symptoms.

One woman had such severe breathlessness that she feared she was choking to death. She knew the cause was polyester because the symptoms were so striking that she was able to find a common factor. What made her case particularly interesting was that this breathlessness was just the latest in a string of symptoms going back over forty years.

First she had suffered from hayfever, then headaches, then nausea and finally, only after about thirty-five years, the breathlessness that brought her to me. At one stage the picture was so confusing for her that she believed she was suffering from several illnesses, before she made the discovery that they were all caused by polyesters and that the symptoms had just changed over the years.

DRY-CLEANING ■

Dry-cleaning causes a lot of problems for the chemically sensitive. All the solvents used by dry-cleaners can produce intolerance through their outgassing. Traces of them remain in the clothes for weeks, even months if they are stored away in a closed cupboard or drawer.

The common solvents used are carbon tetrachloride and the trichloro- and tetrachloro-ethylenes (white spirit, a petroleum fraction, though effective, is rarely used by dry-cleaners today because of its disconcerting habit of catching fire and burning down the cleaner's premises).

Some dry-cleaners add moth repellant to their solvents whether it is requested or not. If you are bothered by dry-cleaning chemicals (some people cannot walk past a dry-cleaner's shop without feeling violently ill and it is hard to imagine a more unhealthy place to work), then pin a note to your clothes or curtains saying that you want no insecticides, mould inhibitors, dirt or water repellants or any other unsolicited chemicals added to the already potent cleaning brew. It will probably have no effect, but it might just prompt a caring dry-cleaner to at least tell you that the recipe can't be changed for one customer.

Closely related to the dry-cleaning solvents are the chlorofluoro-methanes and -ethanes that are used as the refrigerant gas in refrigerators and air-conditioners, as well as in aerosol propellants.

SOAPS AND DETERGENTS ▮

Soaps, washing powders, detergents and cleaning agents are very smelly reminders of how even the most basic household substances can lead to all the symptoms of intolerance and to some very sick patients. There are many people who cannot walk down the detergent aisle in the supermarket without feeling mildly nauseous or experiencing the first stirrings of a headache.

Soaps containing naphtha, cleaning powders with bleach, window-washing compounds, and brass and silver cleaners are just some of the products that constantly bring people to my rooms with severe symptoms of ecological illness.

The original all-purpose cleaning agents were soaps, which were little more than salts of organic acids. To make soap, caustic soda is added to animal fats or vegetable oil, most commonly to beef tallow and palm oil. Sometimes caustic potash is substituted for caustic soda to produce a softer product like shampoos.

If that was all that went into soap, there wouldn't be a problem of the magnitude that exists today. But the manufacturers then go on to add an array of other chemicals, any one of which can produce a softer soap. There are now virtually no unscented washing powders or abrasives on the market and it can take some effort even to find toilet soap that is unscented. Even simple Sunlight soap seems to have a scent in recent years.

Trouble in the Laundry The addition of blue restores the "white look", and modern optical bleaching agents act by absorbing ultraviolet light and re-emitting it as blue light, which makes clothes look whiter. These are the agents that encouraged advertisers to claim that their washing powders were "whiter than white", before they were told to stick to the truth.

Dishwashing detergents, or washing-up liquids, contain alkyl-benzene detergents (benzene is also used in paints and paint strippers, see Chapter 20) that have been neutralised with caustic soda or triethanolamine, as well as perfumes and water softeners. Any one of these chemicals on its own is capable of causing intolerance and, as the labelling is very rarely complete, the search is very difficult. Most manufacturers will eventually produce a complete list of ingredients of their chemical products, if the alternative is that they are going to be accused of wilfully compromising the health of their customers. Incidentally, the poisons information centre in each state, an obvious place to turn to, believes that it is bound *not* to disclose the ingredients of any product.

Because they are not supposed to come into contact with anyone's skin dishwasher detergents are much more powerful than dishwashing liquids. They are very strongly alkaline, as a result of their chlorine content, which is included to remove stubborn stains, and this releases large amounts of free chlorine. They should never be used for ordinary washing-up in the sink.

Keep all these heavily outgassing powders and liquids in a place where their molecules cannot escape into the environment that the family has to live in. If necessary, put them in the garage, which is already hopelessly contaminated by the car's fumes.

AIR FRESHENERS ■

The way air fresheners are marketed, you could be excused for thinking that they get rid of unpleasant bathroom and kitchen odours. In fact, most of them do nothing of the sort. What they actually do is add yet more chemicals to the air where they either overwhelm our olfactory nerve endings with an even stronger smell, or actually poison the nerve endings so that they can hardly smell anything.

It is no wonder that some of the people who pack and store these products suffer chronically from environmental illness. Yet because not all of them suffer (perhaps because their total stress does not predispose them to intolerance, or because of individual susceptibility) workers and employers alike refuse to concede that air fresheners can be responsible. So they go on working in this unhealthy environment, their symptoms get worse and gradually encroach on every facet of their lives. Only when they *understand* clinical ecology and how even the most prosaic of substances can affect their health, do they have the slightest chance of getting better, unless fortune takes them to another, cleaner job. You have to know what you are looking for.

PERFUMES AND COSMETICS ■

Perfumes and hair sprays are often the most troublesome of all the chemicals in the home. They are responsible for acute and chronic, mental, physical and behavioural disorders and symptoms. Cosmetics may be close behind in their effects, usually because they are so close to the nose and are being constantly inhaled.

Every woman knows perfumes that she can never wear without suffering a blinding headache, often accompanied by a very disturbing feeling of anxiety and nausea. Which perfumes will have this effect on her seems to be largely a matter of individual susceptibility to one or more of up to 300 different ingredients in most expensive perfumes. Certainly the cost of the perfume has nothing to do with its ability to produce these unpleasant symptoms, although cheap, sickly, cloying scents seem to be unacceptable to most people.

Cosmetics can have the same effect as perfumes, though usually on fewer people. For the sensitive and the intolerant, travelling in a lift can be an ordeal if they happen upon the wrong perfume or cosmetic. The same applies with men's deodorants and aftershave lotions.

We have already mentioned that some wives cannot stand being near their husbands because of their aftershave. There are also men who shouldn't be near themselves. Unfortunately for them, adaptation and masking often leave them oblivious of the fact that their own smell is causing them to function at less than their true potential or is leaving them feeling exhausted almost before they have finished breakfast.

Threatened by a Hair Spray An airline hostess who was a patient of mine couldn't tolerate hair sprays of any kind. Several times she was taken acutely ill on a flight, to the point of having to be helped off the aircraft, and there was a real danger that she might lose her job, which she loved. The trouble usually came when she brushed against a passenger or another hostess who had just sprayed her hair, and who was surrounded by a fog of molecules. It was even worse if she happened to come close to a woman who was actually spraying her hair.

In her case, no detective work was needed to establish the cause of the trouble. Desensitising drops were only a partial help because different brands of hair spray contain different ingredients, but we were able to bring it under control enough for her to be able to continue with her job.

Once an intolerance of that severity has developed to chemicals, it is difficult to neutralise it unless the victim can also get away from the source of the trouble. I have repeatedly found that reactions to cosmetics usually occur in people who have a considerable overall susceptibility to other chemicals. It seems to be comparatively rare for there to be intolerance to only one chemical.

Interestingly, the corollary of this is that if patients are not troubled by perfumes, there is every likelihood that they will not be chemically sensitive at all. This is often a useful guide.

For those who do suffer, it becomes a matter of shopping around for cosmetics, ointments and creams that have entirely natural ingredients, without artificial colours, scents, or preservatives. Some of these, available in health food shops, are described on the label as "hypoallergenic", a rather clever word that is still no guarantee that the particular product will not cause adverse reactions.

PHARMACEUTICAL DRUGS ■
Clinical ecology makes minimal use of pharmaceutical drugs. One of the ironies of ecological illness is that it can be triggered and then perpetuated by the very medicines that doctors are prescribing to make the patient better.

Most people know that drugs often have potentially serious side effects, even if they never suspect just how serious those effects can be (see p. 8). Often the side effects are acute, bringing on an immediate and unmistakable reaction; but just as frequently they are the chronic reactions of intolerance to some ingredient in the drug, usually unsuspected by patient and doctor alike.

Few people realise the complexity of most drugs, or the number of ingredients that they contain. These are seldom detailed, even in the information provided to pharmacists. They are the same flavourings, colourings, preservatives, excipients and all the other aids to manufacture that have to be meticulously listed when they are present in food. In drugs they are excluded from labelling regulations.

Even relatively straightforward over-the-counter mineral and vitamin supplements contain ingredients that are never suspected by patients or doctors, unless they are being specifically looked for. As I write, I have on my desk a popular brand of synthetic vitamins and minerals, which lists a total of seventeen of these supplements. It looks like very commendable truth-in-labelling, but what I know, and what the label doesn't state, is that in addition to the supplements listed each tablet contains calcium stearate (as a lubricant), gelatin, sugar, sodium benzoate (a preservative), calcium sulphate, acacia, white wax, carnauba wax, sesame oil (for polishing), blue dye no. 2, yellow dye no. 5, yellow dye no. 6, titanium dioxide, polyvinyl pyrolidine and edible white ink.

The chemically sensitive person may be intolerant to any of these substances and, if that intolerance is severe enough, there will be an adverse reaction. If the medicine is taken regularly enough (as is likely to be the case with vitamins or minerals), there is the added danger of masking occurring. This then not only conceals any cause and effect between the medication and the symptoms, but ensures that there will be withdrawal symptoms when the tablets are *not* taken. The great majority of prescribed drugs are synthetic and almost all of them contain petrochemical derivatives which are a notorious source of intolerance for many people.

Drugs That Make Us Worse What happens all too often is that the patient goes to the doctor, say, for something to relieve a severe headache. What neither he nor the doctor (who probably isn't even aware of the potential risk of intolerance developing from anything he prescribes) knows is that the headache is the result not of stress, as the doctor diagnoses, but of intolerance to petrochemicals and salicylates.

The doctor prescribes a mild tranquilliser to help the stress and a pain-killer to relieve the headache. Unfortunately, the tranquilliser contains petrochemical derivatives and the pain-killer has aspirin, which is a salicylate. Inevitably the symptoms get worse, so our patient comes back a few weeks later. This time the doctor prescribes even more potent tranquillisers and stronger pain relievers, and so the vicious circle is perpetuated.

As long ago as 1952, Dr Theron Randolph found that, among his own patients, 50 per cent of those who were chemically susceptible reacted adversely to aspirin (as well as to sulfonamide). Yet this continues to be widely prescribed and self-prescribed, regardless of whether the patient can tolerate salicylates or not.

Even biological drugs, which are pharmaceuticals made from natural materials such as insulin, liver extract, and epinephrine, are not entirely free of risk. When they are taken, the reactions that follow in some patients can be traced to the preservatives in these drugs, a real problem in some cases. Epinephrine, for example, a hormone of the adrenal glands, rapidly disintegrates without preservative.

The Medicine Cabinet   We can't leave pharmaceutical drugs without mentioning the medicine cabinet. Medicine cabinets are notorious for causing more problems than they ever cure! In most homes, they gradually acquire an array of smelly, outgassing products, out-of-date medicines whose original purpose people have long ago forgotten, and generally harmful junk. They are one of the most serious health hazards for young children in the home. Either their ingenuity and curiosity will eventually get them into the most securely locked cabinet, or the day will inevitably come when someone leaves it open by mistake.

Get rid of everything from the medicine cupboard that you can do without, anything that is out of date, or that you are keeping on the off-chance that one day you might go down with the same illness that it was bought for last time. In particular, throw out all the prescription medicines that are left over from an illness. Quite apart from their danger, because they look very tempting to small people, most of them have a shelf life that has probably long passed, whatever is on the label, and your doctor may have a much better drug to offer you next time you suffer from the same illness.

After this purge if anything is left with a very strong smell, banish it to the garage, or somewhere where the outgassing will not be a constant problem.

The first statement that needs to be made about smoking is that it kills people and leads to an array of smoking-related diseases that are entirely avoidable. The second is that the easiest way to improve any community's health and bring down the mortality and morbidity rates, is to stop people smoking.

In 1982, a remarkable seven-month review of 11,800 studies into the effects of smoking was carried out by the respected American Institute for Biological Research. It found that with a single exception (which claimed that smokers perform better than non-smokers), every study that was not funded by the tobacco industry linked cigarettes to degenerative illness in man.

Smoking is probably the most widespread source of indoor pollution and among the hundreds of different compounds in tobacco and cigarette smoke are many that are known to be harmful, among them carbon monoxide, nitrogen dioxide, hydrogen sulphide, hydrocyanic acid and the highly active enzyme poison, hydrogen cyanide. Long-term exposure of about ten parts per million of hydrogen cyanide is considered to be dangerous; the concentration in cigarette smoke is 1600 parts per million. Carcinogens, including certain hydrocarbons, are also present in the tar.

Nor does it make much difference whether you are smoking yourself, or breathing in someone else's smoke ("passive" smoking). It is only a matter of degree. In fact, smoke from a burning cigarette left in an ashtray contains almost twice the tar and nicotine inhaled from a cigarette and so may be twice as dangerous.

Passive smoking poses special hazards, in spite of the attempts by the tobacco industry to downplay them. It increases carbon monoxide levels and carbon dioxide, and it increases the exposure to about twenty-six known carcinogens and some 300 additional additives. We should not tolerate others smoking in our presence.

Smokers often argue that the amount of these substances taken into the body is so small as to have no consequence. It is a foolish argument. The individual amounts absorbed with each cigarette may be small, but the cumulative dosage is appreciable. Cadmium, for example, which in excessive doses affects the neocortex (which is what you are measuring when you look at the verbal scores in an IQ test), has a half-life of between twenty and thirty years in the human body and it has also been closely linked with hypertension and high blood pressure.

Tobacco is a very powerful addictant. In May 1988 the Surgeon-General in the United States declared that nicotine is "as addictive as heroin or cocaine", which prompted a member of Congress to charge the tobacco companies with being involved in a "multi-million-dollar drug-pushing racket". Studies of various groups of smokers who have tried to quit show that about 30 per cent are able to stop if there is sufficient motivation coupled with a genuine desire to stop, and if they are told to stop — perhaps after suffering a heart attack. A further 30 per cent are able to stop provided there is energetic follow-up and encouragement; 20 per cent can be included among the successful group when other more involved techniques are included such as psychotherapy and hypnotherapy.

There remain, however, a hard core of 20 per cent who resist every attempt to stop smoking, even if they came voluntarily for help. No matter what approach is taken with them, they resist it and are unable to overcome the addiction habit of smoking. By varying the initial therapeutic approach, therefore, to take advantage of hypnotherapy or psychotherapy, for instance, means that between 30 and 60 per cent of motivated people wanting to stop smoking can be easily helped. Most, indeed, would have successfully stopped even without any special therapeutic intervention. The remaining 40 per cent are more resistant to therapy — any therapy — and half of them will be unsuccessful. If there is no proper motivation — typically because they come for help only because their spouses insist — the results are usually poor and predictably it is the treatment that gets the blame for being inadequate.

This is therefore one of the most compelling reasons for discouraging people from starting to smoke and for banning any deliberate attempt to encourage people to start, most obviously through advertising.

Many people are allergic to tobacco, although the nausea, dizziness and coughing experienced with the first cigarette after a break from them is probably more a reaction to the drug nicotine.

For parents to smoke in the presence of their children is inexcusable: if they want to commit slow suicide by smoking, they have no right to try to pass this death-wish on to anyone else, least of all their children. Some of the facts from recent research are that

- Non-smoking wives are twice as likely to die of cancer if their husbands smoke than if they don't.
- Half the beds in most public hospitals are taken up by patients with smoking-related diseases.
- The babies of smoking mothers are lighter than other babies. They have significantly smaller heads, arms and legs and are shorter. The mother's smoking stunts the growth of every tissue in her baby's body.
- Long-term smoking dramatically increases the risk of stroke. Investigators at the Veterans Administration Medical Centre in Texas, USA, studied the effects of long-term smoking on bloodflow to the brain. They found that cigarettes cause a very significant cut in bloodflow to the brain and that the greater the number of cigarettes smoked, the larger the cut in flow. They also found that if there were any other risk factors, such as high blood pressure or high cholesterol, the risk went up still further.
- In terms of heart attacks, smoking is three times as dangerous as being overweight. A smoker of twenty cigarettes a day, aged between 45 and 74, has a 64 per cent greater chance of dying from heart attack than a non-smoker. And even more telling, no matter what led up to or predisposed a person to heart attack or coronary occlusion, a smoker has a 150 per cent greater chance of dying at the time of the attack than a non-smoker.

An interesting study at the University of California in 1984 showed that if a child is deprived of zinc, it is more likely to have learning problems. Intriguingly, children also show learning impairment if their mothers don't get enough zinc during pregnancy even though their mothers' diets may be entirely adequate in every other way.

Zinc is a very easy nutrient to lose during the processing of food, and as well it is vulnerable to some other substances.

Cadmium, for instance, is an antagonist to zinc; cigarettes contain cadmium; mothers, in increasing numbers, are smoking cigarettes; and their children are more prone to have impaired learning abilities.

Most fascinating of all, is that the animal research clearly shows that if the mother is low in zinc, the first generation (that is, the first offspring) will have learning impairment; the second will not; and the third and fourth will. Not until the fifth generation are the effects of the zinc deprivation (that is, the mother's smoking) straightened out.

In another study, 16,900 students and their mothers were questioned to see if they could find anything which might predispose the mother to have hyperactive children. They looked at forty possible factors, including whether the mother was educated, whether she was healthy at birth and so on. Only one thing out of this enormous sample was significantly correlated to hyperactivity: the mother had smoked during or prior to pregnancy.

Although the tobacco industry would like the world to believe that no adverse effects result from smoking, there is overwhelming evidence linking lung cancer to smoking, and, of course, bronchitis and smokers' cough are expected and normal in chronic smokers. How many of the 5000 deaths from lung cancer in Australia each year would occur if no-one smoked? Very few. Very disturbingly, of those 5000 deaths, 4100 are men and 900 women, but the number of women dying from lung cancer is rising sharply, while that of men is falling.

There is an inescapable and direct cause and effect between this increase and the thrust of the tobacco industry's advertising, as it struggles to compensate for the fall in cigarette smoking among men. Just as Marlboro directed its macho advertising unabashedly (and highly successfully) at children and teenagers, the ideal age group to lure into lifelong addiction, so they court the women's market. It is always the man who is lighting the cigarette, or holding the cigarette, but rarely smoking them; while the woman is in a submissive, smoking role. In the Alpine cigarette billboard advertisements, it is always a female body that appears and the cigarettes are sold fifteen to a pack, targeted at the teenage female market.

The pharmaceutical industry would never be granted marketing approval for a drug that caused even one death in a year; yet here we have an industry marketing a product that kills

5000 people from just one of many causes. It is an obscene double standard.

Since smoking, especially in those who have any difficulty giving it up, is an addiction, stopping it will lead to withdrawal symptoms. It is the unpleasant withdrawal symptoms, so readily turned off by another cigarette, that make it so difficult for so many to become non-smokers. What then can be done to reduce or minimise these withdrawals?

For those who are genuinely seeking help to stop smoking (and anyone else is wasting their and everybody else's time), I recommend the following which are all well-proved aids:

- Cooperate with yourself. Make it easier to tackle what is never an easy task. Get rid of every cigarette in the house, at work, in the car, in your handbag — everywhere. And with them, send cigarette lighters and all the other trappings of smoking.
- Get other members of the family and colleagues at work to cooperate. This is likely to be difficult if they insist on continuing to smoke, because you will have to suffer the consequences of being a passive smoker at a very vulnerable time.
- Exclude from your diet members of the deadly nightshade family to which tobacco belongs — and that includes potato, tomato, green and red peppers and eggplant — to reduce cross-reactivity within the same food family.
- Take bicarbonate of soda (4 grams or one teaspoonful) three times a day in 100 millilitres of warm water, one hour before meals. The ideal is a mixture of two parts sodium bicarbonate to one part potassium bicarbonate, though carb soda (sodium bicarbonate or baking powder) will suffice. This appears to work by increasing the rate at which nicotine is excreted from the body, so it reduces the pharmacological effect of the stimulating agent in the cigarettes which feeds the addiction and reduces the withdrawal symptoms.
- Take up to 10 grams of vitamin C per day in divided doses, but as a powder (calcium ascorbate). If diarrhoea occurs, it may be necessary to reduce the dose. This has been shown to reduce withdrawal symptoms. Even

higher dosage may be worth trying: up to 80 grams has been used to reduce significantly the withdrawal symptoms of heroin addicts.

- Because many who smoke do so to relieve tension, techniques of relaxation and meditation should be learnt and practised. These can also be used to reduce the symptoms of withdrawal.
- Diet must be essentially healthy, excluding junk foods because of their frequently high fat content, and excessive refined carbohydrates. Low cholesterol levels have been shown to be associated with a low incidence of lung cancer in those who smoke.
- Nicorettes, the chewing gum fad of the times that contains 2 milligrams of nicotine, transfers the addiction from the polluted and dangerous source of cigarettes to a pure form. But it does not remove the addiction, so that it is no surprise that so many people slip effortlessly back into smoking.
- Physical exercise and particularly aerobics improve muscle tone and cardiovascular fitness and increase the level of endorphins which results in a better sense of well-being.
- If there are underlying anxiety, tension and stress problems, professional help may be needed in addition.

These tips are intended mainly for smokers who are finding it difficult to break their habit. Remember that a large percentage of smokers can overcome their addiction by no more than wanting to and by making a concerted effort.

For all that it is often boring and unfulfilling, office work has usually been thought of as at least safe and environmentally unthreatening. The asbestos scare meant that expensive housekeeping had to be carried out to remove it from ceiling spaces and ducting, but that was a construction fault, not a flaw in the design of the office.

It comes as a genuine surprise to most people when they find out that most offices are in reality an environmental minefield, sometimes more hazardous than the industrial factories banished to the outer fringes of towns and cities.

Some of the problems have been known for a long time. The hazards of bad lighting and excessive noise, for example, are well recognised and office designers now give much greater consideration to both. Similarly, the health dangers linked to video display terminals and computer keyboards are receiving much more attention, even though there is still a great deal of ignorance about their ill effects on many people. These include cataract, eyestrain, backache, headache and migraine, and repetitive strain injury (RSI). Led by the insurance companies, who see themselves facing enormous total pay-outs from repetitive strain injury claims, there are still many people (though never the victims themselves) who insist that RSI doesn't exist at all.

The office is also a trap for many of the worst kinds of indoor chemical pollutants, partly because of the products themselves, but also because the ventilation of most office buildings is so poor. The assumption that office buildings could pose no threat to anyone working in them meant that prime consideration was given to their aesthetic appearance and how functional they were.

To conserve heat and minimise heating costs, the buildings were virtually sealed up. Windows were rarely able to be opened; building materials were required to prevent heat escaping through small cracks; and lift shafts and fire stairs, the obvious point of entry for fresh air, were isolated from the working areas.

Office buildings then relied almost entirely on air-conditioning for their air circulation — and just how much they rely on it becomes quickly evident when the air-conditioning breaks down. Even when it is working, the air-conditioning all too often does little else except circulate the same stale air and keep the temperature constant.

Someone sick sneezes, the germs get into the air-conditioning and are circulated throughout the building, or at least on the same floor. By the time it is time to go home, half a dozen other people have felt a tickle in their throats and are sneezing. Sometimes the filters are not properly serviced or are missing altogether, so that the dust, molecules and particulate matter are not only being constantly circulated, but they are always airborne. The effect is much like running a vacuum cleaner without the bag.

Open-plan offices, incidentally, need greater care than they are often shown, because the air movement is rarely sufficient below partition level. All that is necessary to improve air circulation considerably is for the partitions to be lifted about 15 centimetres from the floor, although even some office designers seem unaware of this.

THE SMOKING HAZARD ▮

Smoking and stuffy air are two of the most common causes of complaints in many offices. There is no doubt that smoking, in an atmosphere as cloistered as that of most offices, is a very serious health hazard indeed.

In a highly important and courageous move, the Australian Public Service Board imposed a total ban on smoking in all government offices. This was coupled with a requirement that non-smoking become a condition of employment. In 1987 smoking on most domestic air routes was banned, ending the farce of allocating seats to non-smokers a metre and a half away from smokers.

As the dangers of passive smoking have become even better understood, the problem of smoking in offices has become so serious that it must rank as the most unnecessarily hazardous practice of all. Even passive smokers are exposed to the full spectrum of diseases, including lung cancer, facing smokers, and both suffer intolerance symptoms if they are sensitive to tobacco, as many people are. Both the diseases of smoking and the symptoms of tobacco intolerance are serious clinical ecology problems.

As I write this, a pathologist has just reported that he carried out a drug screen by mistake on a patient's urine, instead of the urinalysis for infection that was ordered. The patient was rightly given the information from this unsolicited test and was even more rightly appalled. It showed an alarmingly high nicotine level in her blood — and neither she, nor anyone in her immediate family, were smokers! She was the victim of passive smoking in an office where the majority of people smoked.

There is no reason why people should have to put up with this kind of assault on their bodies. The children of smokers shouldn't have to put up with it, and nor should those non-smokers who go to work and happen to share space with smokers. Smoking kills people and injures them grievously; passive smoking also kills people and injures them grievously. How, in a sane society, can we tolerate a situation where people who understand this and who have elected not to smoke because they don't want to die or get ill because of cigarettes, have to have other people's cigarette smoke inflicted on them?

TROUBLE WHEREVER YOU LOOK ■

Basement garages also cause problems in offices, particularly on the lower floors of high-rise buildings. The fumes drift upwards — carbon monoxide has been identified ten storeys above an underground car park, getting progressively less dense at each floor, but still posing a threat. More efficient air-conditioning and more fresh air are the solution to this problem.

These are just the start of the pollution problem in the average office. One glance will reveal a veritable Pandora's box of items likely to be outgassing chemical molecules, many of them being constantly renewed so that the outgassing has no chance of abating. From the carpet on the floor to the last rubber band, there are many notorious troublemakers around!

As always in chemical intolerance, only a minority of people are likely to be affected by any one of these items, so that a frequent response, even if something is suspected, is that nobody else is suffering, so it must be your imagination. Nobody understands that this is the very nature of chemical intolerance and that others are certainly also suffering from their exposure to other molecules.

So where are the problem areas in the typical office? Everywhere! Most office carpet and underlay, and frequently the adhesives used with them (see Chapters 20 and 21, "Glue and Adhesives" and "Carpets"), are still outgassing strongly when they are replaced. The adhesives used in the manufacture of office furniture are also often a source of trouble. Particle board, which outgasses formaldehyde strongly, is used in shelving, furniture and space dividers. There is plastic everywhere: even the plants are likely to be plastic!

Inks, ink pads and rubber stamps, typewriter ribbons, felt pens and even the silencing material in many typewriters (which gets warm, increasing the outgassing under the typist's nose) may well cause problems, as will rubber bands and carbon paper. Not many people can hold a sheet of carbon paper, fresh from the box, to their noses and inhale deeply without feeling nauseous. The worst offender is the new carbonless, "automatic" carbon paper, which is heavily impregnated with chemicals, especially formaldehyde. I have one patient who actually gets a high from sniffing this paper, as well as a lot of very unpleasant symptoms.

Oil evaporating from typewriters and other equipment can cause difficulties for anyone intolerant of it. What is more, all the problems associated with office machines are worse when the equipment is not serviced properly or is allowed to get dirty. Photocopiers are frequently tucked away in an out-of-the-way corner of the office where ventilation is probably the last consideration, yet they are the office machines that are most in need of air space around them.

OZONE AND OFFICE CLEANERS ■

Ozone in polluted city air is a frequent cause of intolerance, but this gas is also produced by high-voltage machines, including photocopiers. A German study found that people exposed to ozone suffered chest cramps, headaches, dizziness and severe fatigue — all symptoms that are quite commonly encountered in people working in offices.

On the plates used in many photocopiers there is a layer of ozone which is released into the air when the machine is charged with high voltage — that is, when it is working. Ozone emission levels should never exceed 0.05 parts per million, or one part in twenty million, but the atmosphere around many photocopiers and other high-voltage equipment can be many times this, if ventilation is inadequate. Office designers cannot claim that they have not had the time to incorporate the findings of the German study into their designs: it was published in 1931!

The chemical carbon black, incidentally, that is found in the toners in many photocopiers, is strongly suspected of being responsible for causing skin cancer. It poses no threat at normal times, and none at all, of course, from handling the photocopies themselves; but it does require care by anyone servicing these machines.

Office cleaners tend to use the strongest cleaning agents they can find. Not only does it make their job easier, but cleaners have explained to me that their clients tend to assume that the stronger the smell of disinfectants and cleaning agents the following morning, the better the cleaners have done their job. (This poses a very real problem in schools where children are even more susceptible than most adults to chemical intolerance.)

The victims of all this outgassing are the people who must come and work in it the next day. If, at the end of your working day, you feel your eyes itching or irritated, your sinuses congesting and your head aching; or if you suffer from sore throat, shortness of breath, an unpleasant taste in your mouth, dizziness, nausea or wheezing, and there is no logical explanation for any of these symptoms, and your doctor says he can find nothing wrong — then suspect that you are the victim of your office or workplace. And don't put up with it in silence!

One would imagine that self-interest would spur any employer on to reduce this problem as far as possible, because of the increased productivity, reduced absenteeism and improved morale that would certainly follow. An immediate 75 per cent improvement is definitely possible in most offices by improving the air circulation. That this is not done is presumably only because of the widespread ignorance that exists about the problem. There should not be ignorance. The problem affects executives and the youngest office junior with complete impartiality. Increasing seniority bestows no immunity to any kind of intolerance.

FLUORESCENT LIGHT ▌

It is more than ten years since an American photobiologist, Dr John N. Ott, specialising in the effect of light on living creatures, alerted the world to a previously unsuspected factor in childhood hyperactivity, which he called "malillumination". Ott, then Director of the Environmental Health and Light Re-

A SUFFERING SECRETARY

Ruth was 27 and a secretary when she was referred to me for what her family doctor was convinced was some kind of intolerance. After some years of working in bright, airy offices, she found that she was leaving work every afternoon feeling far more tired than the work she had done warranted (one of the most telling signs of chemical intolerance in an office). By Friday, she was suffering from mild depression and she was aware that her concentration had deteriorated. She was even having difficulty focusing on the page. Yet by Monday morning she was usually feeling much better.

Most alarming, though, was that she had begun to suffer epileptic seizures. At least one day a week, she had to leave work early, often as early as mid-morning, because she thought she was experiencing the symptoms of prodrome, the prelude to an epileptic fit. The medication that her doctor prescribed for her seizures did not prevent her experiencing one at least every three weeks.

Chemical testing revealed that she was very intolerant of benzenes, but the significance of this only came to light when she completed a list, in minute detail, of every task that she carried out from the moment she walked into the office in the morning. Even then, it eluded us for a while.

The man she worked for, it eventually transpired, trusted Ruth's judgment. Every day, he received numerous reports from his employees in the field, and one of her tasks was to read through these and highlight with yellow highlighter any passages she thought he ought to read. What neither Ruth nor her boss were aware of was that highlighters give off not only a very strong aromatic smell, but molecules that can have a disastrous effect on anyone hypersensitive to them.

And so it was in Ruth's case. The weekend allowed her to get over her symptoms, but from Monday to Friday, they got progressively worse, manifesting themselves not only in her tiredness and lack of concentration, but in epileptic-type seizures. The cure could not have been more painless: she threw away the highlighters, underlined the reports in red pencil, and all her symptoms disappeared!

search Institute, was interested in the novel theory that certain types of fluorescent light might have a profound effect on behaviour and learning.

A fluorescent light is electric light which consists of a glass tube containing a small amount of mercury and a chemically inactive gas. The most commonly used gas today is argon, but originally it was neon and the name has stuck.

Fluorescent lights produce only a fifth as much heat as incandescent lamps (the common light bulbs) and, for this reason, they are sometimes called "cool" lights. They also use about a fifth as much electricity as an incandescent lamp once they are switched on and they last much longer. This is why they have become hugely popular, to the point where they are the standard form of industrial and office lighting throughout the world today.

The inside surface of the glass tube is coated with chemicals called phosphors and at each end of the tube, there is an electrode, a coil of tungsten wire coated with other chemicals called rare earth oxides.

There are three main types of fluorescent light in wide use. The principal difference between them is the time that it takes after they are switched on for the fluorescent tube to be fully working. The cheapest, and so the most commonly used, are "preheat" lights, the type mainly found in offices and factories, where there is the familiar delay and flickering as the gas warms up, before the light is fully working. The alternatives are "rapid-start" and "instant-start", which give exactly the same light, but, as their name implies, take less time to be fully functioning.

When any fluorescent light is switched on, the electricity flows through the tungsten wire in the coil and heats it. The earth oxides on the coil then give off electrons, some of which strike the argon atoms and ionise them, meaning that they give them either a positive or a negative charge. When it has been ionised, the argon gas can conduct electricity and a current flows through it from electrode to electrode, forming an arc, or a stream, of electrons.

When an electron in this arc strikes a mercury atom, it raises the energy level of another electron in the atom and, as this electron returns to its normal state, it gives off invisible ultraviolet rays. The phosphors coating the tube absorb these rays and change them into visible light. The colour of the light depends on the phosphors that are used.

Fluorescent Lights and School Grades   Ott conducted his study in four year-1 classrooms in a school in Florida. None of the rooms had windows. In two of them, the artificial lighting consisted of the standard, "cool", white fluorescent tubes, fitted with solid plastic diffusers (the "shades" that cover the light and prevent you actually seeing the tube). This was the lighting used in the majority of schools in America and indeed probably the world.

In the other two rooms, the "cool", white tubes were replaced with full-spectrum tubes, which are more expensive but which produce light across a much broader spectrum than the white tubes, so that their light more closely duplicates natural daylight. Ordinary light bulbs emit full-spectrum light.

Lead foils were wrapped round each end of the tubes, where the cathodes were located, to prevent any leakage that might influence the results of the test; and aluminium "egg-crate" diffusers replaced the usual solid ones.

For forty days, Ott then filmed the behaviour of all the students in the four classrooms, using time-lapse photography. What he was looking for was evidence of behaviour changes, for better or worse, in the classes with the full-spectrum light; and what he found was a dramatic improvement in the behaviour even of hyperactive children and in learning ability.

Year 1 pupils settled down and paid more attention to their teachers in these rooms and overall classroom performance improved. The time-lapse photography allowed hours to pass in seconds, so that Ott had a unique opportunity to watch and record the movement of the class and individual children.

One child, for instance, in a classroom with the full-spectrum fluorescent lighting, had a severe learning disability and was quite unable to read when the experiment began. After forty days under the full-spectrum lighting, he gained a full year in reading ability and his hyperactivity had disappeared.

Similar results were subsequently reported in another school district in California, and later studies in Russia confirmed Ott's findings. The implication was unavoidable that for many children the conventional fluorescent lighting used in schools is directly involved in behaviour disorders, as well as in hyperactivity and learning difficulties.

Other studies have looked at the effect of fluorescent lighting on adults and these results are also worrying, revealing that people working in conventional fluorescent lighting become tense and irritable. Exactly how much mental stress we can blame on our increasingly artificially lit environment is not known, but there are disquieting signs that it may be considerably more than we have ever suspected.

The full-spectrum fluorescent lights that Ott and others used in their studies are also employed to provide normal growth for indoor plants in commercial nurseries. Under this light, the plants grow well and have healthy foliage. Expose the same plants to the more commonly used "cool" fluorescent lighting, however, and they quickly die. If nothing else, this ought to sound a note of warning in the minds of humans!

Melanoma and the Fluorescent Light But this is only a part of the hazard that is being increasingly attributed to fluorescent lighting and the story only gets worse. The most alarming possibility was revealed in a roundabout way when scientists were looking for something completely different.

Two questions have long puzzled epidemiologists looking at the incidence of melanoma, one of the most malignant of all cancers. The first is why the world incidence of melanoma has more than doubled in the last thirty years; and the second, why the incidence of malignant melanoma is increasing particularly on areas of the body that are not normally exposed to the sun. Excessive exposure to the sun is known to be the principal cause of melanoma, which is no doubt why Australia has the worst incidence of it in the world.

The further north one travels in Australia, the higher the incidence of melanoma (although it dips in Queensland probably, it is thought, because Queenslanders have a healthier respect for the dangers of excessive exposure to the sun, or more likely, because the climate is so hot that they need bigger hats and more protective clothing).

Some answers came from unexpected directions. A study was carried out in America in 1978 to explore the possible relationship between melanoma and the use of oral contraceptives. In the course of this project, women were asked about their work environment and any other possible sources of radiation, which included exposure to fluorescent light, both at home and at work, as well as to television.

The researchers frankly admitted afterwards that they had not expected to find a link with any kind of lighting, but they had asked the question only because emission from fluorescent light can sometimes extend to the ultraviolet range. Ultraviolet radiation causes the changes in the skin which in turn can initiate the malignant change.

What they found was no apparent link between melanoma and oral contraceptives and none with television, but a quite remarkable link between the cancer and exposure to fluorescent light. Those who were exposed to fluorescent lighting had twice the risk of developing malignant melanoma, and the longer the exposure, the greater the risk.

Women who had worked outdoors in the sun, without fluorescent exposure, had a lower risk of cancer, than those exposed to fluorescent lighting. Least at risk were women who worked indoors and had never been exposed to fluorescent lighting. (Only women were sampled, of course, in this study because it was originally concerned with oral contraceptives.)

Fluorescent lighting exposure in the home alone was not associated with melanoma, possibly (as we shall see shortly) because a diffuser, or shade, is almost always used in the home.

Australian Women at Risk   Another unexpected finding was the large number of lesions, or sites of the melanoma, on the bodies of women exposed to fluorescent lighting at work, and particularly on areas of their bodies covered by clothing. There has been a disturbing increase in recent years in malignant melanoma on parts of the body that have historically never been associated with melanoma, and in part this has been attributed to changing social habits, particularly nude sunbathing, which has resulted in an increase in melanoma of the genital areas — but why should there be this high incidence in body areas normally covered up at work?

Researchers believe that a likely explanation is that the light-weight summer clothes worn by Australian women can transmit between 20 and 50 per cent of ultraviolet radiation and so may be no protection at all. Indeed, paradoxically, the head, neck and arms may actually be less susceptible to radiation because they are permanently exposed to all kinds of radiation and are usually tanned, which in moderation provides some protection.

It is important to keep melanoma in perspective. The incidence of the malignant form is very low. Other forms of sun cancer, such as solar keratosis and squamous and basal cell carcinomas, are much more common. But rare or not, a doubling in the number of cases in a very short period is highly significant, particularly because malignant melanoma is almost invariably fatal and claims the lives of many young people.

I believe that there is one very basic precaution that can be taken with fluorescent lighting. The presence of plastic diffusive covers over the light strips reduces the spread of ultraviolet light. This may well explain why there appears to be a clear-cut relationship between melanoma and exposure to fluorescent lighting at work (where the lights are often unshielded), and none at home, where most people use shades. Naked, unshielded, unshaded fluorescent tubes should never be used, a lesson that ought to have the support of law in the workplace.

Flickering Fluorescent Fits   There is one other, quite different reason to be concerned about fluorescent lighting, which, though not dangerous, causes a lot of unnecessary suffering. Many people complain of headaches when they have been in a room lit by fluorescent lights (though they rarely make the association unless they know what they are looking for), and a few suffer epileptic-type fits as a result.

For these people, the cause of the trouble is not the radiation, but the fifty-cycle-per-second flicker peculiar to fluorescent lighting. This is not normally consciously noticed by the human eye, but it is no less real for that, and it can lead to symptoms of headache and epilepsy, as well as probably being associated with many of the reports of irritability and nerviness experienced by people working in fluorescent lighting. The problem is worse if there are ceiling fans under the fluorescent lights. This results in flickering on the flickering, and produces exacerbated symptoms, particularly migraine.

As frequently happens in ecological illness, other sensitivities, which may be to chemicals or food, may complicate the picture. Dr Laurence Dickey, one of the most experienced American clinical ecologists, reported the case of a patient who worked in a large plant under fluorescent lighting. Dickey established that she was markedly sensitive to beef — but only while she continued to be exposed to fluorescent light. Under full-spectrum artificial light, or in open sunlight, she was not noticeably sensitive to it at all.

In summary, then, we find fluorescent light affecting people adversely in three quite distinct ways. The disturbed behaviour in John Ott's research was probably caused by the positive ions generated by the "cool", white light. As we will see in Chapter 24, an excess of positive ions over negative ions frequently causes behaviour disorders, poor concentration, irritability and so on.

In the case of malignant melanoma, it is probably the ultraviolet light emitted by the fluorescent tubes that causes the changes to the skin that develop into the cancer. Then there are the problems caused for some people by the constant flickering of the tubes.

It is a subject that needs a great deal more careful study, for almost certainly it is a much more widespread cause of many of the unpleasant symptoms experienced by office and factory workers than has ever been suspected.

24 Negative Ions — Help or Hindrance?

A whole industry has grown up around negative ions and negative ion generators. Lavish claims have been made, invariably accompanied by well-documented published studies, about the benefits of negative ions in areas as diverse as assembly-line productivity, security guard alertness, motoring safety, human performance, allergy and the prevention of infection. Secretaries are claimed to work more efficiently, frayed tempers are soothed, headaches disappear as though by magic. Yet for all those thousands who swear by their generators, or ionisers as they are popularly called, there are many detractors who are just as vocal.

Ionisers have been variously described as a cheap and effective godsend for millions of sufferers from numerous symptoms, and as a complete waste of money benefiting nobody except the people who make and sell them. Even people who have bought them are divided, with many swearing that they are everything they claim to be, and others ridiculing them as a gimmicky waste of money.

In Europe, notably in Hungary, Germany and Russia, where some of the most solid research has been carried out, they have been extolled for years, not only as personal units in homes, offices and cars, but as huge installations that ionise entire hospitals and public buildings.

In the United States, on the other hand, there was such scepticism that for a time the Food and Drug Administration banned them altogether. Even today, they can only be sold in the USA on condition that no claims are made of any specific health-giving properties. As a result, American promotion tends to be along the lines of "purify the air you breathe by removing dust particles before they end up as soot in your lungs".

How useful, then, are ionisers in reducing ecological illness, which ought to be one of the areas that most benefits from ionisation, if the claims are right? The answer seems to be that for many people in fairly limited situations, they are very beneficial. Clinically, I have seen them produce excellent results with many patients, although in some cases there may well be a placebo effect (where the patients either want to please their doctor, or have convinced themselves that ionisers are beneficial, to the extent that it is *this* factor, rather than negative ions, that produces the improvement).

WHY WE ARE CONCERNED ABOUT IONS ■

Air consists chiefly of oxygen and nitrogen, with small quantities of other gases including carbon dioxide. Each molecule of air comprises one or more atoms, each of which has a central core — or nucleus — of positive charges surrounded by an equal number of moving negative charges, which are known as electrons. An ion is a molecule of any substance that has either gained or lost an electron.

The majority of molecules (all but about 4000 in every 3000 million) are electrically neutral, meaning that they have an equal number of positive and negative charges. If a molecule loses an electron, however, it is no longer electrically balanced. The positive charge now predominates and it is referred to as a positive ion, or "posion" in the industry jargon. On the other hand, if the molecule gains an extra electron, the negative charge is dominant and it is known as a negative ion, or "negion".

Ions occur naturally in the atmosphere, but the theory behind the present enthusiasm is that everyday environmental situations can also produce an unnatural number of ions, or more particularly a notable lack of them. It is claimed that the negative ions contribute to human well-being, while positive ions have the opposite effect, resulting in illness and unpleasant symptoms.

These adverse reactions, it is maintained, can be reversed by deliberately boosting the number of negative ions to counter the surplus of posions; and even when excess positive ions are not a problem, there is therapeutic value in being exposed to large quantities of negions.

Most of the research suggests that negions lower (and posions raise) the blood levels of serotonin, a powerful neuro-hormone that plays an important role in transmitting nerve impulses and in our moods and sleep patterns.

Unfortunately for the negative ioniser industry, it faces a substantial credibility gap in that the claims have so far not been supported by the irrefutable proof that science requires. The ionisers can be made to sound extremely appealing to a scientifically ignorant market, but it is quite another thing to convince cynical scientists that negion generators achieve most of what is claimed for them.

The degree of acceptance varies from country to country, and I should expose my bias from the start. Many of my patients have benefited immensely from ionisers and, as with all aspects of ecological medicine, there is no way that I am going to advise against their use when, with one or two easily avoidable exceptions, they are as safe as they are effective. The scientists can come later and explain to me precisely why ionisers work.

THE EVIL WINDS ■

Probably the best documented cases of ions affecting human behaviour are the notorious winds that we have already discussed (see Chapter 5, p. 49), such as the Santa Ana in California, the Föhn in Austria and Switzerland, and the Sharav that sweeps across Africa and the Sinai Peninsula twice a year. In Syria, there is the simoon, which appropriately means poisoning, for these winds bring distress and violent mood swings. In Australia, the northerly winds in Victoria and sometimes the westerlies in New South Wales may have the same effect.

These winds are often caused by a warm upper air mass sliding down over the top of cooler air and becoming a hot, dry, ground-level wind. The wind is often charged with dust and debris from far away and the ratio of positive to negative ions can rise as high as ten to one.

The most important work into the effects of these winds has been done in Israel, which suffers from the Sharav. Professor Felix Sulman, of the Department of Applied Pharmacology at the School of Pharmacy of Jerusalem's Hebrew University (Sulman is a medical doctor, among his many qualifications), is probably the world's foremost authority on the ionising effects of these highly antisocial winds. He has no doubt that the harm attributed to them is fully justified.

For example, writing of the very high incidence of headaches and migraine associated with the winds, Sulman said:

> *Attacks of migraine resulting from heat stress are a common occurrence in 20–30 per cent of a population exposed to hot, dry winds. The electrical*

charge (positive ionisation) engendered by every incoming weather front
produces a release of serotonin. In addition there also exists a syndrome of
adrenalin deficiency which may produce headache . . .

The Föhn is a steady, warm, dry wind, which blows from
the ridges of the Alps and has a very similar social effect to the
Santa Ana and the Sharav: crime rates soar (by as much as 20 per
cent), suicides rise, police leave is cancelled and car accidents
increase. Some surgeons refuse to do elective surgery during
the Föhn. All this is because of excessive positive ions in the
atmosphere.

Up to a day and half before the winds actually arrive, the
level of positive ions increases and many people begin to react. It
may well be that the well-documented ability of animals to sense
natural disasters like storms and earthquakes before they occur is
related to ionisation, as might be the ability of people with
arthritis to forecast when a change of weather is coming. If positive ions achieve all this, then negative ions have a very strong
case!

NEGATIVE IONS MAKE BETTER DRIVERS ■

Another area that has been well researched is the effect of ionisation on drivers. Again, the results are totally convincing to those
who have benefited from ion generators in their cars or trucks,
but not to scientists looking for hard, replicable evidence.

In an Australian study, for instance, truck drivers were
tested over an average of more than 3200 kilometres a week. Increased alertness and awareness while driving were reported by 87
per cent of drivers; 80 per cent said they slept better, more deeply
and for shorter periods; 73 per cent said they were calmer, and
less irritable and short-tempered with other drivers; and 93 per
cent found their cabs fresher and cleaner. Similar studies in
Europe produced much the same responses.

Now whether the research was scientifically flawless or not
— and it obviously was not, because there are too many extraneous factors involved — the reality is that a great many drivers do
believe that they are safer, more relaxed and more alert when they
have an ioniser in their cabs. So what can possibly be gained
from criticising ionisers to the point where their use is ridiculed?

Again, the theory is that the electrical systems of motor
vehicles tend to produce positive ions, so that car heaters, fresh-

air ventilation systems and air-conditioners all upset ionisation. At the same time there is friction between the air and the vehicle as it is moving, which sets up a positive charge on the metal bodywork. This in turn acts as a magnet and attracts to the metal any negative ions that may be in the car. All in all, coupled with the high level of pollution that is always associated with traffic fumes, an environment is created that reduces alertness and makes the driver a hazard.

I don't know if this will stand the close scrutiny of scientists, but I do know that many tens of thousands of drivers feel much better from having an ioniser in the car and are rid of many symptoms that resisted any other treatment.

THE IONIC ASHTRAY ▌

There is a second use for ionisers that attracts much less dispute. Free negative ions projected into a room attach themselves to particles of dust, pollen and smoke, which are then attracted to neutral or oppositely charged surfaces in the room.

A very simple experiment will show how effectively they perform this task. Take an ioniser into a room full of tobacco smoke and switch it on. In an instant the smoke disappears! The final rather undesirable proof of this is the area immediately round the ioniser. If you stand the machine on a metal surface, the result is like electroplating. Because the ioniser is positive, it attracts the negions and the particulate matter on to it, but the matter doesn't dust off. Choose the surface carefully!

There are several different ionisers on the market, and they are sold in various sizes and strengths. They produce the negative ions through a series of fine needles, the tips of which carry a very high voltage at low currents. As they stream out of the machine, a slight breeze can be felt. They are sold through health stores, electrical retail chains and frequently by mail order, and the industry seems to devote a good deal of energy to warning potential customers to stay clear of the opposition.

The dangers are not great. The main risk is that some older models emit annoying quantities of ozone, which can be bad for you. It may be that some, at least, of the sensation of cool, fresh air that is often experienced near an ioniser (it is usually compared to the marvellous freshness that follows a thunderstorm, or standing near a waterfall) comes from the ozone as well as the negative ions. Ionisers can often quickly clear a headache, simply by sitting close to them and letting the ions waft over you, although it is not a good idea to do this for lengthy periods with some older models if the ozone emissions are high. Chemically intolerant patients may also find that they help in reducing the background levels of outgassing.

In spite of some manufacturers' claims, most ionisers that are sold are only useful for personal use at short range, for example on a desk, a bedside table, in the kitchen, or in a car or truck. The pyramid-type ionisers are good because the needles point in different directions. Ionisers that are big enough to improve the atmosphere significantly in a whole room are available, but they are considerably more expensive.

Finally, I come to the most hazardous form of chemical contamination and the source of untold suffering for the chemically
intolerant, quite apart from the gross poisoning for which it has
been responsible.

Environmental poisoning takes many forms. Dying from
lead poisoning has long been a euphemistic joke to describe being
shot to death, but it has taken on a new twist in countries where
hunting and fishing are popular. It is estimated that each year
American hunters alone deposit some 3000 *tonnes* of lead pellets
in lakes, ponds and marshes.

Waterbirds then ingest these pellets when they are eating
and die from lead poisoning. The US magazine *Sports Illustrated*,
which is no enemy of the hunters, estimates that between 2 and 3
per cent of the autumn population of all species of waterfowl die
in this way — which means that between 1.6 and 2.4 million
ducks die each year from true lead poisoning.

On several rivers in England, the swan population has been
decimated from poisoning by small lead weights used by fisher-
men and abandoned on the river beds. Again, the birds pick
them up unwittingly as they feed.

LIVING IN A PESTICIDE SMOG ▮

The poisoning caused by pesticides and herbicides (which kill
plants, particularly weeds), however, is much more insidious and
takes place across a far broader arena — almost the entire land
mass on earth that human beings occupy, and much of the ocean
as well. We live in a pesticide smog and it is no exaggeration that
there is probably not a corner of the globe that has not been penetrated by pesticide residues.

As the only purpose of pesticides and herbicides is to kill

some form of life by poisoning it to death, one would imagine that the first priority of any community using them would be to treat them with the utmost wariness, applying them conservatively and keeping them as far removed from stock and people as possible. The trouble with pesticides is that there is no point at which they stop killing.

Yet so far are we from achieving this goal that we now use about 500 grams (1 pound) of pesticide for every human being on earth each year. It is sprayed with such little regard for life that Oxfam has estimated that 750,000 people around the world are annually poisoned by pesticides. More than 14,000 of these die as the result of acute pesticide and herbicide poisoning, and this figure is known to be greatly understated in undeveloped countries, where records are scanty and autopsies rarely performed.

Nor do these awful statistics take account of the millions of victims of chronic pesticide poisoning, where there may be no immediately identifiable cause and effect between exposure and symptoms, but where the price that must be paid includes cancer, birth malformation and all the symptoms that are part and parcel of ecologically induced sickness.

What is more, as though the price that we pay in terms of ill health and suffering were not enough, there is the actual cost to society of these products in terms of livestock loss, pollution of the soil, water and air, contamination of food and the bottom line of the profit and loss account at the end of the year.

In the United States one study of some of these unwanted side effects placed their cost in that country alone at $839 million in 1980 — about 20 per cent of the value of annual sales of pesticides by American companies. That was also, by coincidence, approximately the profit that the pesticide and herbicide manufacturers earned the same year, which means that Americans are subsidising the industry's annual return almost dollar for dollar! In Australia, where the industry is almost entirely controlled by foreign companies, the equation is even more unfavourable for Australians.

GOOD FOOD THAT HARMS US ■

We have already seen that more than 400 synthetic chemicals have been identified in human tissue, some of them clearly pesticides, yet, in spite of this, people are still not educated to consider chemical poisoning as a possible cause of their general lethargy and other symptoms.

Because we are brought up to believe that fruit and vegetables are always beneficial and healthful, few of us eating an ordinary diet are likely to suspect that our daily apple or banana is probably so contaminated by chemical sprayings, almost none of which can be removed, that it is the direct cause of the headaches, arthritis or fatigue that so many of us have come to take for granted. Masking means that there is no immediate cause and effect relationship that might lead us to suspect this, unless we have been told about the link.

A 1984 study in San Francisco which sampled ten different fruits and vegetables in the city's markets, found that 44 per cent of the samples contained detectable residues of nineteen different pesticides; and seven of these were known or suspected carcinogens. The situation would probably be almost identical in Australia, but comparable research is all but non-existent here.

Apples, as we have seen, are likely to have been sprayed up to fourteen times between the orchard and the checkout counter. Once the crop has been sprayed with a combination of pesticide and kerosene, or any other chemical solvent used as a vehicle for the pesticide itself, neither washing, rubbing, peeling or even cooking can be guaranteed to get rid of the residues of any of these sprayings.

Even when fruit and vegetables (vegetables get just the same treatment) have been harvested and are ready to go to market, they are not left alone. The cardboard containers and boxes that are used to transport them are usually sprayed to prevent insects or mould.

One of the obstacles to pinning down the chronic effects of pesticides and herbicides is that the damage may show up long after the chemical has left the body. Like X-rays, they are capable of triggering genetic damage or cancer while they are in the body, and then of disappearing without trace as the disease process relentlessly gathers momentum. It might be years before this legacy of damage manifests itself; or sometimes just months before a malformed baby arrives.

The herbicide 2,4-D (with 2,4,5-T, an ingredient of the notorious defoliant Agent Orange), for example, is rapidly eliminated from the body, but people exposed to it only very briefly on their skin have weeks later developed nerve damage in their arms and legs, which has then persisted for years.

The enormous, and enormously profitable, trade in pesticides and herbicides (worth $4 billion a year in the US alone), is dominated by a tiny number of multinational corporations based in Europe, America and Japan. The five biggest — Bayer of West Germany, Ciba-Geigy of Switzerland, Monsanto of the USA, Shell of Holland and ICI of Britain — together account for about 25 per cent of the total world agrochemical sales, which in 1985 were worth some $13 billion a year. Less than three dozen firms control 90 per cent of that global market, making it easy for them to speak in unison, to close ranks when they are threatened or to bully governments into compliance.

THE INDISCRIMINATE KILLER ■

Pesticides are a relatively new phenomenon. Only after the Second World War did they come into prominence, when the World Health Organisation began to use the organochlorine DDT to wipe out malaria-carrying mosquitoes.

At first the campaign was unprecedently successful and malaria was all but eradicated, saving millions of lives; but the euphoria was short-lived. It became apparent that an awful price was paid in the damage that DDT did to the rest of the environment. Worse still, the sacrifice of the environment had all been for nothing, because the mosquitoes, through natural selection, developed resistance to DDT.

The manufacturers recommended spraying the mosquito survivors with even stronger and more toxic amounts of DDT, but by then they seemed to have acquired heightened resistance, not only to the original DDT, but to many other chemicals. Today, with a trail of havoc left behind in the environment, malaria is again on the rampage. The mosquitoes are too resistant.

Sometimes there is the added irony of the natural predators and pests alike being destroyed, for the organochlorines are non-selective. Often the pest, through natural selection, manages to survive against all the odds, but in an adapted form which the re-introduced natural predator does not recognise as prey. The pest thrives and the predator itself now probably becomes a pest, turning its attention to some beneficial species.

What was hailed as the organochlorines' greatest advantage, the need to use them only occasionally because the chemical remained active for years, turned out to be their greatest curse. Nature has no way of degrading them, so they remain in the biosphere for years, killing not only their target pests, but hosts of beneficial and harmless species as well.

Less than one in a thousand species of insects are harmful to humans, crops or animals, but pesticides are totally non-selective in many cases and kill them all. The chemicals get into the food chain, killing or damaging the young and the eggs of many species along the way. Birds eat the insects and die or cannot reproduce properly; animals eat the birds; and we may eat the animals.

Fish are hypersensitive to many chemicals, as are bees, and only a few parts per billion may kill them. The unexplained discovery of a dead fish in a waterway should be as great a cause for alarm as the sight of a dead canary down a coal mine. Fish-kill is often a predictable consequence of run-off from sprayed fields, in spite of mock surprise and regret from manufacturers, sprayers and (all too often) local government and health officials.

The droplets of spray are often so small that 20 per cent can escape into the air to drift away on the wind, never reaching their target at all, particularly when they are sprayed from the air. The powerful downdraught of the blades of helicopters, which are being used increasingly for agricultural spraying, propel the spray for a long way, even on a calm day. The pesticide droplets sometimes turn up thousands of kilometres away from the area where they were sprayed, to begin the contamination process all over again, coming down in the rain or snow, polluting waterways and pastures.

It often takes a disaster or the prospect of losing a lot of money to stir Australian governments into action. This was certainly the case with DDT. While most other countries in the developed world have long viewed DDT as a totally unacceptable hazard, Australia has continued to permit its use on pome fruit (apples, pears and quince, for example) and stone fruit. Although its use was not permitted on crops in Australia, the level of residue was very high. In 1987, when alarming amounts of DDT began turning up in beef being exported to the United States, which threatened the entire beef-exporting business, action was finally taken to ban its use altogether. It could now be claimed that DDT was banned over the whole continent.

THE PROMISE THAT TURNED SOUR ▐

The new pesticides, along with a new generation of fertilisers and "superseeds", were to be the solution to the chronic food shortages afflicting much of the world, particularly the Third World. Most of these products are petrochemical-dependent, opening up a gold mine after the Second World War for the handful of huge multinational chemical and petroleum corporations who alone could afford the multimillion-dollar research and development costs.

Instead, pesticides quickly proved that they were not the miraculous panacea, the wonder means of expanding agricultural productivity, that had been promised. Even putting aside the ecological turmoil they were causing, they were not even in many cases cost-effective.

On the bottom line — the argument most likely to appeal to most farmers — there was rarely any improvement in overall profitability, especially viewed over five years or more. As productivity increased, so did the bill for agrochemicals. Then, even though the heavy input of chemical fertilisers produced lush crops, these in turn fed increased numbers of pests requiring ever greater and more potent amounts of pesticide to control them, unless farmers were willing to try to get off the pesticide roundabout altogether. Failing that, the bill for pesticides and herbicides would get larger every year.

It is the ultimate irony that after more than forty years of increasing reliance on pesticides, insect damage to major crops is as great as ever. Indeed, repeated studies have shown that crop losses from insect damage have actually risen since the 1940s. United Nations figures show that there was a sixteen-fold increase in the number of pests resistant to one or more of the common pesticides in the twenty-five years ending 1980.

Once pests have outmanoeuvred a particular pesticide, they seem able to develop resistance and to adapt much more quickly and easily to other chemicals. Even weeds are becoming resistant, with thirty common annual weed species now reported to be unaffected by the most commonly used herbicides that once effectively killed them.

The inevitable response from the people who manufacture and market agrochemicals is to spray still larger quantities, more toxic, more potent and usually more expensive. Always it is the farmer and the consumer who ultimately pay, and it is a treadmill from which it is very difficult to escape once one has stepped on to it.

Pesticides, by design, are rarely specific to one species of insect or pest. It costs between $25 and $30 million to launch a new pesticide. Given the ability of many insects to develop resistance, and the need for as broad a market as possible for the product, there is economic sense in ensuring that it is *not* specific to one species. The great loser when this philosophy is adopted is the ecology.

EXPLOITING THE VULNERABLE ■

In her 1962 best-seller, *Silent Spring*, Rachel Carson sounded the first well-documented alarm about the concentration of pesticides in the food chain, and the dangers to the ecology that this posed. After publication of *Silent Spring*, many Western governments did begin to set maximum permissible levels of a pesticide; and then, much more slowly, they controlled the actual application and availability.

As public awareness of the health and environmental hazards associated with herbicides, and especially with pesticides because of the quantities used, has grown, governments in America, Japan and Europe in particular have imposed restrictions and in some cases total prohibition of their use. It was very significant that the countries that were the first to act were also the home bases of the major agrochemical manufacturers.

Even when their products were banned, however, the manufacturers, often with the blessing of their governments, continued to manufacture and export them, in exactly the same way that the pharmaceutical manufacturers did, even when it was illegal to use the chemicals in their own countries. In many cases, their methods of selling were on a par with those of the tobacco companies, which have sought for a long time to make up for their dwindling sales in many Western countries by deliberately marketing in developing nations cigarettes with a tar and nicotine content so high that a high percentage of quick addicts, and so a continuing market for their product, was guaranteed. Such cigarettes would be illegal in the parent company's home market, yet in these new markets there is rarely any consumer awareness of the dangers of cigarettes, any more than of pesticides.

Today, the fastest growing markets for pesticides are in the undeveloped countries of the Third World, where highly toxic chemicals are often used in conditions that in most Western countries would be criminally dangerous. Instructions for their safe use are often inadequate and are written in a language the people do not understand, even assuming they are not illiterate.

Those who can read come across American labels calling for mandatory safety equipment, which they cannot afford and is rarely provided. They read that if poisoning does occur, they must see a doctor immediately, but in all probability a doctor is neither available nor affordable.

Even when the pesticides are manufactured in Third World countries, the safety standards imposed fall far short of those demanded in the company's country of origin, as the 1985 Bhopal tragedy with methyl isocyanate vividly illustrated.

FROM WEAPONS OF WAR TO INSECT KILLERS ■

Organophosphorus compounds (OPs) have largely replaced the discredited organochlorines. DDT and the other organochlorines (such as pentachlorophenol, PCP, which causes cancer in laboratory animals and is easily absorbed by the skin, the lungs and the gastrointestinal systems of humans) were proving so persistent in the environment that they had became politically unacceptable.

Organophosphorus compounds were first synthesised by German chemists in the 1930s, not for agricultural purposes, but as potent weapons of war. They were never used as weapons and after the war many more OPs were developed for use against aphids and other insect pests.

Compared with organochlorines, most OPs have relatively low stability in the environment, in that they do not persist for so long (although those which end in "-thion", like malathion and parathion, are more resistant to degradation, or decomposition, and break up more slowly in the soil). OPs deteriorate rapidly in water, plants and animal organisms. At the same time, they generally have limited cumulative properties, again unlike the chlorinated hydrocarbons, which stay in the soil and accumulate in plants through the animal chain. However, OPs are not safe, and they are often just as disastrous as organochlorines in the food chain because they are in most cases far more acutely toxic.

Just how deadly OPs would have been in war can be judged from the fact that the new agrochemical OPs were a hundred times less toxic than the nerve weapons from which they were developed, yet were still so highly toxic that, in some cases, two or three drops on the skin were sufficient to kill humans. As pesticides, they act either by contact (parathion, methyl parathion and malathion, for example); or on the insects' systems (demeton,

demeton-o-methyl, OMPA). They are used for the control of numerous insect pests; as fungicides to control plant disease; to control vermin in fruit and vegetables, cotton and cereal crops, ornamental plants and tree nurseries; and to kill parasites in domestic animals.

The most undesirable feature of many organophosphorus pesticides is their very narrow zone of safety — the difference between the dose that gives rise to the first signs of poisoning and the lethal dose. The signs of acute poisoning by OPs usually appear rapidly and vary according to the size of the dose and the route by which the poison enters the body. The central nervous system is affected, and this may manifest itself in a number of ways, ranging from slurred speech and loss of normal reflexes, to convulsions or coma.

Paralysis can also occur, and in the most serious form, extends to the muscles of the respiratory system and results in death. Even mild inhalation causes a feeling of tightness in the chest and increased nasal and bronchial secretions. Ingestion often results in severe gastrointestinal disturbances, even after the smallest exposure, including nausea, cramp, vomiting and diarrhoea. There is evidence that OPs also cause spontaneous abortion.

HOW OPs HARM US ■

Organophosphates all act in the same way on the human organism, by destroying the enzyme cholinesterase, which is vital for the transmission of nerve impulses within the brain and central nervous system. In cases of severe poisoning, death may occur within a few minutes to a few hours, if the dose was large enough for that particular victim.

It is important to know this, so as to understand the true nature of the chemical that we are spraying over our land, often with complete disregard for the most basic safety requirements, and that is even widely used inside many homes.

In chronic illness (that is, illness that is the result of smaller doses than are needed to trigger an acute reaction), the symptoms can also be very severe, and there is evidence that one massive single dose of an OP, rather than frequent and regular exposure, can sensitise the victim not only to that particular poison, but to a host of other chemicals that may not even be organophosphates.

Repeated exposure to organophosphates, even in minute

traces, breaks down the ability of the vital organs to handle them. Professor William Ray, a cardiac surgeon in Dallas, Texas, has now identified the long suspected link between exposure to dichlorvos (an OP) and coronary occlusion.

Yet dichlorvos, in spite of being one of the most toxic OPs, a carcinogen and a mutagen (an agent that causes mutation), is the active ingredient in Shelltox Pestrips and in animal flea and tick collars, outgassing into kitchens, bedrooms, nurseries and wardrobes in millions of homes around the world. A number of greyhounds have died from the effects of pesticide collars and presumably many other dogs have met the same fate, although their owners are unlikely to have had autopsies carried out on them to prove the cause of death.

Remember how close children often get to pets, and how they grab dogs or cats around the neck and hug them, often with bare arms. If the pets are wearing pesticide collars, the children will have them close to, or actually touching, their faces and bare arms and they will breathe in the vapours of the pesticide — a carcinogen and a mutagen — and absorb it through their skin.

Having products containing dichlorvos at home is like having a little time bomb ticking away. It may never go off, but nobody knows for sure; and if it does, nobody can predict the damage that it will cause, much of it years later.

DESIGNED TO KILL PEOPLE — AND THEY DO! ■

We have become so cavalier about the way we use pesticides and herbicides that many are now being sprayed when there is no evidence that the pests are even in the district. It makes about as much sense as taking a preventative drug for a heart attack when there is no suggestion that there is anything wrong with your heart. All it achieves is to needlessly contaminate the environment a little more and put at risk a few more people's lives and welfare.

There are very many chemicals polluting our environment. What singles out the pesticides and herbicides, and particularly the OPs, is that they are chemicals that were introduced and are manufactured for the very reason that they *are* poisons intended to kill. With most chemicals that damage the environment and account for so much ecologically triggered illness, the harm comes as a by-product of a substance that was not intended to injure any living organism.

WALTER AND THE FUMIGATED OFFICE

Walter is a patient who has been fighting for years for what he sees as justice. The general manager of a Sydney communications company, he learned in a very unpleasant way of the shattering effect on a healthy person's life of sudden exposure to a high dose of pesticide. In his case, the villain was again dichlorvos. He arrived for work at 8 a.m. as usual one April morning, and shortly afterwards, for no reason that he could immediately identify, he felt very ill. Among the symptoms that he was experiencing was a very frightening feeling of impending doom.

He put up with it for a few hours and then, sensing that he was on the point of collapse, had to ask a colleague to drive him home. On the way out, he called at his managing director's office to tell him that he was leaving, but found a note on the door warning that the room was being fumigated and that no-one should enter it.

Until that day, Walter had always enjoyed excellent health. Only the year before he had passed a Health Commission medical to enable him to take up a physically demanding appointment, and had held a commercial pilot's licence.

He very soon began to suffer all the symptoms of asthma, which he had never had before, and he became highly susceptible to many other substances that had never bothered him before — among them traffic fumes, air-conditioning, tobacco smoke and a variety of other things many of which are unavoidable in a city environment. The very air in Sydney seemed to be corrosive to his chest.

In the end, after trying unsuccessfully to carry on with his job, he was forced to resign and leave Sydney, going to the country where he thought the clean air would help him recover. Instead, his respiratory condition actually grew worse. He also began to suffer from a variety of physical problems that he had never experienced before, including colitis, mouth ulcers, excruciating headaches that lasted for a long time, dizziness, ringing in the ears and fluid retention. Finally, before the year was ended, he was granted an invalid pension.

As if that was not enough, an allergist and a clinical ecologist found that Walter had become sensitised not only to chemicals, but to many common foods and other substances that he inhaled. He modified his lifestyle even further. Then about two and a half years after the original incident in the office, he suffered a coronary. His family doctor, by now very familiar with his problems, blamed Walter's coronary on the stress induced by all the intolerances from which he was suffering.

From the first day, Walter never had any doubt that all his symptoms originated from his first exposure to a massive dose of the chemical that was used to fumigate the managing director's office at work, which he quickly identified as dichlorvos. Many of his symptoms are typical of acute dichlorvos poisoning. To rub salt into his wounds, he had to subject himself to examination by a number of doctors before he qualified for an invalid pension, and some of them seemed to

delight in insinuating that he was making the whole thing up.

Ironically the country town that Walter selected when he opted to get as far away as possible from the polluted city turned out to be in the centre of one of the most pesticide-contaminated regions of the whole of Australia. He was forced to move on again.

As I write, nearly six years later, he is still fighting for recognition that the dichlorvos made him the man he now is, so that at the least he might get some financial compensation. Those who will have to pay that compensation and who are most anxious to ensure that no precedent is set are vigorously opposing him. He is a good fighter, but it seems set to become a long war of attrition.

The difference may be academic for the victim, but it should be sufficient to require that the most stringent controls be in place before these substances are released into the atmosphere, usually by people who have no real understanding of their dangers. The regulations and recommendations may exist on paper, but they certainly are not followed in real life. As to actually taking them into one's home and using them near children, it defies credibility!

It ought to be a universally acknowledged scandal that there isn't a single animal species on the planet, including humans, that is free of traces of DDT. Instead, entire populations, even in highly developed, highly educated countries such as Australia, have been gulled into believing that broadcasting these chemicals carelessly across the countryside is a necessary and acceptable price that must be paid for living in a nation that relies heavily on its primary production. Some organisations even imply that it is almost unpatriotic to criticise the chemicals that produce the crops that made Australia great!

It is bad enough that up to 64 per cent of pesticides applied to wheat may end up unaltered in bread; or that sometimes 20 per cent of pesticides being sprayed on crops never even reach their target, but are carried away on the wind and escape to play havoc far away; or that residues of pesticides that are known to be carcinogenic are being found in human tissue in increasingly large amounts in people sometimes living far away from the site of the nearest spraying — without turning it into a national virtue!

The populations of many towns in the areas that are being most heavily treated with pesticides are committing slow suicide. The Coffs Harbour region of New South Wales has become notorious for the high incidence of birth deformities, possibly linked to a very high usage of pesticides in the area. Instead of a priority program to ensure that the risk is immediately removed until the truth can be established, the authorities rely on statistical arguments to make their point that nothing has as yet been proved positively and that, until it has, nothing will be done to ban or even restrict the use of pesticides that are falling on innocent people in the town.

Yet it is a statistical fact that in 1984 mothers living near Coffs Harbour gave birth to babies with an incidence of deformity that was six times the national average. It is also a fact that this same region is intensively sprayed with extremely toxic pesticides, which drift over the area, and some of these are known to result in birth deformities in laboratory animals. The pesticides are sprayed aerially and from the ground.

Preliminary investigation showed that seven of the twenty-two chemicals regularly used in the Coffs Harbour region have been proved to be either mutagenic, meaning that they cause genetic damage, or teratogenic, meaning that they damage the unborn child.

In particular, a new fungicide came under suspicion. Doctors have also linked the pesticide smog to which residents of the area are exposed to hundreds of cases of gastric illness for which there was no other explanation.

In 1986, it was announced that Coffs Harbour would become Australia's first "pregnancy control area", with every pregnant woman in the district being closely monitored both before and after the birth of her baby. Hopefully this will pin down the cause so irrefutably that neither local authorities nor the pesticide manufacturers and suppliers can any longer rely on "lack of firm evidence" to deny responsibility. In the meantime, the spraying goes on!

AERIAL SPRAY — DEAD BABIES ■

A case in New South Wales will illustrate the effects of this reckless spraying. Similar cases occur wherever aerial spraying goes on and will continue to occur, in spite of token legislation now being proposed by a number of state governments to restrict the distance from homes where aerial spraying can be carried out while the inhabitants are still in their homes.

The pilot of an agricultural aircraft was spraying the OP Folimat to rid a property of wasps. He had put down the same spray the previous year. At one corner of the property there was a house which the pilot assumed belonged to the farmer, who knew what the pilot was spraying and so would be well out of the way. He therefore made no attempt to switch off the spray as he passed low over the house. What he did not know was that this house had been subdivided from the farm and that a woman lived there.

By ill coincidence, the woman was in the house on both occasions when the aircraft was spraying; and on both occasions she was three months pregnant. Both babies died, one at birth, the other soon after birth.

In the uproar that followed as everyone tried to defend themselves when the tragedy became known, the unhappy woman actually found herself being accused of "sitting on her husband's tractor while he sprayed". When the truth emerged, it transpired that her husband didn't own a tractor, didn't have enough land to spray and never used chemicals anyway.

Most people are not recklessly stupid if they have the information on which to base a decision. Many children born today will suffer health problems all their lives, not because their parents were careless or irresponsible, but because they were not given enough information to allow them to make an informed decision on how to protect themselves. They are the victims of the ongoing pesticide dispute, which will inevitably end up with these dangerous products being as roundly condemned as cigarettes and asbestos are today. In the meantime there will be many victims of intolerance and much suffering.

SPORTSDAY IN TASMANIA ■

Another example, typical of Australian officialdom's response to pesticides and herbicides, is the use of a pesticide called diazinon, which is sold under a number of trade names, including Diazamin, Basudin and Gesapon. In its warning to users of diazinon, the US Environment Protection Agency states, "Do not breathe spray, mist or dust. Do not get into eyes, skin or on clothing. Do not use on humans, or allow people to enter the treated area until the spray has dried. Keep out of bodies of water and do not use near or in water that will be used for any purpose by humans or livestock." In Australia diazinon is used as a sheep dip!

Early in 1986, DDT was sprayed on a council oval in Tasmania shortly before a school was due to hold its athletics day there. A number of parents who found out about the spraying were understandably alarmed by the potential danger and asked the state's Registrar of Pesticides and Herbicides if there was reason for concern.

The registrar's office replied that it was perfectly safe — "You could scoop the sprayed grass up in handfuls and eat it." The answer seemed so improbable that the parents then asked their local member of parliament to investigate further. Before they received a reply, the athletics day took place, with many parents accepting the word of the Registrar of Pesticides and Herbicides' office and allowing their children to play on the grass.

Two days later a letter arrived at the school from the Department of Education, which had by then heard from the Department of Health. At all times, the letter cautioned, children must wear shoes and socks to protect them from the effects of the DDT and under no circumstances must they sit on the ground or allow any bare skin to come into contact with the grass.

Fatalities from acute poisoning by DDT, unlike the OPs, are rare, but it has been proved to cause cancer in test animals and it is associated with both brain and nerve damage in human beings. It accumulates in the body fat of humans and it has been found in significant and sometimes dangerous levels in mothers' milk. Yet the office of a state Registrar of Pesticides and Herbicides, the people's watchdog, can say, "You could scoop the sprayed grass up in handfuls and eat it"!

AUSTRALIA — THE DUMPING GROUND ■

Laying claim to be among the deadliest of all the chlorinated hydrocarbons are the so-called "-drins" — aldrin, dieldrin and endrin, all three acutely toxic, but also posing serious chronic dangers. They have produced cancer in test animals as well as adversely affecting human reproduction.

All the -drins are associated with birth defects in animal studies, and endrin and dieldrin are embryo-toxic in animals, causing spontaneous abortion. They are also environmentally very persistent (residues of aldrin remain for up to seventeen years) and can be found in rainwater, ground and surface water, soil and food crops.

In normal concentrations, like DDT, they kill birds and fish, as well as beneficial insects and the predators of the pest they are supposed to be wiping out. Endrin has been classified as "supertoxic", the worst rating that a chemical to which people are exposed can be given. With aldrin, it is linked with brain and nerve damage in humans.

It requires only a few drops to kill a healthy adult, and both aldrin and dieldrin have been suspended from use in agriculture in the United States since 1974 (aldrin is considered to be a human carcinogen in the United States). In spite of this, they have continued to be marketed actively by their manufacturers throughout the Third World, as well as in the handful of so-called developed nations which continue to allow themselves to be used as a dumping ground for them. These include Australia.

Aldrin and dieldrin in combination (as they often are) are so highly mobile that once they are released into the environment, their dispersal is uncontrollable. The World Bank has recommended that these pesticides should never be used at all, yet aldrin is still widely used in Australia for termite control and is sprayed under new houses, often compulsorily before local councils will allow a building to be lived in, and then resprayed annually. Endrin is even used on crops in some states.

BRAIN TUMOURS IN CHILDREN ■

Two other organochlorines that the US Environmental Protection Agency took steps to phase out in 1974 for all domestic and agricultural uses are chlordane and the closely related heptachlor.

They are now banned in the USA. So concerned are they, for example, in the state of California, that at government expense the US Air Force has moved every family from houses that might be contaminated with chlordane after being sprayed against termites.

Both chemicals have long been suspected of causing cancer in humans (they are known to be carcinogenic in animals), and there is strong suspicion that they are associated with leukaemia in humans. There is an association between both pre- and post-natal exposure to mixtures of chlordane and heptachlor, and the development of malignant brain tumours in children. The World Bank has recommended that they should never be used as pesticides. They persist for a long time in the environment and they are highly toxic to beneficial insects, fish and other wildlife. They also accumulate in human fat tissues and can be transferred across the placenta from mother to unborn child.

In Australia, the federal Department of Health says these chemicals are safe if the directions are followed, an absurd proviso when they are frequently used by people who are demonstrably careless about their own safety, let alone anyone else's, and who work without close supervision. Even if the directions were scrupulously followed on every occasion, most responsible governments have decreed that the chemicals are far too hazardous to be used for almost any application.

The principal manufacturer, Velsicol Chemical Corp. of the United States, markets them vigorously wherever they can still legally be used, regardless of the US government's restrictions and the warnings of the World Bank and the World Health Organisation. Among the countries where they are still sold are the majority of Third World nations and Australia.

THE PROBLEMS OF A DAIRY FARMER ■

Jim is a dairy farmer in Kempsey, in northern New South Wales, who became not only a victim of heptachlor, but of the kind of bureaucratic bungling that makes pesticides so hazardous in Australia.

In 1983, he was faced with a weevil problem in his lucerne paddocks, 15 hectares of which provided him with the feed he needed to keep his seventy milking cows in top condition. The most recent recommendation he could find from the state Department of Agriculture for the northern coastal district where he lived was to use heptachlor, so he bought enough to control the weevils according to the recommended dose.

When he got the heptachlor back to the farm, he read the label carefully and decided that half this recommended rate would be sufficient to control his particular weevil problem. He applied it correctly and during that winter his award-winning Jerseys and Friesians grazed the lucerne, which was now free of weevil.

The first hint of the disaster that was about to strike him came in September of that same year, when a routine factory test of his cow's milk detected unacceptable levels of heptachlor residues. It made no sense to him: all that he had done was use heptachlor in strict accordance with the instructions issued by the department — in fact at only half the recommended strength — yet he was being told that the milk was unfit for human consumption.

He immediately closed off the 15 hectares of lucerne that had been sprayed. This itself posed serious problems because he had no other paddocks of good quality for his cattle to graze in. Milk production dropped by between 10 and 20 per cent.

He also had in his shed 4000 bales of lucerne hay that was contaminated with heptachlor and so unsellable for any purpose, as well as being unfit for feeding to his cows. Much more worrying was that his 2-year-old son must also have been drinking unacceptable levels of heptachlor for months in his milk. Jim lost three full days' milk production before the heptachlor left the cows' systems and his milk was pronounced safe again.

Just how damaging to dairy farmers this kind of incident can be was shown soon after Jim's experience, when eight other New South Wales dairy farmers had their milk and herds impounded for several weeks, this time because of dieldrin residues in the milk. It had been acquired by feeding the cows legally bought grain that had been illegally treated with dieldrin. Consumer milk sales promptly plummeted by 20 per cent.

Jim's problems were far from over. His initial shock turned to anger at what he understandably saw as the injustice of what had occurred. Why hadn't the department warned him? Why hadn't the manufacturer, Velsicol Chemical Corp., or its agents warned farmers? Above all, why wasn't its use banned on pastures for grazing livestock, if there was a risk even when the chemical was applied at half the recommended rate?

NEVER USE ON CROPS — EXCEPT IN AUSTRALIA ■

What Jim found out as he delved deeper only increased his fury, even if it should have come as no surprise to those who deal regularly with the agrochemical companies and the bureaucrats charged with controlling their activities.

In 1975, eight years previously, Department of Agriculture officers had indeed been briefed on the dangers of heptachlor residues in milk, meat and eggs. The warning read:

> *Heptachlor is chemically and biologically similar to other members of the cyclodiene group (of chemicals) including dieldrin. It is even more intractable than dieldrin and is translocated from the soil by quite a number of plants, giving rise to residues which can persist in animal fat and can be excreted in milk for particularly long periods.*
>
> *Care is needed when heptachlor is used for the treatment of seed or soil in the establishment of crops, lucerne, legumes and maize. Under no circumstances should it be used for the treatment of pasture or fodder crops.*

Yet for four years after the warning was given, the Department of Agriculture printed agronomic recommendations for the New South Wales northern coast that suggested "on lucerne, incorporate heptachlor for white-fringed weevil control". After that, the only notice that the department sent to farmers concerning the potential dangers of heptachlor use was in May 1984, six months after Jim began to complain. But the situation was even worse than that.

Australia is unusual in that all state Departments of Agriculture are not only responsible for advising farmers how to use chemicals, but are also in charge of approving which chemicals can be used and of authorising registration. Inevitably, because of their resources and skills, they have to rely heavily on data provided by someone else, usually the manufacturer. Each state sets its own rules, so that the deadly endrin, for instance, is permitted in Victoria but banned (as it is in almost all developed nations) in the states adjoining Victoria, which are still exposed to large doses of it as it drifts across the borders on the wind.

In October 1981, as part of the process of restricting the use of organochlorines, a pesticide order was issued by the New South Wales Department of Agriculture banning the use of heptachlor in the state, for everything except pest control in houses and other buildings. Any other use became illegal.

Incredibly, however, the regulation apparently placed no obligation on anyone to attach warning notices to any of the chemicals or fertiliser preparations that contained heptachlor. What happened many times was that chemical suppliers continued to sell heptachlor, or heptachlor-containing products, to farmers with a label that stated that the chemical was registered for use in crops and lucerne, when in reality it was a banned and dangerous substance. Jim purchased heptachlor with such a label on the package.

A single general notice, which made no mention at all of heptachlor or the commonly used heptachlor-containing chemical G5+, was distributed by the department in 1983 (still eight years after the original warning of the dangers). However, it was not until the memorandum of May 1984, after Jim's disaster, that a specific warning was sent to farmers. After that, with the stable door long since opened, fresh labels giving heptachlor bans were attached to the products.

The explanation of the New South Wales Department of Agriculture to the State Ombudsman, called in by Jim, was almost immoral in its implications. It explained that it had not carried out a program warning farmers of the withdrawal and dangers of heptachlor because "it was considered that heavy emphasis on its danger or misuse would have played into the hands of the local environmental lobby".

Instead the Department of Agriculture chose to leave the farmers in ignorance; it put at risk their families and particularly their children and pregnant wives; and it exposed the sprayers, and everyone else who unwittingly came into contact with the spray, to a high risk of being poisoned. All this was in addition to the financial loss that Jim and certainly others actually suffered or were exposed to.

At the time of writing, Jim too has set off on the lonely and expensive road to secure some kind of justice and compensation.

SUSPICIONS IS NEVER ENOUGH ■

In Australia, as in some of the most exploited Third World countries, suspicion is not enough for a product to be banned, or even in many cases meaningfully restricted.

Even when the dangers are known and recognised, the use is allowed of products that are widely banned or restricted elsewhere. These are dangers that affect not only the users: the spray is carried away on the wind, the residues remain in food, and the chemically sensitive and intolerant are exposed to the full spectrum of ecological illness.

Parathion, a non-specific insecticide that is widely used on crops such as tobacco and cotton, as well as on fruit and food crops, is just such a chemical.

Parathion is so poisonous that the World Health Organisation believes that it may be responsible for half of all the pesticide poisonings in the world today. In Central America it accounts for 80 per cent of all poisoning cases. It is so toxic that a teaspoonful spilt on the skin may be fatal to humans.

According to records held by the Environmental Protection Agency in the United States, between 1966 and 1980 thousands of people were poisoned by parathion in that country alone, of whom "at least several hundred" have died. Yet in the USA control is far more rigorous than in Australia. When the use of parathion is permitted at all, no worker, for example, is allowed to enter a field that has been treated with the chemical sooner than forty-eight hours after the spraying.

In Australia, parathion is registered for use in all states against aphids, and in Victoria and New South Wales for use on fruit trees. Personal protection is often scorned.

WHEN THE EXPERTS LIE ■

Because research is so voluminous and complex, most countries rely heavily on information provided by manufacturers to determine whether a product should be approved for marketing. This implies a large measure of trust in the manufacturers, but how justified is that trust? And how much importance can we attach to the data on which governments base their decisions?

There are many reasons why taking the word of the chemicals industry that a product is safe is likely to lead down a very dark and dangerous path. Just a handful of these reasons include the corporate philosophy that allowed asbestos to be so widely used without warning to either workers or users of its dangers, when the chemicals industry had known for more than half a century that it was highly carcinogenic; the continued marketing of thalidomide for a full year after it was known to cause birth defects; the persistent efforts of the tobacco companies, even in a so-called enlightened country such as Australia, to trap the young, and particularly young women, into becoming addicted to nicotine to ensure their next generation of consumers; and the proven falsification of more than 20,000 tests to allow expensively developed chemical products to get on to the market.

The *Journal of the Royal Society of Medicine*, in an October 1985 article, noted that the pesticide industry's constant assurances that "careful and extensive testing results in a rarity of significant pesticide residues in our food" is simply not true.

A 1984 report from the National Research Council in the United States carefully documented the lack of toxicity data on most commercial chemicals. It stated that because of inadequate scientific testing and data, complete toxicity and health exposure assessments are possible for only about 10 per cent of pesticides and 5 per cent of food additives in commercial use in the USA — and US testing is considered to be superior to that of any other country in the world! In Australia, most of the thousands of commercially important chemicals in use have not been thoroughly tested at all.

One of the most important testing facilities in the United States, which acted for many of the major chemical manufacturers, was Industrial Bio-Test Laboratory. So important have the findings of Industrial Bio-Test been, that data from Canada and Malaysia, for instance, indicate that more than a quarter of all the pesticides registered for use in those countries were licensed exclusively on the basis of IBT's tests, and the number in Australia is probably just as high.

Executives of Industrial Bio-Test Laboratory, however, have now been convicted of falsifying the results of more than 22,000 critical safety tests performed for their clients. When a team of US federal inspectors, alerted by some very distinguished scientists who had become increasingly suspicious of some of the laboratory's findings, arrived at IBT's offices, they were met by the company's president, who said blandly, "Gentlemen, there has been an unfortunate misunderstanding: we accidentally destroyed all our records last night".

There is no practical way in which Australian health authorities can hope to establish whether the tests that were carried out on many of the products approved by Industrial Bio-Test were genuine or phoney. Neither is there any possible way that the Australian National Health and Medical Research Council, underfunded and grossly overworked, can begin to evaluate them. Just as alarming was the observation of one of the

American inspectors after the trial of Industrial Bio-Test executives, that "what happened here is not at all exceptional".

INDEFENSIBLE PRACTICES ▮
Sometimes manufacturers are caught off guard and shown in a most compromising way to be capable of behaving just as appallingly as most of us suspect in our blackest moments. Ciba-Geigy was hoist with its own petard when an internal memorandum from the company's Australian technical regulatory manager to the director of agriculture was leaked to the *Sydney Morning Herald*.

The memorandum, whose authenticity was not denied by the company, discussed eight products and activities "which Ciba-Geigy Australia would have the greatest difficulty defending". It was no exaggeration. The contents make it very difficult for Ciba-Geigy ever again to claim that its primary concern is always the safety of its products.

For example, the memorandum confirmed that the company had failed to destroy crops in plots that were used to test illegal chemicals. It also confirmed that monitoring procedures for the dangerous chemical chlordimeform, which causes cancer, were conducted up to forty-eight hours after workers had been exposed to the chemical, instead of within twelve hours, the maximum time elapse permitted in order to establish whether any harm has been caused to them.

The memo discussed a cattle spray called Tifatol, which contained a solvent, Dutrex oil, that had been proved to be a carcinogen in laboratory animals. It noted that "In 1979 we agreed with [the New South Wales Technical Committee on Veterinary Drugs] to replace this solvent, but after an early unsuccessful attempt to develop a new formulation, we dropped the project". Ciba-Geigy went on using the Dutrex oil, in spite of being specifically ordered to change it and in spite of knowing of its potential for causing cancer. Seven years later nothing had been done. Either the Technical Committee on Veterinary Drugs was ineffectual or had no inclination to force Ciba-Geigy to act; or perhaps it had no information.

Ciba-Geigy was no stranger to controversy over the chemical chlordimeform. Earlier it had been discovered performing tests on teenage Egyptians — a new twist to the exploitation of

Third World countries — to determine whether chlordimeform (whose most common trade name is Galecron) affected humans in the same way as laboratory animals, in which it was known to cause cancer. It had already been shown to cause bladder damage in humans.

WHAT HAPPENS TO THE CHILDREN? ■

There is still much that is not known about pesticides. We have no real idea, for example, what the long-term effect of pesticides is on the non-human organisms that become their victims. By living weight, soil organisms — the creatures that live under the ground — account for half of all the living matter on earth, yet the effects of pesticides on them are almost completely unresearched. Earthworm populations are known to be decimated by most carbamate pesticides, such as Baygon, Baysol, Ficon and Mensuorol, but the significance of this within the ecology is still unknown. It *must* be significant

Like OPs, the carbamates work by inhibiting cholinesterase, and the toxicity of some of them, already very high, has been shown to increase by a factor of 6.5 when they are ingested or inhaled by laboratory animals on a low-protein diet. It is a finding of great significance, because carbamates are extensively used in Third World countries where malnutrition is endemic, and in Australia where frequent users are Aboriginals and poor whites, many of whom are often poorly nourished.

Studies of the specific effect of pesticides on children and other vulnerable groups, including the elderly or those suffering from disease as well as malnutrition, are not required before a chemical can be released and in consequence are rarely done.

There is also a complication that some pesticides, already highly toxic, turn into completely different poisons, sometimes becoming even more toxic, when they are in the presence of other chemicals that are not necessarily themselves pesticides.

Parathion, for example, deadly in its own right, becomes four times more toxic when it comes into contact with oxygen. Similarly, the toxicity of malathion is greatly enhanced when it is combined with a common industrial plasticiser, TOTP, even when the TOTP exposure comes two weeks after that with malathion.

The opportunities for this kind of interaction may not be

many, but how many of those working with plasticisers are even aware that accidental exposure to this popular pesticide in their own gardens, a fortnight later, exposes them to great potential danger?

THE KILLER UNDER THE FLOOR ■

One of the most alarming uses of pesticides that we are only too well aware of, and which causes interminable and often very debilitating intolerance reactions, is the routine spraying of homes. Many local authorities require all new buildings to be sprayed, usually with one of the chlorinated hydrocarbons such as aldrin, dieldrin, chlordane or heptachlor. Afterwards spraying takes place at regular intervals, regardless of whether it is needed or not.

The Shell Company has stated that some of its most frequently used pesticides persist for up to thirty years, particularly when the soil under the house has a high clay content, which prevents the agent being leached away. In consequence, some of the most persistent chemicals in the environment, known to be carcinogenic and mutagenic, and causing untold misery and illness to those who are chemically sensitive, are a part of our home environment.

According to the standards laid down by the Standards Association of Australia, 200 gallons of chemical are routinely sprayed before the floor goes down in new homes, and again the standard makes no allowance for different soil types, so that in clay areas, the poison stays on the surface of the ground. Not only are many tradesmen, and particularly the pesticide operators, heavily exposed, but so are all the inhabitants of the house, their visitors and sometimes their next-door neighbours.

It is not necessary to go underneath the house to be exposed, although the risk there is clearly higher because of the danger of skin penetration. The active ingredient is usually highly volatile and seeps into the rest of the home. If there is carpet between the dirt under the house and the rest of the building, then this too becomes contaminated and continues to outgas for years.

There have been countless cases of chemical poisoning reported by pesticide sprayers and by tradesmen who have to go to work after the spray has been put down. Common symptoms include headache, nausea, double vision and sometimes collapse.

These symptoms are so frequently experienced by those who work with pesticides that they are often considered an unavoidable part of the job.

One woman in Melbourne felt so desperate after her house had been sprayed with an organochlorine (a feeling of impending doom is a common symptom), that she spent a night in a tent in her backyard to get away from the fumes. In the end, she had to leave her house.

Pesticide firms rarely ask people to leave their homes for more than half a day after spraying, yet the exposure can continue for years. One of the largest operators uses an ether-based chlordane, spraying huge quantities underneath the floors of homes — indeed spraying anything likely to be affected by soft-wood borers: pantry shelves, pianos, kitchen sideboards, even wooden toilet seats; and because many people mistakenly associate a pleasant smelling substance with a safe substance, the chlordane is scented.

THIS ONE'S NOT POISONOUS! ■

Australian researchers Linda Cawcutt and Catherine Watson, whose book *Pesticides — the New Plague* should be mandatory reading for every Australian, reported a case of a pest control company that sprayed a house with between 200 and 300 gallons of an aldrin–dieldrin mixture.

The house had a slab foundation, so the operator pulled back the carpet, drilled holes in the concrete and then ran a hose through the house from his truck. What he intended to do was to pressure-impregnate under the house. What he didn't know was that there was only a 12 millimetre gap under the slab. Immediately, the pesticide blew back and the house was flooded with enormous quantities of this carcinogenic brew.

Instead of ordering the family to get out of the house immediately and stay out until a certificate had been granted that it was safe to live in, the operator told the occupants that they had no cause to worry. There was no danger, he assured them — the chemical could be washed out with water.

In fact, as they found out later, both aldrin and dieldrin are insoluble in water and need solvents to wash them out. They contacted the Health Department, who sent a doctor round, who turned out to be as wrong, and even more foolish, than the operator had been. He said the chemical was neither too bad, nor too widespread, and then, presumably to reassure them, crouched down on the floor and did a taste test of the poison watched by the occupants. It was about as sensible as looking for a gas leak with a lighted match.

Still unconvinced in spite of this bizarre performance, they retained an independent laboratory to test the pesticide levels in the house. Apart from confirming that the house was a potential death trap in its present condition, the laboratory showed that the doctor had ingested a 3.7 per cent mixture of the pesticide, more than seven times the maximum safe level. He could easily have ascertained that aldrin–dieldrin had been known since 1959 to attack the central nervous system of humans, and that it is a proven carcinogen and mutagen.

Later Shell, the manufacturer of the chemical, agreed to help in the clean-up and sealing of the slab, but there will be traces of the poisons for twenty years and more.

Those who live most dangerously with these pesticides are building inspectors, who spend much of their working lives crawling around recently sprayed houses, sniffing to see whether the work has been carried out. It is not surprising that many have become fearful of dying of leukaemia or cancer, and get out of this hazardous occupation at the earliest opportunity.

AGENT ORANGE IN YOUR GARDEN ■

Herbicides kill weeds and in the process kill a great deal more as well. Anyone who had doubts about their potential for disaster had those doubts cast aside after seeing the devastation wrought by Agent Orange in the Vietnam War, not only on the environment, but on tens of thousands of hapless humans.

Agent Orange was a dirty concoction that included the phenoxy compound hormone weed-killers, 2,4,5-T (2,4,5-trichlorophenoxy acetic acid) and 2,4-D (2,4-dichlorophenoxyacetic acid). It was particularly dirty because of the abnormally high content of dioxin, an unavoidable by-product in the manufacture of both these herbicides, which is one of the most deadly and carcinogenic chemicals known.

The herbicide 2,4,5-T is particularly effective against woody weeds (it is widely used for the control of blackberries); 2,4-D destroys broad-leaved plants and most leafy weeds, making them ideal in combination for defoliating great tracts of forest and jungle in South-East Asia.

Apart from the danger of the dioxin, 2,4,5-T is of particular concern to humans because it crosses the placental membrane, so that unborn babies are vulnerable to all the damage that the chemical can inflict on the mother. Hardly any safer, 2,4-D is not just sprayed but hosed on vegetation by many council employees, who rarely wear proper protective clothing, never advise people when they are coming to spray and certainly never inquire about the possibility that pregnant women may be within range of the drift.

The herbicide 2,4,5-T is marketed under at least twenty-five different trade names, and 2,4-D under more than forty. Although both are embryo-toxic, foeto-toxic, teratogenic and carcinogenic, they are freely available in shops and supermarkets in Australia and there are no meaningful restrictions as to their use.

They are frequently implicated in chemical intolerance which may quickly become masked after even a brief exposure to a sufficiently large dose, and symptoms are likely to include nausea, aching legs, headaches, shaking and sometimes numbness in the lower limbs, followed by depression and crying, and a burning sensation in the throat.

WORKERS AT RISK ■

Agricultural and council workers are most at risk and most in need of protection against their own carelessness and ignorance by their employers. Some may not have had the level of education that allows them to fully comprehend the dangers of many of the products they are using; some are aware in an abstract kind of way, yet can't be bothered to take the necessary precautions; and some are just uninformed.

Perhaps there is something perversely odd in the Australian make-up that makes it seem macho to deliberately flaunt regulations even when they are there for our own protection; or to be seen exposing themselves to danger. As many will surely learn, there is nothing very manly about acquiring the cancer that may surface perhaps fifteen or twenty years later.

Never, incidentally, under any circumstances, burn the empty packet of a herbicide that contains 2,4,5-T or 2,4-D (or any other pesticide or herbicide for that matter) because they change their chemical form when they are subjected to extremes of heat and become even more dangerous. This heating can occur during manufacture or prolonged storage, or unsuspectingly during waste disposal by burning and, very dangerously, during bushfires in areas which have recently been sprayed with it.

On the subject of burning, by the way, treated logs, such as Koppers logs, may be impregnated with arsenic which is extremely dangerous if it is burned. Never burn the off-cuts of green-coloured treated logs, even on an outdoor bonfire; and never under any circumstances inside the house.

If you come across roadside spraying of noxious weeds, or pests, close the car windows and any direct air vents immediately, and if you can see the spray being blown back across the road, turn the car around and drive the other way. The alternative is that your car will fill up with the spray molecules (there may be no colour or smell to give away their presence), and you will finish the journey breathing in chemicals that will include dioxin if the spray happens to be 2,4,5-T or 2,4-D.

Interestingly, in the United States 2,4,5-T had been all but drummed off the market by public pressure before it was officially withdrawn. Hopefully the same thing will happen in Australia with both 2,4,5-T and 2,4-D before many more victims of their deadly molecules have to suffer.

One of the most senior Australian public servants charged with overseeing the use of pesticides and herbicides said publicly not long ago that critics of 2,4,5-T and 2,4-D spraying programs were quite wrong in linking these herbicides with the high rate of birth abnormalities in people frequently exposed to them, even though both had long been known to be teratogens. "Such abnormalities", he said, "could equally well occur in a group living in the vicinity of a pizza parlour or a telephone box."

Earlier, he had declared that the whole herbicide controversy had been drummed up by the marijuana growers, afraid that their crops would be wiped out by spraying.

I think we still have a long, long way to go.

26 Testing for Chemical Intolerance

Establishing the source of chemical intolerance poses a different set of problems. In food testing, a relatively long time is needed for the fast and the individual challenges to identify the problem foods, but at the end of the test, they have usually been pinpointed. Relief from the symptoms and illnesses may then just be a question of avoiding those foods.

With chemicals, on the other hand, the test to establish intolerance takes a very short time and requires no fast at all, but it can require weeks and sometimes months of painstaking detective work to identify the source of the outgassing, so that it can be eliminated from the patient's environment. Even then, complete avoidance may not be possible, and the doctor must resort to safe desensitising drops.

Testing, for example, may reveal a strong positive reaction to aldehydes, which immediately puts formaldehyde under suspicion. But formaldehyde is so pervasive, turning up in anything from crease-resistant clothes, vitamin A and paper (to improve wet-strength), to shampoos, deodorants and wood veneers, that detecting each source of formaldehyde outgassing can be difficult and frustrating.

The history the doctor takes when he first sees the patient and the detailed questionnaire that must be filled in (Appendixes III and IV) establish whether chemicals are likely to be involved in intolerance reactions. Chemical intolerance is usually found in association with food intolerance, so that food testing may still have to be carried out.

The chemical questionnaire takes patients through a long list of chemicals to which they might regularly be exposed. They are asked whether they like the smell of a chemical, have no feelings one way or the other about it, or positively dislike it, even to the point of being made physically sick, or left with a headache after exposure.

Liking a smell does not necessarily mean that people will

not be affected by it, any more than liking a food means that it is always a safe food for that person. If addiction is involved, as it usually is, there is every chance that the food responsible for the unpleasant reactions is one that is enjoyed. If patients mark up two or three chemicals, on the other hand, that make them nauseous, then almost always, they have a quite significant chemical problem.

HOW WE TEST FOR CHEMICAL INTOLERANCE ■

Unlike in food testing, it is not necessary to fast before the test, although no foods or drinks are taken during it. Fasting appears to have no effect on whether an acute reaction follows exposure to the chemical. In the majority of cases, it is not even necessary to have a chemically free environment to conduct the tests, although it is certainly desirable for the air to be as clean as possible, to eliminate any extraneous out-gassing that might complicate the results.

Only in the most intractable cases of severe chemical intolerance to multiple substances, usually where patients are so affected that they cannot be freed of symptoms for long enough to carry out the test, is the Environment Control Unit needed. In the unit, there are virtually no chemicals, even to the point of excluding synthetic sheets and felt-tip pens. Every aspect of the environment is controlled in the unit, from the air to the food and the drinking water. Testing booths are used where the patient sits and inhales chemicals as they are released into the booth. The patient's reactions and symptoms are noted by staff watching from outside. The chemicals are then removed by exhaust fans.

For the great majority of patients, the procedure is much simpler. The doctor places one or two drops of the chemical to be tested, at a predetermined dilution, under the patient's tongue and then waits for a short time — rarely longer than ten minutes — to see what develops. The drops have no taste, no smell and produce no reactions at all unless there is chemical sensitivity.

The same results would be obtained by injecting the drops, but putting them under the tongue causes less discomfort to the patient, is usually faster and has no disadvantages. Because a chemical cannot be altered by digestion, as foods can, all that matters is introducing them into the body in some way. It is irrelevant whether they get there by ingestion, injection, inhalation or being held under the tongue, which is one of the fastest ways of getting them into the circulation.

The patient first swallows, to remove any saliva from the mouth, then places his tongue on the roof of the mouth as a single drop is placed under the tongue. The tongue is kept on the roof of the mouth for thirty seconds, then rested for a further ninety seconds. The patient swallows only after two minutes. If there is to be a reaction, it may have already started before the two minutes have passed.

The main reason why the reaction is much faster than in food testing is that the molecules go straight into the bloodstream, unlike the protein in food which has to make its way down the gastrointestinal tract before it is digested and enters the bloodstream.

Although there are hundreds, even thousands, of possible causes of chemical intolerance in most people's lives, testing is not complicated, because most chemicals implicated in chemical intolerance fall into a surprisingly small number of broad groups. It is necessary to test only a handful of chemicals to cover the spectrum of perhaps 90 per cent of those most commonly implicated in intolerance. The drops that we use for testing are preparations of stock chemicals of these main groups. A negative result means that there is probably no need to look further at any of the chemicals within that broad group.

Phenols, alcohols and aldehydes cover many of the most common sources of trouble. Phenols and alcohols essentially bridge all the petrochemical derivatives, the coal-tar derivatives, petrol, gas, plastic, newsprint and so on. I usually add tobacco drops and, for patients from the country, any pesticides and herbicides that are regularly sprayed in the region where they live. Even if the patient doesn't know, local authorities can provide this information.

With most of the herbicide and pesticide sprays, there is an all-or-nothing response: either the patient reacts, or he doesn't and the dose often seems to have minimal effect on the reaction. With other chemicals, however, such as phenols and alcohols, the reaction is much more variable, and the level of exposure and the time that the patient is exposed to the outgassing largely determine the severity of the symptoms.

We take account of this in chemical testing by the use of what is known as serial dilution end-point titration (SDET), a longwinded name for a technique that is familiar to many patients being treated for true allergy.

SERIAL DILUTION END-POINT TITRATION ■

In SDET, a stock solution of a substance, in this case a chemical group, is progressively (or serially) diluted in a predetermined way, and different dilutions are then given to the patient to establish the precise dose (the end-point) that triggers the symptoms. (Titration refers to the actual process of progressively diluting the stock solution.)

The stock solution of a chemical is strong enough to cause a toxic (or poisonous) effect in its own right. The dilutions, on the other hand, are of a strength that affect only hypersensitive people. With phenol, for example, the stock is 0.4 per cent phenol, as a dilution with water; with formaldehyde it is 40 per cent; and alcohol mixtures (methyl, ethyl, propyl, isopropyl and butyl) 50 per cent. (Even though initially we normally test only for main groups of chemicals, it is possible to test specifically for any of the individuals within those groups, as for formaldehyde within the main aldehyde group and, frequently, for car exhausts and diesel fumes. I often test for chlorine.)

Dilution 1 is one-fifth of the stock solution; dilution 2 is one-fifth of dilution 1 (or 1/25 of the stock), and so on, as listed below.

DILUTIONS AS FRACTIONS OF STOCK SOLUTION

Dilution 1	1/5
Dilution 2	1/25
Dilution 3	1/125
Dilution 4	1/625
Dilution 5	1/3125
Dilution 6	1/15,625
Dilution 7	1/78,125
Dilution 8	1/390,625
Dilution 9	1/1,953,125

Dilution 9 is normally as far down as you need to go, with patients suffering reactions from chemicals at dilutions of nearly one two-millionth of the stock solution. But with some exquisitely sensitive individuals, we need to go even further to find the smallest dose that will produce a reaction — down sometimes to dilution 12, which is one 240-millionth of the stock solution!

Dilution 10   1/9,765,625
Dilution 11   1/48,828,125
Dilution 12   1/244,140,625.

What we are aiming to do is to establish the smallest dilution, using this formula, that will bring about a reaction. I normally use dilution 5 as the starting point, although experience of most chemicals measured against the symptoms and signs in the patient may lead me to vary this. (A symptom is the reaction a patient feels subjectively: a sign is a reaction observed by another person.)

The patient's replies to the questionnaire are very relevant to the choice of dilution. The number of "dislike" and "made sick" replies on the questionnaire determines the initial dilution number. For patients suspected of having only mild sensitivity, I begin with dilution 5. If the first dilution produces no response, then I give progressively stronger doses about every ten minutes until I find the one — the end-point — where there is a reaction. On the other hand, if there is a reaction at the first attempt, I wait for the symptoms to pass and then go, perhaps, to dilutions 8 or 9, and work upwards. Each time I place the drop under the patient's tongue and then wait for up to ten minutes for the reaction.

If there is no reaction at dilution 1, the patient is not hypersensitive to that particular chemical. Testing is never taken to stronger than dilution 1 because the stock is toxic in its own right.

No reaction to a test, which means that there is no intolerance, does not automatically rule out a direct reaction to the chemical. Tobacco smoke, for example, can affect almost anyone if there is enough of it, and perhaps produce coughing or a headache.

BECOMING A HOUSE DETECTIVE ■

If an SDET test proves positive, indicating that there may be chemical intolerance to a particular group of chemicals, then we proceed with testing for more specific substances within that group, gradually narrowing the field. At the same time, the patient must search his or her own environment, at home and at work, to try to identify whatever it is that is outgassing and causing the illness or symptoms. It can be a slow and frustrating

TESTING FOR TOBACCO INTOLERANCE

Smokers are challenged to see if they have intolerance reactions as well as direct effects from their habit. They stop smoking for at least three days, preferably for five accompanied by a full five-day fast. Unlike other chemical hypersensitivities, smoking intolerance reactions appear to be heightened by the fast and it is, in any event, an excellent method of beginning to break the addiction.

The test takes one of two forms. The most usual is for patients to chain-smoke three cigarettes of their normal brand within fifteen minutes. It is remarkable how often the symptoms alone are so unpleasant that smokers not only swear that they will break the habit, but weeks later are still keeping their word!

The other method of

testing, which I prefer because I do not think it is desirable to encourage anyone to smoke even three test cigarettes, is with sublingual drops, as with any chemical test for intolerance.

The drops are prepared from a commercially available stock solution and in the case of the ones that I use, from a hundred cigarettes of different brands, at least twenty cigars, and pipe tobacco. The reactions that these drops can produce vary from mild headache in the hypersensitive to violent aggression and frank psychosis. It is essential during the fast and test that the environment is kept entirely free of tobacco smoke, which means there should be no visitors whose breath or clothes smell of tobacco, if that is possible.

process, and the help of a skilled and experienced clinical ecologist is invaluable in drawing up a list of likely suspects.

If the problem is tracked down to the home, it may be possible to resolve it by simply getting rid of a piece of furniture or changing the curtains or bed linen. The problem may be more difficult to resolve if the source is, for example, the gas supply, the carpet in a rented unit, or an unavoidable chemical at work. In such cases, the effects of the chemical can usually be neutralised by taking advantage of a peculiarity of the SDET technique that is not unlike the turn-off reaction in food intolerance.

SDET makes it possible to establish with considerable precision the dose of a particular chemical that is required to trigger a reaction. But it is also possible, by going back in strength one step from the symptom-producing dilution, to produce a dilution that *prevents* symptoms from occurring.

If dilution 4, for example, is the strength required to bring on the symptoms of intolerance to formaldehyde outgassing, then just one or two drops of dilution 5 taken each day under the tongue will prevent those symptoms from occurring at all. Nothing could be simpler.

There is one reason, however, why drops are not automatically used to prevent the symptoms, instead of spending time looking for the source of the trouble: in time their efficacy does weaken. It is also a fact that the drops do not strictly desensitise patients, but only give a type of protection. Even though the symptoms are removed the sensitivity remains, and it may be a stressor. It is better to remove the problem altogether, whenever this is possible, and so get rid of this stressor, rather than merely cover it up.

At the very least, the drops give patients a break from the symptoms, sometimes for years, while they try to find a more permanent solution. They are especially useful for chemicals that are almost impossible to avoid completely, such as car exhaust fumes.

CHEMICAL ADDICTION ■

It is interesting that, once the chemical has been pinpointed, during the initial period of avoidance patients often experience symptoms that are apparently identical to the withdrawal symptoms of food intolerance. This suggests that even with chemicals a significant component of addiction is involved. If this is the case — and I believe that it is — it means that even when people *do* suspect that a substance is causing trouble, they are likely subconsciously to do all that they can to avoid being deprived of it, a commonly encountered difficulty in food addiction.

Once a person has developed intolerance to a particular chemical, just as to a specific food, he or she will always be vulnerable to it. Avoidance will prevent the symptoms and illness, but like most alcoholics, if that person slips back either accidentally or by design, the hypersensitivity to the chemical will return.

In one sense, those who react quickly and unpleasantly to a chemical are fortunate, in that they *know* they are environmentally sensitive and, more importantly, know what they are sensitive to. If every time you go into the garage and start the car, you feel weak in the knees and want to vomit, it doesn't take much imagination to associate the symptoms with the act of starting the car, and then presumably with the petrol fumes.

Usually, however, it is not so simple and, because of masking, the cause and effect are not associated. Typical is the man who potters about with his lawn-mower on Saturday, cleaning the engine with petrol when he isn't actually cutting the grass.

He experiences no reaction at all on Saturday or Sunday, but when he gets to work on Monday, he has an annoying headache that stays with him for much of the morning. Logically he blames this on the fact that he is back at work for another week, or on the sun, or on anything but the truth, which is that he is suffering a masked reaction from his exposure to the petrol fumes two days earlier. With an understanding of ecological illness, he might be able to arrive at the truth: with none, he has no chance, any more than his doctor has if the headache is bad enough to take him to his doctor's surgery for relief.

THE ONLY APPROACH THAT OFFERS HELP ▌

The 1 or 2 per cent of the population who might react to formaldehyde doesn't involve very many people — perhaps 30,000 in Australia. However, were it not for clinical ecology, it is almost certain that these 30,000 people would not get any relief or help at all, and would have to live with their symptoms for the rest of their lives.

What is more, another 1 per cent of the population is likely to suffer from the effects of exposure to petrol, paints and adhesives, as well as from food intolerances and, as we shall see, intolerance of many things around the house. All these people need understanding and knowledge about their problem.

PART FOUR

Some Common Disorders

Although food and chemical intolerance can cause any of the symptoms that any of the organs or tissues are capable of manifesting, there are a few diseases and disorders that should be looked at in a little more detail than the others. They have a special relationship with intolerance, to the point, in most cases, where many clinical ecologists look on them as being primarily ecological illnesses. What most of them have in common is that the prognosis is uniformly bad unless an ecological approach is taken; and uniformly good when they are tackled in this way. They are the disorders that must be treated as ecological illnesses.

Enough has been written about the havoc wrought by the effects of alcohol and alcoholism for no-one to be in any doubt about the gravity of the problem. It is said to be a conservative estimate that the adverse effects of alcohol cost Australia some $3 billion a year, with 600,000 Australians classifiable as alcoholics and as many again as problem drinkers, who are candidates to become the next batch of alcoholics.

On a per capita basis, Australians consume 20 per cent more alcohol than Americans, which puts them twelfth in world ranking, and 47 per cent more than the British. In the early 1980s, Australians were drinking ten litres of alcohol — not alcoholic beverages but straight alcohol — per man, woman and child every year.

The effects of this abuse are well documented and even in the womb a price must be paid. Drinking any amount of alcohol during pregnancy can damage the unborn baby. Heavy drinking at this time can cause mental retardation and slow growth patterns in the baby, or even miscarriage.

The lifespan of alcoholics is 10 to 12 per cent shorter than the average, and 40 per cent of all marriage break-ups result at least in part from problems associated with alcohol. Seventy-three per cent of men who commit violent crimes have been drinking. In the terrible damage that it is doing to the Aboriginal people, alcohol is tearing a whole race apart.

The children of alcoholic mothers as well as fathers are four times more likely than other children to become drunks (alcoholism in women has been on the increase for years). In many cases, even when the children of alcoholics are adopted by non-drinkers from an early age, they still develop the symptoms of alcoholism at a much higher than average rate, suggesting that there is some inherited factor involved.

One estimate is that 140,000 school children aged between 12 and 17 get "very drunk" at least once a month. More than

1175 young Australians, aged between 15 and 34, die every year from causes that are directly attributable to alcohol, compared, for example, to 371 who die from illegal drugs in the same age group. Hundreds die and thousands are injured on the roads every year because drivers have been drinking.

DRUG ADDICTION OR FOOD INTOLERANCE? ■

Alcohol is a powerful drug — a depressant, not a stimulant as many people think — and the alcoholic is a drink addict in the way that a food intolerant person is a food addict. Like many drugs, it is also toxic, poisoning the body if it is taken in large quantities, or in comparatively modest quantities in combination with other drugs. It can damage all the major organs of the body.

There have been numerous theories to account for alcoholism and as many attempts to find a cure. None has had any notable success in reducing the incidence of alcoholism or the fearful toll that it takes.

A theory of special interest to clinical ecologists is that alcoholism appears to be linked to the foods and food fractions in the drink as well as the ethyl alcohol itself. All alcoholic beverages consist of some usually common food, plus other ingredients, plus alcohol. The conventional thinking is that it is the alcohol component that is responsible for all the ills of alcoholism.

We frequently find that those who are intolerant of the food from which the drink is made actually prefer that drink. Those whose drink of choice is beer or whisky, which are grain-derived, are usually found on testing to be intolerant of solid foods made from cereal grain.

Some alcoholics find that they lose their addiction to alcohol and can control their drinking without difficulty by avoiding drinks prepared from substances that food testing has shown they cannot tolerate.

In reality it is a good deal more complicated than this, because very few alcoholic drinks contain only a single food. Whisky, for example, contains so many ingredients that it is impossible to positively identify any one of them as a problem, even if there were no synergistic effect involved (the heightened effect of two or more ingredients reacting together), which there often is. One popular brand contains ninety-four separate ingredients!

Gin is almost as complex and so too is vodka, for all that it is usually marketed as the purest of drinks.

Another hypothesis is that addiction to an alcoholic drink is simply a worsening symptom of an existing food intolerance. Like sugar, alcohol needs no digestion, but passes straight through the gut wall into the bloodstream. Many of the food fractions go with it and are absorbed very rapidly, and so produce a more immediate (and a more severe and noticeable) reaction than when they are ingested as solid food.

Rye, for example, is absorbed much more quickly when it takes the form of whisky than as rye bread, which is why the rye-intolerant alcoholic reaches for the bottle and not a sliced loaf.

Alcohol is produced by fermentation, which is the action of yeast on liquids that contain sugar and starches, so that here too one would not be surprised to find a close association between excessive alcohol consumption and excessive yeast in the body. It may be that some of those alcoholics who show no improvement at all when we identify addictant foods in their most frequent drink are actually addicted to and intolerant of the yeast. Others may similarly be addicted to the alcohol itself.

The blood glucose levels of alcoholics are invariably a mess, and almost every alcoholic I have treated has been hypoglycaemic. The diet many of them live on must contribute to this, but it may be that the low blood glucose is itself contributing to the alcoholism, perpetuating the vicious circle, rather than merely being a symptom of it.

Alcoholic beverages are a food–drug combination, always a dangerous situation in food intolerance. It gives them much in common with coffee and Coca-Cola, both food–drug combinations that cause endless problems in many people. Maybe it is the terrible social consequences of alcoholism that make it appear to be different from any other food–drug intolerance.

A DIET FOR ALCOHOLICS ■
None of this necessarily resolves the problems of alcoholics because alcoholism is a very powerful form of addiction. Like all addicts, the alcoholic will consciously and unconsciously resist any attempt to wean him or her away from the addictant, and alcohol is a very freely available addictant.

Alcoholics make very unsatisfactory patients at the best of

times, not least because you cannot believe a word they say. When I have to treat them, I invariably trust their blood alcohol levels rather than their solemn assurances that "I haven't had a drink in a month".

If they can be persuaded to go on to a sensible diet, and there is some indication that the food content of the alcoholic beverage they are addicted to is at least partly responsible for their condition, I have had a fair degree of success. The difficulty is that even if former whisky addicts find that they can safely drink gin or vodka, whisky remains the addictant and the craving for it is not being satisfied. Almost inevitably, they slip back, have "just one" drink of whisky, and the whole frustrating exercise has been in vain.

The diet I recommend for anyone with a drinking problem is the four-day rotation diet, and this needs to be observed for drink as much as for food. Patients cannot have any wine or brandy, for example, except on those days when they are allowed to eat grapes.

Some of the methods used for helping alcoholics fall down in the most basic ways. As long ago as 1979, to take a good example, there was a conference in Italy that brought together experts in alcoholism from all over the world. They looked at anything in people's lifestyles that might be influencing the development of alcoholism.

The consensus of the conference was that caffeine, sugar and nicotine were the three factors that they most felt were in some ways directly contributing to an increased need for alcohol. Yet if you go to a typical meeting of Alcoholics Anonymous, what do you almost invariably see them doing? You see them drinking a lot of coffee, putting sugar in it and smoking! It is no wonder that so many alcoholics leave AA meetings craving a drink even more than before they went in!

Many doctors become so frustrated with the alcoholics they try to help that they give up what they see as a perpetually one-sided battle. It is easy to sympathise with them, but the cost to the country of alcoholism and of all excessive drinking is so appalling in financial and human terms that anything that might reduce its incidence deserves consideration.

Taking an ecological approach is certainly no guarantee of a panacea around the corner, but it is one option that does promise to pay worthwhile dividends.

Arthritis is one of the most common and debilitating systemic physical diseases in the Western world. It is entirely a disease of so-called civilisation and is almost unknown in those countries that do not exist on a typical Western diet.

Some fifty or more types of arthritis have been described (the word comes from the Greek *arthron*, meaning a joint, with the suffix "-itis", which denotes inflammation), but rheumatoid arthritis and osteo-arthritis are the most common. Probably third in the list is gout, which is essentially a metabolic disorder involving the metabolism of uric acid. Excessive amounts of uric acid accumulate in the blood and precipitate out into the tissues, especially the tissues that are adjacent to the joints, and this results in the arthritis. The classic location is the big toe.

Rheumatoid arthritis can begin at any age. It is an auto-immune disease, which means that the body destroys itself instead of wearing out. Osteo-arthritis, on the other hand, which is perhaps the more familiar form, is a degenerative disease and is found more in older people and in joints that have been damaged. It is possible for both forms to be present in the same patient.

In osteo-arthritis, the weight-bearing joints and the spine tend to be most affected. Rheumatoid arthritis affects the smaller joints such as the fingers and wrists, although the bigger joints, especially the knee and the hips, can also be affected.

Sufferers of arthritis do not need to be told that orthodox medicine is short on explanations and therapy for the disease. Because nobody actually dies from it, there is an odd belief, in spite of the sometimes excruciating pain, among those who are not its victims that it is a disease that we do not need to be quite so concerned about.

A BETTER TREATMENT FOR ARTHRITIS ▮

Clinical ecology is acutely involved with muscle and joint aches and pains and from its earliest days, its practitioners suspected that diet was implicated in arthritis. There has to be some better solution than a therapy consisting solely of ever stronger drugs, some with alarming side effects including cataract, followed by the physical removal of the affected joints and their replacement with synthetic ones.

The normal five-day fast so often relieves the symptoms of arthritis that it was inevitable that food and diet would be suspected. Food is not, however, always the cause of arthritis. Some patients showed no improvement at all when the disease was approached from this angle, but when it *was* implicated it was so potent a cause that other environmental factors were also suspected when it failed.

Cause and effect in arthritis are highly individualised and require sometimes long-term study, until the pieces of the jigsaw finally drop into place.

As long ago as 1949, the cause and effect relationship between certain foods and the onset of acute arthritis symptoms was shown. It is only in the last ten years, however, that it was realised that chemical intolerance accounted for almost all those cases that failed to respond to the food approach. Foods are probably more important than chemicals as the cause of arthritis, at least in bare numbers, but the number of those who respond to the chemical approach and not to food is significant.

DEADLY NIGHTSHADE AND ARTHRITIS ■

Over almost forty years, sufficient arthritis patients have been seen and successfully treated ecologically that we are able to say categorically that the approaches and techniques of clinical ecology offer great hope to the great majority of sufferers.

Although any foods can be implicated if there is regular and frequent exposure, the group that should immediately be suspected and tested for consists of members of the deadly nightshade family: tomatoes, potatoes, red and green peppers, capsicums and eggplants. Tobacco is another member of the same family, which is yet another good reason to avoid it.

Just because there is no response to the exclusion of these foods, however, does not mean that other foods may not be implicated. The deadly nightshades are an easy group to exclude and to observe the outcome of this exclusion. Partial benefit may result, which is a strong pointer to look further; or there may be no benefit at all, in which case it is still necessary to begin investigating the rest of the patient's diet before excluding food as the cause.

One case history should be enough to show what clinical

ecology has to offer the arthritis sufferer. Emma was 68 when she came to me, the victim of painful arthritis, mainly osteo-arthritis but mixed with other types. It was so severe that she hobbled into the clinic supported by a niece and a four-pronged walking stick.

She went on to the five-day fast and by the fourth day most of the pain had gone from her joints and most of the swelling had settled. (It is now possible to use devices to measure both the progression and regression of joint swelling during food testing.) By the end of the fifth day, Emma was markedly improved.

Testing showed that she reacted adversely to a number of foods, particularly tomatoes and potatoes, though interestingly not to other members of the deadly nightshade family. This re-inforced the belief that there is not automatic cross-reactivity to other members of a food family, only a greater likelihood that intolerance to them will also develop. Coffee, wheat and eggs also produced unpleasant reactions in Emma.

She walked out of the clinic without any assistance — she almost danced out she was so overjoyed — without even needing her walking stick. Follow-up has shown that, provided she keeps to her diet, her arthritis remains a thing of the past and she is free of all its symptoms. If she does deviate from the diet by eating "unsafe" foods, the symptoms still begin to return almost immediately, in spite of the fact that four years have passed since she first came to me.

It is to be hoped that the time will come when she can tolerate these foods again (Emma misses her coffee and her potatoes). If this happens they will be included on a four-day rotation basis to prevent the intolerance re-emerging.

Asthma is potentially very serious, even life-threatening, to many of those who suffer from it, and very frightening in its more severe forms, particularly for children. It is normally considered to be one of the classic symptoms of true allergy, caused by exposure to house dust, mites, pollens, moulds, or animal danders. But it is also frequently caused by intolerance to many foods, chemicals and even drugs; as well as by infection, a chill, a row or any other emotional upset and stress. Allergists insist that in these cases there is no allergy involved, because there is no elevated IgE (see p. 39). The patients, however, don't need to be told by anybody that what they are suffering is asthma.

Certain foods and drinks, in their own right, are capable of provoking an asthma attack in sensitive people. Nuts, seafoods, eggs and dairy products are the foods that are most implicated. Much more common as provokers of asthma are certain chemical additives in foods, put there as colouring agents, preservatives, or flavour enhancers. Three in particular — sulphur dioxide and its derivatives, monosodium glutamate (MSG) and the yellow food dye tartrazine (code 102) — are notorious troublemakers for asthmatics.

SULPHITE ▌

One of the worst offenders is sulphite and the various sulphite-based synthetic chemicals widely used as fruit and vegetable preservatives as we have already seen in Chapter 10. Sulphite stops potatoes going brown after they have been peeled, so that it is likely to be present in every potato bought in a restaurant or takeaway outlet; and sulphite is sprayed on salads in salad bars to keep the lettuce fresh. There is a strong suspicion that sulphite bleaches are commonly (and illegally) used in food shops to prevent fruit salads from turning brown.

Sulphite also prevents undesirable bacterial growth, particularly in acidic foods and drinks, and it helps to preserve the vitamin C level in fruit juice.

The two forms that are most troublesome to asthmatics are sodium metabisulphite (code 223) and potassium metabisulphite (code 224), neither of which occurs naturally. The active agent, sulphur dioxide (code 220) is liberated over a period of time so that dried fruits, for example, may contain 3 grams per kilogram at the beginning of the year, but only 1 gram per kilogram after being stored for several months. Some metabisulphite is lost in cooking — as much as 50 per cent in cooking sausages — but it can never be completely cooked out.

Some asthmatics are so sensitive to sulphur dioxide that the fumes given off during cooking alone are enough to provoke a severe attack. Typical symptoms are a tightness in the throat and a wheeze within minutes of eating, say, a pickled onion, or a glass of white wine or orange juice.

Although metabisulphite is the most troublesome form for asthmatics, all sulphites are potentially harmful and all have been known to bring on unconsciousness in the most sensitive patients.

Sodium bisulphite (code 222) is another synthetic preservative (it is often used with uncooked prawns and shrimps). A dose of 115 milligrams per kilogram by bodyweight of sodium bisulphite killed 50 per cent of a group of rats in one study. Sodium sulphite (code 221), a common food preservative and anti-oxidant, is also used for fixing photographs!

The following foods should be expected to contain meta-bisulphite and treated with great caution by asthmatics and anyone else who suspects that they are intolerant of sulphides. The list is extracted from the *Asthma Welfarer*, the journal of the Asthma Foundation of New South Wales:

VEGETABLES
Dried vegetables
Instant mashed potato
Pre-cut, pre-peeled or commercially prepared chipped potatoes
Potato chips (some brands)
Pickled onions
Pickles

MEAT, FISH AND POULTRY
Sausages
Sausage meat
Frankfurters
Chicken loaf
Devon
Brawn
Uncooked fresh prawns

DAIRY PRODUCTS
Fruit yoghurt
Cheese spreads

FRUIT
Dried "tree" fruits (e.g. apples, apricots, pears)
Fruit bars
"Fresh" fruit salad from commercial outlets — (Adding metabi-
    sulphite to salads to maintain their appearance may mean
    that so-called "fresh" fruit salad is far from fresh. There is
    no way of telling by looking at it.)
NB: *Sultanas, currants and raisins do not contain metabisulphite and
    prunes are not preserved with it.*

BEVERAGES
Orange- or yellow-coloured soft drinks in glass bottles
Cordials
Commercial chilled fruit juice, with the exception of canned,
    pasteurised juices or drinks in "tetra-brick" packs such as
    Poppers)
Bottled drinks containing fruit juice
Champagne
Wine, especially sweet white wines, which can contain as much
    as 35 milligrams per glass. Even dry white wines contain
    10 to 15 milligrams per glass
Cider — (Some unpreserved brands are available. Look at the
    label.)

MISCELLANEOUS
Vinegar
Vinegar-containing foods, such as salad dressings and sauces
Dessert toppings
Flavouring essences
Jams

MONOSODIUM GLUTAMATE (MSG) ▮

Monosodium glutamate, or MSG (code 621), is bad news for a lot
of people including many asthmatics. As in all the symptoms
provoked by MSG (see Chapter 10, p. 133), the amount of MSG
consumed plus the degree of individual sensitivity to it determine
the severity of the symptoms. The more MSG that is eaten, the
worse the symptoms will be — which is not invariably the case

with most of the substances that cause food and food-chemical intolerance.

Another peculiarity of MSG is that the onset of the symptoms may not occur until up to twelve hours after it has been consumed, instead of the almost invariable four hours with other substances. This makes it even more difficult for the patient or the doctor to recognise it unless it is being specifically suspected and tested for. This is not necessarily because of masking, but simply a sequel to the time that it takes for this particular chemical to have its effect.

It is almost always added as a flavour enhancer, notoriously in Chinese restaurants in fried rice, foods with batter or crumbs, and foods with spicy sauces. At the 1988 Australian and New Zealand Association for the Advancement of Science (ANZAAS) conference, a warning was given that MSG in quantities up to fifteen times the World Health Authority's maximum recommended levels are being routinely added to food by some Chinese restaurants in Australia. The latest estimates suggest that 20 per cent of people are adversely affected by MSG.

Curiously, when MSG is present as a naturally occurring substance (mainly in tomatoes, mushrooms, chicken and corn), it rarely has the same unpleasant effects as it does when it is synthesised and added to food. The exception to this is that the three cheeses containing MSG naturally — parmesan, camembert and blue vein — all frequently evoke the same reaction as synthetic MSG.

Avoiding MSG is relatively simple with packaged and tinned foods, because it must be listed among the ingredients, either by name or by its code number, but almost impossible when eating out in restaurants or takeaway outlets, or in other people's homes. In many cities there are Chinese restaurants that specialise in cooking without MSG, but on the whole it must always be assumed that any Asian food restaurant will make generous use of MSG to bring out the flavour of its product.

MSG has no distinctive taste in cooked foods (though a few hypersensitive people claim to be able to detect it by smell). Its only purpose is to improve the taste in the food to which it is added. Bland and boring food is probably safely free of MSG, and there are, of course, a great many other ways of bringing out the flavour of food, even if they do require a little more effort than tipping up a bottle.

Avoid also any product that lists vegetable protein among the ingredients, because this may contain MSG. If the vegetable protein is delivered to the final manufacturer with MSG already added, as we have seen, the manufacturer has no obligation in Australia to include it in the list of ingredients. Only those substances the manufacturer itself adds need to appear, and imported foods may not mention MSG at all, no matter at what stage it was added.

Foods that are likely to contain MSG and that asthmatics and anyone else sensitive to MSG should beware of, include:

Takeaway pizza, especially when it is spiced or seasoned
Takeaway seasoned chicken
Commercial savoury soups
Packet and tinned soups
Pies
Sausage rolls
Frankfurters
Tinned meat and luncheon meat
Meat and fish pastes
Frozen prepared meals
Canned vegetables in sauce
Flavoured potato chips
Savoury biscuits
Cocktail onions
Gherkins
Soya sauce
Mixed seasonings and spices
Gravy makers and stock cubes
Tomato purée, paste and sauce
Commercial breadcrumbs
Stuffing mixes
Meat tenderisers
Yeast and meat extracts

TARTRAZINE FOOD COLOURING ▮

The third food additive that asthmatics need to take special care to avoid is the ubiquitous yellow food dye, tartrazine (code 102). It has been known for many years that tartrazine, and to a lesser extent other azo dyes (see p. 136), provoke asthmatic attacks. It is one of the most common food additives, turning up not only in food and drink, but in many pharmaceutical drugs and medications. There is, however, a positive trend to remove it from the latter. The antidepressant Serepax is a very widely prescribed drug that used to be coloured with tartrazine, but no longer is. This is an entirely desirable trend.

Labelling requirements make it mandatory for tartrazine to be identified either by name or code number on all Australian-made foods. However, similar requirements are not mandatory for any drugs, whether ethical (requiring a prescription), over-the-counter items, or vitamins and health food products. In consequence, asthmatics must suspect any items that are coloured yellow, orange, brown or green, unless they know the product is safe.

SALICYLATES AND OTHER ADDITIVES ■

Salicylates, which include all pain-relievers that contain aspirin, are well-known provokers of asthma. Appendix IX includes the most commonly encountered natural sources of salicylates.

Among the additives that have been branded as unsafe or dangerous to asthmatics, there are twenty-one in particular that must be treated with the greatest suspicion and normally avoided. These are listed below, with their code numbers. Some have not been approved by the National Health and Medical Research Council for use in Australia, but this may be because no request has been received by a manufacturer for their use.

Potassium benzoate (212)
Calcium benzoate (213)
Ethyl 4-hydroxybenzoate (E214)
Ethyl 4-hydroxybenzoate, sodium salt (E215)
Propyl 4-hydroxybenzoate (E216)
Propyl 4-hydroxybenzoate, sodium salt (E217)
Methyl 4-hydroxybenzoate (E218)
Methyl 4-hydroxybenzoate, sodium salt (E219)
Sodium sulphite (221)
Sodium bisulphite (222)
Sodium metabisulphite (223)
Potassium metabisulphite (224)
Propyl gallate (310)*(Also suspected of causing reproductive
        failure and liver damage.)
Octyl gallate (311)*

Dodecyl gallate (312)*

Sodium hydrogen L-glutamate (621) (Also known as monosodium glutamate.)

Potassium hydrogen L-glutamate (622) (Banned for children
under 12 weeks old.)

Calcium dihydrogen di-L-glutamate (623)

Guanosine 5'-(disodium phosphate) (627)

Inosine 5'-(disodium phosphate) (631)

Sodium 5'-ribonucleotide (E635)

*Products 310, 311 and 312 are banned in foods for young children and babies

Any chemical that outgasses has the potential to trigger an asthmatic attack and must be suspected once all the above chemicals
or foods have been excluded. During testing it is important to
remember that, although asthma is the problem that is being
treated and indeed may be the only symptom of intolerance that
is causing any trouble, it may not be the symptom that is evoked
in the test. The fact that testing produces another symptom,
which might affect a completely different part of the body, does
not mean that the substance causing the asthma has not been
identified. It can be very confusing even to an expert, let alone to
someone coming to ecological illness for the first time.

30 Candida — the Troublesome Yeast

Candida albicans is a yeast that inhabits the bodies of all adult humans and most children by the time they are six months old. Many babies are actually born with a well-developed candida colony in place: we call it oral thrush when it is in the mouth. Even if it is not present at birth, candida is everywhere and the baby will certainly acquire it very quickly.

Because candida is found in all humans, its presence must be compatible with living a normal, healthy life, and indeed it is part of the normal bowel flora. This means that the yeast organisms coexist with other bacteria in the gut, especially those in the lower digestive tract. As long as the immune system is functioning normally and other factors, such as ingestion of antibiotics, have not upset the balance, candida is entirely harmless and under control — fortunately.

If you could feed a yeast colony adequately, it would grow from one teaspoonful until it filled an average size room from floor to ceiling, in six hours! You only need to look at how yeast bubbles in a fermenting vat to get some idea of the power that is at work. The miracle is that it doesn't take over our bodies.

The trouble comes when the immune system, which normally ensures that candida stays in its correct place, in the gut, malfunctions for some reason. Candida is extremely opportunistic and it never misses a chance to spread if the immune system, which is its only real control, becomes too weak to perform this task and drops its guard.

There are a number of predisposing factors which play a role in triggering the "overgrowth", as it is known when yeast runs amok. We will consider them one by one shortly. The effect is that it spreads through the digestive tract, forming new colonies, as well as causing infection in the throat, mouth and nasal passages, on the skin and in the prostate, even in the lungs as well as the very vulnerable vaginal area. After upper respiratory infections, vaginal thrush is the second most common infection in general practice.

A BEWILDERING DISEASE ■

It is difficult to describe the mechanism by which candida infections, which collectively are known as candidiasis, cause the bewildering array of symptoms for which they are responsible. Because *Candida albicans* is present in everybody and the yeast can be found everywhere in the body, even in a healthy person, there are no diagnostic tests that can identify candidiasis separately. The yeast organism looks the same under a microscope and behaves the same, whether it is in its proper place in the gut, or causing havoc somewhere else in the body.

One means by which candida produces symptoms is certainly sheer overgrowth, which leads, for example, to vaginal discharge or oral thrush, as well as symptoms in the gut such as constipation or diarrhoea and anal itching. All these are local effects of the overgrowth.

When the symptoms spread beyond the gut, it is presumably because of toxins or toxic products from the yeast itself. One author has described seventy-nine different toxic products in candida that infect humans! They are absorbed into the system and in their own right place a load on the immune system. As the efficiency of the immune system is further reduced, other problems emerge so that the picture gets progressively worse.

It is also probably the case that candida can directly affect — or attack — the immune system, the very thing that is supposed to keep it in order. The likely mechanism here is more c nplex. Candida causes suppressor-cell disease, which results in there being insufficient of these cells, whose role is to slow down the production of antibodies by the B-cells. The immune system then goes overboard, as it were, without proper controls, producing excessive antibodies to everything, however trivial and at the slightest provocation.

As a result, there is a greatly increased likelihood of patients developing an intolerance response to numerous substances, including foods and chemicals, that would normally cause no problems. This in turn leads to yet more symptoms in any part of the body.

Finally, there is a concept that the bowel wall itself, which is normally a protective membrane keeping the products of digestion safely enclosed in the bowel, is disturbed by the presence of candida. The notion is that the yeast colonies dig into the wall and grow there, damaging the wall itself — the "leaky bowel" syndrome put forward by Dr David Buscher. The incomplete products of digestion escape from the bowel into the blood, where they can cause often serious symptoms in whichever organ or tissue the blood happens to carry them to.

This is an extremely difficult thing to prove one way or the other in the laboratory, but microscopically, colonies have been shown to grow in the gut wall. The theory has now been extended to include the notion that the damage caused by the leaky bowel allows peptides and polypeptides to be absorbed. This, coupled with the damage that can be caused to the immune system itself, because of suppressor-cell disease, produces antibodies, so that when food is next ingested an intolerance reaction occurs.

THE SYMPTOMS OF CANDIDIASIS ■

All of this because a yeast, that seems to perform no useful function at all, grows in excess, then escapes from its proper place. It is really no wonder that this is yet another disease that many members of the medical profession refuse to take seriously, because it fits into none of their preconceived ideas of cause and effect dictated by the law of parsimony.

Candidiasis can affect both men and women, and men can become extremely ill, especially with neurological problems. But it is women who suffer far more frequently, presumably because their bodies have more appealing places in which a colony of yeast can flourish.

Any attempt to compile a definitive list of the symptoms of yeast-provoked infection, which is as long, or longer, than those of food and chemical intolerance, must be inadequate. There are some symptoms, however, that are particularly important in helping to identify candidiasis and they include the following:

Fatigue or lethargy
A feeling of being "drained"
Poor memory
A "spacy" or unreal sensation
Depression

Numbness
Burning or tingling
Muscle aches and weakness, or "paralysis"
Pain or swelling in the joints
Tenderness and abdominal pain
Constipation, diarrhoea and bloating
Vaginal discharge and persistent vaginal burning or itching
Prostatitis
Impotence and loss of sex drive
Cramps and other menstrual irregularities
Premenstrual tension
Spots in front of the eyes and erratic vision.
Genital itch and redness in males (jock itch)
Otitis externa (inflammation of the external ear)

It is possible to list the major symptoms by age groups as well, because symptoms change as a child grows into adolescence, and then adulthood.

In infants and toddlers, rash and wind problems are likely to predominate, while older children are more likely to have abdominal pain, headache, bed-wetting, dermatitis and behaviour problems that range from restlessness to hyperactivity; argumentativeness, poor concentration, short attention span and tantrums. Any of these symptoms can be caused by other factors, but if the doctor already suspects that candida might be implicated, they are a valuable pointer.

In adults, fatigue, headaches, depression, irritability, dandruff, indigestion, flatulence and flatus, and thrush are major symptoms.

In institutions where large numbers of women live in close proximity, such as a women's prison or an army mess hut, vaginal thrush or monilia is often rampant.

SEVEN SITUATIONS TO AVOID ■
Denied any useful tests for establishing the presence of candidiasis, the doctor must rely heavily on the patient's history. Exposure to one or more of seven situations in particular has been repeatedly shown to predispose people to candidiasis. All can lead to an upset in the balance between the yeast and the host.

1. Antibiotics Antibiotics are probably the chief culprit in upsetting the balance. They do not in themselves cause candidiasis, as many writers claim, and indeed they have little, if any, effect on the yeast at all. What they do is kill off the normal bacteria in the lower gastrointestinal tract that keep the candida in check. It is this that allows the candida to multiply excessively.

Once this has happened, if it is not reversed, the yeast can persist in excess, not only in the gastrointestinal tract, but it can grow in other areas often far distant from the gut where normally it does not occur in significant amounts, such as the vagina, oesophagus, throat, ear and even a baby's bottom — not so far removed from the gut! It invades the deep tissues only when the immune system is extremely weak.

Treatment, as we shall see shortly, is a course of the drug nystatin, which eliminates candida in the bowel and is even more remarkable in a most unusual way: it is a drug that is extremely safe.

Multiple antibiotic use is something that the doctor must ask about, especially in young children. Broad-spectrum antibiotics, such as the tetracyclines, for all that they may be needed, are the worst troublemakers so far as yeast is concerned. The longer that they, or any other antibiotics, have been taken, the more likely they are to be causing problems. Anti-acne treatments, for example, often require two tablets of tetracyclines to be taken daily for months at a time.

2. *The Birth Control Pill and Pregnancy* This may seem like a contradiction, but birth control and pregnancy have much in common, and both predispose women to have candidiasis. The pill contains progesterone, the female sex hormone, and candida thrives on it. Women's natural level of progesterone hormone rises steadily in the premenstrual phase and remains constantly elevated during pregnancy. Many female problems with candida begin with repeated pregnancies, and especially involve vaginal thrush, with its itching and white discharge.

Yeast problems are most likely to occur in the latter half of the normal menstrual cycle. The length of time on the pill and the number of pregnancies are both important. After a birth, when the progesterone level falls, the yeast symptoms may temporarily disappear, but later they will almost certainly return, and next time they will require far less stimulus to trigger them.

3. *Other Drugs* Although antibiotics are the worst offenders, they are not the only drugs to be associated with heavy

yeast activity and infection. Steroids in particular, such as cortisone and prednisone, and the immuno-suppressant drugs that are used in the treatment of cancer, for example, also predispose people to acquiring candidiasis.

4. Other Yeast- and Fungus-associated Infections The danger here is that there will be cross-reactivity between one yeast-related infection and another. Vaginitis in women, prostatitis in men, are both common and may well leave them vulnerable and exposed to other yeast- or fungus-provoked symptoms that might be as unrelated to the first symptoms as athlete's foot, ringworm or any fungal infection of the skin or nails.

5. Diet High in Refined Carbohydrate The whole problem with yeast is believed to have started 10,000 years ago when humans first began to make radical changes to their diet. Diets that include excessive amounts of sugar and white flour act as fuel to the yeast, in addition to all the other problems that are likely to be caused over a period of years by their excessive consumption. The human body is completely maladapted to cope with this kind of diet.

Carbohydrate (starchy and sugary foods, especially refined sugar) is the main food of candida, which does not appear to be able to digest protein and fat. The last place in the body where you want fungus colonies to be appearing is the brain, which must take about 50 per cent of all blood glucose. Too much alcohol, and particularly beer with its high yeast content, fuels the candidiasis.

The dietary recommendations given for food intolerance, particularly the rotation diet, are suitable here (see Chapter 17).

6. Diets High in Moulds and Yeasts These foods, more than most others, promote undesirable new growth of candida. As far as possible, yeasts and moulds must be eliminated from the diet because of the risk of cross-reactivity.

Yeast is found mainly in bakery products; alcoholic beverages; products that contain vinegar, such as mayonnaise and many sauces; products containing yeast-derived vitamins of the B complex series, including some packaged vitamin-enriched cereals; and black tea, the leaves of which are yeast-fermented. Torula, which is listed in some processed and smoked-food ingredients, is a fungus.

Yeast is found in the following foods, all of which may need to be eliminated, at least in the short term, once candidiasis has been diagnosed or strongly suspected:

Bread

Biscuits (about the only biscuits that are yeast-free are some crackers, such as Cheese Jatz, Sesame Thin, Plaza, Wheat Crispbread, Uneeda and Thin Captain)

Pastries

Hamburger buns

Cakes and cake mixes

Pretzels

Flours enriched with vitamins from yeast

Mushrooms

Cheese

Buttermilk

Vinegar

Mayonnaise (The vinegar in mayonnaise causes the problem, so substitute freshly squeezed lemon in home-made mayonnaise.)

Olives

Pickles

Tomato sauce

All fermented drinks (including wine, brandy, whisky, rum, vodka, gin and beer)

Malted products (including cereals, sweets, malted milk drinks, canned citrus and fruit juices)

Vitamin and multivitamin capsules made from yeast (particularly vitamin B)

Any foods that actually have mould on them should be avoided. Some moulds and fungi appear when the food has been left out for too long, or even during the normal process of ripening.

Rockmelons often collect a thin film of mould, which may be almost invisible against the mottled skin of the fruit.

7. ***Moulds and Yeasts in the Environment*** Airborne mould spores (moulds and yeasts are closely related members of the vegetable kingdom) can also exacerbate candida, particularly during warm months when the humidity rises. The mould spores float around like pollen to be inhaled by anyone within range, and they often lead to both intolerance and conventional allergy.

(As in all ecological illness there must first be individual susceptibility. Not everyone suffers or suffers equally from moulds and
yeasts, any more than they do from foods and chemicals.)

Mould spores cause a special problem for anyone affected
by excessive candida growth, because there is ample evidence that
yeasts and moulds in the outside environment predispose these
people to develop candidiasis *inside* their bodies, and exacerbate
any symptoms of candidiasis that they already have.

The ideal breeding condition for mould requires dampness
and darkness. Even a low-wattage bulb left burning in a cupboard or in the bathroom reduces the mould population, but
mould can thrive anywhere.

It flourishes in wallpaper glue, in vegetables and fruit, even
in the fridge, on a slice of old bread left at the bottom of the
breadbin, in damp shower curtains and behind the base of toilets,
on magazines and old books, on shoes and on top of the soil of pot
plants, in the tray that catches the water in self-defrosting fridges
and in the archetypical haven for moulds, the dark, damp old
house.

A small amount of borax, a natural anti-mould agent,
sprinkled over the area is an effective temporary solution in many
cases and brings none of the undesirable side effects of the potent
concoctions that are sprayed out of aerosol cans for the same purpose and which give no greater protection. The only long-term
solution is to remove the conditions that promote mould growth,
the dampness and darkness.

Some wallpapers, incidentally, contain chemical mould-
retardants, but the outgassing from these can cause as many
symptoms in the chemically sensitive as the moulds themselves.

TREATING YEAST INFECTIONS ■

Diagnosis of candidiasis, as we have said, is very difficult unless
there is the positive evidence of discharge, as in vaginitis or oral
thrush. For all the research that has been done into the disease,
the best authorities are agreed only that you cannot depend on the
culturing or growing in the laboratory of samples taken from any
part of the human body to make a firm diagnosis that will confirm even whether a person has or doesn't have candidiasis.

There are people with high candida levels in the stool
culture who do not have a trace of any symptoms of candidiasis.
There are others who have improved dramatically when they have

been treated for candidiasis, because their symptoms have suggested that this is appropriate, even when not one positive culture was taken from any part of their bodies — saliva, urine, faeces or blood.

In the majority of cases, because yeast is everywhere, a swabbing from any part of the body will grow it. The best that you can do is give a calculated opinion, based on the facts that you do have, on your own experience and above all on the patient's history.

As with so much else in ecological illness, because there is no tangible evidence many doctors still refuse to accept that candida is responsible for any of the myriad symptoms that patients present with. They can diagnose vaginitis readily and correctly as a yeast infection and treat it properly; but when the candidiasis is in the gastrointestinal tract, or anywhere else where it cannot be seen (because there is no visible discharge for example) they often deny its very existence. Long ago I stopped counting the number of patients who arrived at my rooms having been labelled at least once as "neurotic" or "a hypochondriac" by physicians and psychiatrists alike.

What happens is that the illness caused by candidiasis is named according to the organ that is affected — kidney trouble, heart trouble, bowel trouble, skin disorder or even nervous breakdown, for example. Inevitably when doctors look for a cause on this basis, refusing to take candida into account, they find nothing. There is the usual barrage of tests and repeated tests, second and third opinions, before inevitably falling back on the conclusion that the patient must be imagining the whole thing.

Candida must be suspected if there has been exposure to any of the seven situations listed above.

Getting Rid of the Fungus Successful treatment requires the yeast products, the toxins and so on to be cleared from the bloodstream, and this can be accomplished only by ridding the tissues of the fungus. In turn, the starting point for this is to clear the gastrointestinal tract of the excess candida, which is usually the only step in the process that is relatively swift and uncomplicated.

Resistance to infectious agents of any kind, whether viruses, bacteria or fungi, depends ultimately on our immune systems. In the treatment of chronic candidiasis, the aim is to kill or at least substantially reduce the rate of growth of the fungus, and at the same time to stimulate the immune system to be more effective in resisting the yeast.

Treatment includes modifying the diet to ensure that all foods favouring the growth of candida (which means basically carbohydrates) are eliminated as far as possible. Carbohydrate, as we have seen, is the ideal food for yeast to thrive on. The worst carbohydrate is, of course, refined carbohydrate — sugar and sugar-containing foods. If only one food is to be excluded, it must be sugar and, in some mild cases, that may be all that is necessary to free the patient of symptoms. Complex carbohydrates, such as vegetables, may well be tolerated.

Alcohol intake should be reduced to a minimum. Some authorities recommend that it be eliminated altogether until the yeast is firmly under control.

The second factor in the diet is that foods with an unusually high content of yeast or mould (which is tied up with the overall dose load) must be excluded or reduced. These include the more obviously yeasty foods such as mushrooms, aged cheeses and yeast-fermented items like bread, fermented drinks, Vegemite and Marmite. They can also include vegetables that are less than fresh, many of which begin to go mouldy soon after they are picked. Carrots and potatoes are particularly prone to this.

Nystatin — a Remarkable Drug   Any of the other predisposing factors listed above must be avoided where practical, and drugs are also almost always required to kill the candida in the gastrointestinal tract. By far the most commonly prescribed drug is nystatin, marketed under the trade names Mycostatin and Nilstat. As we have said, it is very unusual, in that it is an ethical drug that is almost entirely free of any undesirable side effects.

Nystatin rarely passes through the wall of the intestine and does not enter the bloodstream at all until the dosage is raised to far above the normal recommended level. It remains in the digestive tract and greatly reduces the level of yeast, which it kills by direct contact. Because this contact is required, nystatin is ineffectual against the yeast that is already in other body tissue, unless very high doses are deliberately prescribed for this purpose.

Some strains of yeast are very sensitive to nystatin and yield quickly. Others are highly resistant and, because patients may be carrying several different strains at the same time, the yeast embedded in tissue in other parts of the body may take a long time to be eradicated. The body's own immunity must deal with it, and months and sometimes years may be required for the immune system to rebuild itself enough to be effective. It is imperative that in the digestive system yeast levels are kept as low as possible during this rebuilding process.

Nystatin is available as a tablet or a capsule. I prescribe the latter, recommending that the patient open the capsule and place the powder it contains into a small amount of water. Initially this is taken as a mouthwash, squelching it around the mouth before swallowing it. (Yeast is present in the mouth.)

It is important to begin treatment with a very small dose and then build up gradually, because the sudden destruction of large numbers of yeast colonies can liberate so much toxin, which is absorbed, that the patient feels terrible. He or she is actually being poisoned by the release of the substances in the yeast cell into the bloodstream, where they are carried to all parts of the body.

The dose of nystatin is built up from half a capsule a day (250,000 units) to eight capsules, and in some cases even as many as sixteen (8 million units). Individual patients learn to find the dose that they need to control their symptoms.

Some doctors recommend a new drug, ketoconazole, marketed as Nizoral, which is claimed to be particularly effective in the treatment of vaginitis and systemic (that is, outside the gastrointestinal tract) candidiasis. It is very toxic, however, and if it *is* used it should always be monitored with blood tests. It is also expensive, at the time of writing, and not available under the subsidised pharmaceutical benefit scheme.

I believe that eventually it should be possible to use a yeast vaccine to create resistance to candidiasis, but work in this direction is still in its early days.

Do You Have Candidiasis?   There are ten questions that I find are a very positive guide to the presence of candidiasis. Score 1 for each "Yes" answer. If you score from 3 to 4, it is possible that there is candidiasis present; 5 to 6, it is probable; 7 to 8, it is likely; and 9 to 10 it is highly likely. The questions are as follows:

1. Are you troubled by confusion, depression, fatigue, poor memory?
2. Do you have digestive problems — constipation, bloating, gas, diarrhoea, stomach-aches?

3. Do you suffer from premenstrual tension (PMT) and/
    or recurrent vaginitis, bladder infections or prostatitis?
4. Do you crave sweets, bread and/or alcohol?
5. Do you have recurrent headaches, muscle or joint
    pains?
6. Do you have skin rashes, hives, eczema, itchy ears,
    itchy rectum or anus?
7. Do you have fungus infections — vaginitis, "jock
    itch", thrush, athlete's foot — or thick, yellow, in-
    grown toenails?
8. Are you taking, or have you been treated with anti-
    biotics, birth control pills, cortisone drugs or steroids?
9. Are you sensitive to tobacco, perfume, chemicals (such
    as car fumes, newsprint, plastics)?
10. Are you uncomfortable in mouldy areas?

We still have much to learn about candida and the damage
that it can do to its victims. In the meantime, there is a great deal
that we are able to achieve towards minimising the symptoms. It
is in many ways the quintessential ecological disease, caused originally by maladaptation to our diet and perpetuated at every
stage by some factor in our environment. Simply winning widespread understanding of what it is all about will be the next most
important step forwards.

31 Eyesight, Sunlight and Glasses

I always have my patients read aloud from a book or magazine if chemical intolerance is suspected because often an early sign is blurring of the vision. It can happen in food intolerance as well, though less often. One patient, a doctor, was highly intolerant of garlic and among the symptoms each time he ate it (always unwittingly when he ate away from home) was that the focal length of one of his eyes altered so that everything viewed through it was hazy and out of focus.

I see patients who complain that although they need to wear glasses, the lenses that have been prescribed for them are either no help at all, or even make things worse. What has sometimes happened is that these people were tested by an optometrist or ophthalmologist when their vision was disturbed because of chemical or food intolerance, perhaps even from exposure to chemicals while travelling to the eye specialist — perhaps even in his rooms! In other words, the testing was carried out while they had the abnormality and when the reaction passed off, their vision returned to normal and the glasses in front of their eyes became a positive hindrance.

Anyone who suspects that they are intolerant should fast the night before an eye test, avoid having breakfast and, if possible, stay away from suspected chemical pollutants.

Sunglasses need another note of caution because the harm from the sun can correctly be said to be an environmental illness. Almost nobody *needs* sunglasses! Those who do (and there certainly are some who do, and that has nothing to do with whether they think they look better wearing them) ought to be measured to find out why they have that problem.

About the only time when it is necessary for everyone to wear sunglasses is when they are in snow or on the water on a sunny day, particularly when snow skiing. Mountaineers can burn their eyes (snow blindness) when climbing at high altitudes without sunglasses specially made for that purpose.

I hate to see little children wearing sunglasses. Apart from the fact that most wear them only because their mothers think they look cute, or they want to mimic their mothers, most cheap children's sunglasses are downright dangerous. They encourage the child — and often the mother — to think that it makes it safe to stare at the sun through them.

And they are a bad habit to acquire. If you do wear them, the retina in the eye becomes confused and doesn't work as well. It takes up to twenty-four hours after you take your sunglasses off in bright sunlight for the eyes to be functioning optimally again, with the muscle of the pupil and the iris contracting at maximum efficiency.

We are animals and as such we have been living under the sun since time immemorial. The sun gives life and the real dangers of spending too much time under the sun without proper skin protection should never be twisted to mean that the *correct* amount of exposure is highly undesirable.

Outdoor light provides mid-range ultraviolet light and endocrinologists have shown that allowing this mid-range ultraviolet to enter the eyes, when the skin is also experiencing sunlight, helps in stabilising hormone levels. It is fine that people are exercising more and jogging in the morning and the evening, but you don't get much ultraviolet light until about midday.

People ought to find the time to go outside — ten minutes is all you require — in the middle of the day. In ten minutes you start converting sunlight and the cholesterol in your skin into vitamin D. There is no need for the whole body to be exposed, only your hands and face, and it doesn't matter if it is cloudy. One of the important benefits of vitamin D is that it helps with calcium production and calcium is a tranquillising mineral in the body.

There is no need to sit out in the full heat of the sun. You can get all the exposure you need sitting under a shady tree, but not in the shade of a brick building. The ultraviolet cannot go round corners. Under a tree, it is dispersed and bounces off leaves and the grass. The ultraviolet gets into your eyes in healthy amounts and it goes without saying that you shouldn't be wearing sunglasses.

Most contact lenses, spectacles and sunglasses have ultraviolet inhibitors and keep this valuable ultraviolet light from penetrating, so that people who wear glasses all the time are constantly being deprived of this healthful and free source of energy.

The reason for this inhibitor being put in is ridiculous. During the Second World War a lot of fliers got sunburnt from being in planes with clear bubbles protecting the cockpit and gun positions at relatively high altitudes and some had their eyes badly burnt. The government asked the ophthalmologists and optometrists to develop an inhibitor and this has remained in most glasses ever since.

It is possible to buy glasses and contact lenses without the inhibitors which are ultraviolet transmitting (UVT), but you will almost certainly need to make a point of asking for them from your optometrist.

32 Halitosis — Bad Breath

Halitosis, or bad breath, is quite a common symptom of food intolerance. When we eat foods that we digest and can tolerate, our whole body functioning is clean. The breath is sweet and the mouth tastes pleasant, in contrast to the bottom-of-the-bird-cage taste in the mouth that so many people wake up with.

Of course, if you smoke cigarettes you will always wake up with a foul taste in the mouth and be just as unpleasant to anyone within breathing range. Those "Kiss a non-smoker and tell the difference" advertisements are not fooling.

Even the odour of faeces is markedly reduced when the food we eat is being properly digested and there is no intolerance, and flatus is relatively inoffensive. It is improved still further by reducing the amount of animal fat and protein that is eaten.

One of my patients, Marjorie, complained of an array of symptoms that did nothing for the quality of her life. They included mucus dripping from her nose, blurred vision, conjunctivitis, nausea, stomach cramps, a white coating especially on the tongue and also on the roof of her mouth, itchy and swollen eyes, dry, burning mouth, constant depression and nervousness. All in all, the picture she presented was something less than appealing, but it was another symptom that bothered her most of all. She had bad breath. Indeed, not to put too fine a point on it, her whole body smelled bad and her underarm odour was the worst of all.

Poor Marjorie went through agonies because of her smelly breath. She was fasted for the usual five days and then challenged with all the foods that she ate regularly and frequently enough to make them potential addictants. At the end of the test, the villains had been pinned down — refined sugar, eggs, oranges, tomatoes, milk and all dairy products.

By avoiding these foods, all her symptoms disappeared, but the last to go was the halitosis and body odour. My experience is that it is always one of the last symptoms to clear up, almost as though it accompanies any of the other symptoms, and that it can take three months to be finally rid of it — but don't despair, in time, it practically always does go away.

The one thing that nobody should ever believe, any more than they should believe a word that the tobacco industry says, is the specious advertising of the sugar industry, which maintains that refined sugar (the sugar in the sugar bowl) is a natural product. It is nothing of the sort!

The sugar industry claims that, because sucrose comes from cane sugar and cane sugar is a natural product, by definition sucrose is also entirely natural. By sucrose is meant the refined sugar that we use at home and in processing.

In fact, the sugar the industry is foisting on to us is an artificial, white crystalline substance *manufactured from* a natural product — a very different thing. It is a highly concentrated extract from sugar cane. Only if it was marketed with the cane's fibre, minerals and vitamins all intact could the industry with any integrity describe it as a natural product, reinforcing the message, as they often do in their advertising, with a picture of someone squeezing the juice out of the cane. As we have seen, about the only consumers who see the fibre, minerals and vitamins are the pigs.

WHY EXCESS SUGAR IS SO HARMFUL

Most of us are introduced to sugar almost as soon as we can eat solids, often as a reward in the form of sweets. What a prize! From earliest infancy, we give our babies the sweet tooth they will probably take with them to the grave (assuming they still have any teeth left, of course, after sugar has taken its toll), bequeathing to them all the diseases and disorders associated with refined sugar.

The average Australian consumes more than 45 kilograms of sugar each year (nearly 7 *stone* or 99 pounds!), or about 128 grams (4½ ounces) a day, a huge amount of a food that is nutritionally useless, high in empty kilojoules, tooth-rotting and responsible for one of the most prevalent of all ecological disorders, hypoglycaemia.

After we have eaten sugar, our bodies have to convert it biochemically so that we can get energy from it. This is achieved by passing it through between twenty and thirty different chemical steps. Each of these steps requires a chemical catalyst, or trigger, to make it happen; and these biochemical catalysts are enzymes which in turn cannot work unless they have been activated. *Their* triggers are the B vitamins, particularly B_1, B_2, B_3, B_5 and B_6.

But refined sugar contains no vitamins, because processing has removed them all; and the body itself generally cannot manufacture the B-complex vitamins. We have to eat them every day if we are to maintain correct levels. The liver can store B vitamins, but in the face of constant consumption of refined sugar, it does it increasingly inefficiently.

Any sugar that is not broken down to yield energy, or to be turned into metabolic waste products (and not all of these are always eliminated) must be converted into fat, if more kilojoules are consumed than the body needs. The obesity statistics show how often this is the case.

The same argument could be applied to any food, but the special danger in refined sugar is that it is nutritionally such an empty product, apart from its kilojoules, that you can go on eating sweet things without doing anything to assuage your hunger.

From a processing point of view (and within the home) sugar certainly does sometimes make otherwise unpalatable food enjoyable. Many foods would be very unappetising without it, especially fat-containing foods. It is the quantities that are consumed, which are far in excess of what is needed to make the occasional food more tasty, that cause the problems. This must certainly not be confused, as the sugar industry tries to confuse it, with meaning that sugar is therefore nutritionally useful.

The same caution, incidentally, applies to raw sugar and brown sugar. Raw sugar has some fibre added after processing — added, mind you, not left in from the natural cane; and brown sugar is coloured and taste-altered with caramel, a suspect product in its own right.

Addiction and intolerance to most refined carbohydrates are very common. White flour and all its products, particularly (because they are eaten so frequently) white bread, cakes, scones, biscuits and pastries, have to be the prime suspects in any case of ecological illness. Intolerance to white sugar that manifests itself in all the familiar symptoms of food addiction to a frequently consumed food are less common, but sugar brings with it two other very serious problems indeed, diabetes and hypoglycaemia, the two sides of the same coin.

HYPOGLYCAEMIA ■

Hypoglycaemia is a most confusing and contentious subject, but it is one that is very important in ecological illness. By definition, the word simply means low blood sugar, or blood glucose, to give it its correct name. But that is about the only thing on which the medical profession is agreed. Popular usage has the word also meaning all the symptoms that result from hypoglycaemia, but on that there is no general agreement.

An increasing number of doctors, on the evidence of what they see in their own practices, believe that hypoglycaemia can be a devastating disorder, affecting perhaps 10 per cent of the whole population, sometimes in a very debilitating and unpleasant way. Many books have been written about it. Other doctors — and there are many of them — deny that hypoglycaemia exists at all except as a rare condition associated with a few equally rare diseases.

Thirty years ago, an American physician, Dr S. P. Guiland, told a meeting of the American Medical Association that "there is probably no illness today which causes such widespread suffering, so much inefficiency and loss of time, so many accidents, so many family break-ups and so many suicides as hypoglycaemia". There is no way of quantifying it, but my instinct and that of many of my colleagues, is that Guiland was not exaggerating.

Yet there are doctors who insist that in quarter of a century of practice, they have never seen a case of hypoglycaemia!

It is little wonder that if there is this much disagreement and dissent among the so-called experts, their long-suffering patients are often completely bewildered about what to believe. So what do we know about hypoglycaemia? How does it fit into a book on ecological illness? And if it does exist, what can we do about it?

A Disease That Confuses Doctors My own position is quite clear. I am sure that hypoglycaemia *is* often misdiagnosed — but usually by the sufferers themselves after they have read books and articles on hypoglycaemia, and not by the medical profession. When the medical profession misdiagnoses, it usually either misses the disease altogether or puts the wrong interpretation on the symptoms that *are* found.

Having said that, I have not the slightest doubt, from many years of clinical experience, that hypoglycaemia does exist on the scale that Guiland suggested.

As with much to do with clinical ecology (and hypoglycaemia *is* an ecological illness, as I shall explain) a part of the problem is a semantic one. The whole subject of food and chemical intolerance is complicated, as we have seen, by the lack of a suitable alternative in the English language for the word "allergy", which had a very specific meaning and which the conventional allergists refused to share. When clinical ecology introduced the concept of food and chemical intolerance, which by any rational lay definition involved "allergy" to foods and chemicals, there wasn't a suitable alternative. In consequence, we are still toying with "intolerance" and "maladaptation" and other words which, like "clinical ecology" itself, are often not at all helpful when we are seeking the widest acceptance for something that can offer real benefits and hope to almost every family in the land.

Hypoglycaemia is in much the same boat. The sceptical doctors, who insist that hypoglycaemia is rare, are correct if they are referring only to the hypoglycaemia that is caused by an organic disease. The hypoglycaemia, however, that I encounter a dozen times a day in my practice is extremely common and has no organic cause. It is intolerance to something in a patient's personal environment, only the form that it takes is different from the food intolerance discussed so far. Hypoglycaemia and food intolerance are often inextricably linked.

To differentiate this form from "true" hypoglycaemia, which is most frequently caused by a rare tumour (insulinoma, see p. 399), the term "reactive" hypoglycaemia is used, because it is a reaction to food, particularly to refined carbohydrates and most particularly to sugar. As such, it fits fairly and squarely within the province of clinical ecology.

Reactive hypoglycaemia is almost invariably caused by a diet rich in sugar and sweet food. In other words, too much sugar in the diet results in too little sugar in the blood! It's an odd paradox. To find the explanation, we must look at the mechanism the body has for controlling the level of glucose, or sugar, in the blood.

Maintaining the Sugar Balance Maintaining the delicate balance between too little and too much glucose is one of the most important functions of our biochemical being. Every organ, as well as every muscle, needs glucose to function effectively. The brain, in particular, reacts badly and swiftly to being deprived of it. That is why so many of the symptoms of hypoglycaemia are neurological — symptoms such as anxiety, depression, lethargy, apathy, irritability, argumentativeness and a poor sex life.

When the thalamus, the emotional centre of the brain, is denied sufficient glucose, antisocial behaviour and violent mood swings often follow.

Normally, there are very effective and very complex processes at work to ensure that the balance is constantly maintained and falls within the ideal range for the optimal functioning of all the organs.

Hormones, particularly adrenalin and cortisone, play an important part (which is why stress in any form can interfere with even normally balanced blood glucose levels), but the main responsibility falls on the pancreas, a gland 15 to 20 centimetres long that lies under the stomach. In particular, cells within the pancreas, known quaintly after the German anatomist who first described them as the islets of Langerhans, have a vital role. They produce insulin, the hormone that moves glucose out of the blood and into body tissue.

Most diabetics (diabetes mellitus), whose blood glucose level is high, fail to produce enough insulin and sometimes produce none at all, which is why they have to take regular doses of insulin. Sometimes the pancreas produces the correct amount of insulin, but for some reason the body is unable to use it properly. This may happen, for instance, when blood fats are high, or when the patient's diet is high in fats. This is why it is becoming increasingly common and correct for diabetics to go on to a low-fat diet, as well as to exclude refined sugars.

In hypoglycaemia, exactly the opposite is occurring. Too much insulin is produced with the result that blood glucose falls too low.

In "true" hypoglycaemia, the low blood glucose level is due to excessive insulin from an organic disease such as insulinoma, a tumour of the pancreas. This growth produces excessive quantities of insulin, which is released at irregular intervals, resulting in low blood glucose levels, often extremely low. The same can happen in hypertrophy (enlargement) of the islets of Langerhans. Brain tumours may also be responsible, sending faulty messages to the pancreas. But this is not the hypoglycaemia that we are talking about.

The Price We Pay for Too Much Sugar What probably happens in the very common reactive hypoglycaemia, which is caused by things that we eat, is that its victims have been eating large quantities of sugar and sugary foods over a long period. Eventually the pancreas and the islets of Langerhans are so overworked and overloaded by being constantly called upon to dispose of the excessive amounts of glucose, that they begin to react in an inappropriate way. They anticipate the amount of insulin needed to remove the sugar and almost invariably overreact.

As a result, even when the amount of sugar being ingested is quite small — sometimes no more than the taste of sugar in the mouth — they secrete excessive amounts of insulin that are far more than the blood glucose present warrants. The result is that too much glucose is removed from the blood and the patient becomes hypoglycaemic.

If these people just allowed the situation to correct itself, which would eventually happen unless the pancreas has completely broken down, the problem would not be so serious. Normally, the amount of insulin released increases as glucose increases, which in turn leads to lower glucose and so lower insulin — fine tuning that ensures that the blood glucose does not go too high or too low.

Instead, what happens is that unconsciously (and sometimes very consciously), people with hypoglycaemia recognise that sugar brings rapid relief from the often very unpleasant symptoms of low blood glucose. Within a couple of hours of a meal, they are likely to be reaching for a very sweet snack.

The effect of this is that they very quickly feel refreshed and well. Of course as soon as they eat the sweet snack, the pancreas equally promptly overreacts again by secreting (or releasing) more excessive amounts of insulin. Very soon they are feeling as bad as before — and reaching yet again for another sugary snack. It is no wonder that so many hypoglycaemics are chronic and compulsive sugar nibblers, and that so many of them are obese.

For this very reason, the advice often given to hypoglycaemic patients by doctors, to suck a barley sugar or eat a sweet to counteract the feelings of weakness and lethargy, is completely counterproductive for most of them. The relief this gives is brief before the pancreas once again panics and the blood glucose level is dumped.

Sugar is the quick fix because it passes very rapidly into the blood. Eating a steak also releases sugar into the blood, but it takes a lot longer, because the protein and fat in the meat have to undergo a complex process of digestion, and then still have to be absorbed from the gut and further metabolised before they are finally converted into glucose. It is a much more gradual and healthy process, with which the pancreas could cope perfectly well if this were the main source of our sugar.

Punishing Our Bodies That hypoglycaemia is so prevalent is yet another example of the maladaptation of Western people in their diet. We have already noted that the average Australian and American eats more than 45 kilograms of sugar each year. Our bodies are hopelessly ill-equipped to cope with this kind of assault on our systems.

Our ancestors ate practically no concentrated sugar or starch, but adapted well to coping with the small amounts that did feature in their diet. Today, we are still only adapted to these small quantities. The fact that many people appear to be able to eat as much sugar as they like without risk of hypoglycaemia is only a reflection of the marvellous adaptability of the human body and the punishment that it can take. But it's a lottery. Some people smoke cigarettes all their lives without apparent ill-effects, but most do not. It is the same with sugar.

There are other factors at work as well. Both caffeine and nicotine stimulate the adrenal glands and cause the liver to release glucose into the blood. The pancreas again reacts by releasing insulin, and eventually too much insulin. To relieve the inevitable symptoms that follow, the patient usually reaches for another cup of coffee or another cigarette, and the whole vicious circle is perpetuated.

When the caffeine intake is combined with high sugar in the diet, as with sweetened coffee or with cola drinks (which contain caffeine as well as prodigious amounts of sugar), there is a compounding effect. It is easy to see how closely hypoglycaemia and food intolerance can be enmeshed.

Even when food intolerance and food addiction do not involve sugar-rich foods, they are often implicated in hypoglycaemia because the stress associated with intolerance triggers the pancreas to manufacture insulin. When this stress is constant, the pancreas is again likely to overreact and to produce too much insulin. The result is hypoglycaemia, and hypoglycaemia is usually at its worst in times of stress and distress.

Dr Carlton Frederick, one of the foremost authorities on the disease, has shown how stress, even as minimal as running on a treadmill for a few minutes, can elicit the full-blown symptoms of low blood glucose, typically about four hours after the exercise and in patients who otherwise react normally and have no history of low blood glucose.

Food Intolerance and Hypoglycaemia When food intolerance and hypoglycaemia are involved simultaneously, as they frequently are, the symptoms of both may be very similar, but still be occurring independently. If only sugar is eliminated from the diet, therefore, the symptoms may appear to persist, when in fact these same symptoms result from food intolerance. It is still necessary to identify and eliminate the offending food as well before the symptoms are completely removed.

It is important to know this because many people give up sugar and other stimulants after reading about hypoglycaemia and recognising it as the cause of their own problems. When they find that they feel only marginally better, or even no better at all as sometimes happens, they become downhearted and lose interest. This depression adds to their stress and the symptoms become even worse.

The only mistake they have made is to give up too soon. The effort they made in eliminating as much sugar as possible from their diet was just one essential step. If they had pinpointed their food intolerance and taken care only of that, without dealing simultaneously with the sugar problem, the result would have been the same. That is why I almost always measure patients' blood glucose during testing for food intolerance.

Even when people are obviously eating and drinking unhealthily large amounts of sugar (one of my patients was drinking four litres of Coca-Cola each day, which put nearly 500 grams of sugar into his body, most of it going straight to the bloodstream), or taking too much caffeine or nicotine, this may be a subconscious search for a "high" that will help overcome the symptoms of food intolerance, which is the real problem.

Deficiencies in vitamins, particularly vitamins B_5, B_6, C and biotin, and minerals such as magnesium, zinc and chromium, all of which are closely involved in the mechanism of maintaining normal blood glucose levels, may inhibit this mechanism and contribute to hypoglycaemia.

Even the perennially maligned fluoride has been implicated on the grounds that fluoride has the effect of blocking aconitase, a key enzyme in the metabolism of sugar for energy. To my knowledge, nothing has yet been proved one way or the other, but it may turn out to be one more nail in the coffin of fluoride.

Alcoholics become chronically low in blood glucose because alcohol prevents the release of glucose from the liver into the bloodstream. But I believe there is an even closer link between hypoglycaemia and the cause of many cases of alcoholism, a link that needs to be explored (see Chapter 27).

Mimicking Every Disease Whether hypoglycaemia occurs occasionally after a single meal, where it is of no real concern, or is entrenched and chronic, the symptoms can mimic virtually any disease. As we have seen, the disorders associated with the brain are the most severe and the hardest to live with, but migraine, arthritis and asthma are all common symptoms.

Hypoglycaemia is often missed at medical checkups. Even when it *is* recognised, it is likely to be treated (if it is treated at all) in the worst possible way, by encouraging the patient to stabilise the condition with more sugar. It is often found, not because the doctor is looking for it, but when diabetes is suspected: instead of high levels of blood glucose, low levels are found. The main significance of this is that the patient is *not* diabetic.

Diabetics are only too well aware of the need to keep their blood glucose levels rigidly under control. The hypoglycaemic patient, however, is often not even aware that he *is* hypoglycaemic, let alone of the need to control it. So many doctors dismiss it as being of no serious concern, to be corrected by sucking a barley sugar, that this attitude is entirely understandable.

The consequence is that these people are trying to function, hour after hour, day in and day out, with some of the symptoms that the diabetic is not expected to endure for more than a brief period when he takes an overdose of insulin. Perhaps it is because diabetes is seen to be life-threatening, while reactive hypoglycaemia — for all that many would aver that it is life-destroying — never actually kills. People tend to dismiss diseases that do not actually kill you, no matter how much pain or discomfort they cause, as being not too serious. Ask any victim of arthritis!

Unfortunately, the symptoms are often also the kind of symptoms that doctors with no understanding of ecological illness, choose to dismiss as neurotic.

As an example of how often hypoglycaemia can be misdiagnosed, a recent American study comes as a salutary warning. I have no doubt that the same findings would be made in Australia.

Of 522 patients who were being treated for hypoglycaemia, no less than 514 had previously been misdiagnosed, with no suggestion that low blood glucose levels played any part in their symptoms! The most common diagnosis was "neurotic", followed by "slightly nervous" and "imaginary sickness" (in more than 65 per cent of cases!). These were followed by "chronic asthma", "skin disease caused by nerves" and "psychoneurotic".

Even more worrying were the fifteen who had been wrongly diagnosed as being "mentally retarded", the one who was said to have Parkinson's disease (he didn't), the twenty who were dismissed as alcoholics, and the nineteen who were labelled as suffering from "post-childbirth shock", a handy peg on which to hang cases that defy conventional methods of diagnosis.

Perhaps we shouldn't be surprised, when we remember all the wrong diagnoses of food and chemical intolerance. The doctors responsible were, when all is said and done, merely practising the medicine they were taught in medical school. For 98.5 per cent of that group of patients, what the doctors had been taught was clearly not enough.

TESTING FOR HYPOGLYCAEMIA ■

The standard test for hypoglycaemia is the glucose tolerance test (GTT), which is also the classic test for diagnosing diabetes. In both cases, we are concerned with the body's ability or inability to deal with ingested sugar.

After a short fast, usually overnight, the patient is given a concentrated solution of glucose to drink. I normally recommend 75 grams of glucose diluted in water. Most pathologists use a commercial preparation, artificially flavoured and coloured to improve the taste. How undesirable that is! A blood sample is taken before the glucose is drunk, which serves as a control and is known as the fasting blood glucose level. Then at various intervals in the hours after the glucose has been drunk, more blood is taken and measured for its glucose content. By comparing these subsequent readings with the control, plotted usually as a curve on a graph, the doctor can see how the patient's body tolerates and responds to sugar entering the bloodstream. Blood insulin levels can also be measured.

In a healthy system, where there is no hypoglycaemia of concern, the blood glucose level rises to a peak about one hour after the ingestion of the glucose. Then, over the following hours, it gradually settles down again to approximately the control level.

In diabetes, the control is elevated and then the level rises much higher than normal and only very slowly goes down, not returning to the fasting level for six hours or more, depending on the severity of the diabetes. In hypoglycaemia, on the other hand, the initial rise is usually followed by a rapid drop to below the fasting level, as the pancreas pumps out the insulin: the lower and the faster it drops, the more severe are the symptoms likely to be.

There are a number of "typical" hypoglycaemic curves (see Fig. 3) which are not really typical at all, so great are the number of individual variations. Hypoglycaemia is an extremely personal disease and a hundred hypoglycaemic patients are capable of having a hundred different reactions to the GTT.

Even for doctors who are working daily with hypoglycaemia and who understand many of its quirks, the curve can be very confusing. Doctors without this experience may easily misinterpret the results and read the significance of the curve incorrectly. One cause of the confusion is the standard medical practice that treats levels of blood glucose below a specified figure as being hypoglycaemia by definition. This figure is commonly set at 2.8 mmol/L (50 mg per 100 mL) of blood, but 3.5 and even 4.0–5.6 mmol/L are sometimes used. Whatever the figure (I personally favour 2.8 mmol/L), I do not believe that this is the correct approach.

The Important Factors in the GTT   The simple fact of a fall in the blood glucose level, even an appreciable fall, is not necessarily significant in itself. About a third of the population normally experiences a measure of hypoglycaemia when they are hungry and it is a normal mechanism that tells us it is time to

Figure 3.

TYPICAL RESULTS OF A SIX-HOUR GLUCOSE
TOLERANCE TEST

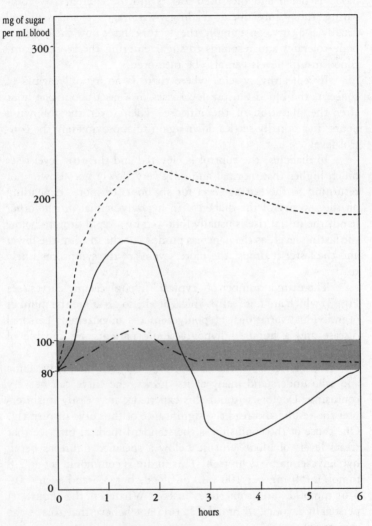

Patient with blood sugar level of 80 mg per cent drinks glucose at zero hours.

Normal span _.._.._.._.._.._.._.._.._.._.._.._.._.._

Diabetic range _ _ _ _ _ _ _ _ _ _ _ _ _ _ _ _ _ _

Hypoglycaemic drops _____

eat. At the end of a six-hour GTT, which has itself come after an overnight fast, almost everyone is likely to be hungry and many will demonstrate a fall in blood glucose level.

What is much more important in hypoglycaemia than any absolute figure is the fluctuation in blood glucose during the test and the speed at which this fluctuation takes place, for these are the two factors that have the greatest bearing on the symptoms.

The blood glucose level may fall to 2.8 mmol/L or below, for example, but if it recovers quickly to the fasting level, it may indicate only mild hypoglycaemia with no noticeable symptoms. On the other hand, the low point on another patient's curve may be at, or even above, 3.5 or 4.0 mmol/L. If the level has fallen rapidly to this point from the initial peak an hour or so after ingesting the glucose to the fasting level and then takes several hours to climb back to the original fasting level, this prolonged and *relatively* low level of blood glucose may result in very severe reactions.

Again, there is often a rapid and short-lived rise to quite high levels, even to the point of resembling diabetes, followed by an equally rapid drop. This fall, too, is often associated with severe symptoms of hypoglycaemia, even if the reading at the end of the six-hour period is relatively normal. It is what has happened in the meantime that is significant.

Because of this need to be aware of fluctuations, frequent blood tests must be made. Some doctors using the GTT, who are looking only for diabetes, test once after two hours. If they find high levels of blood glucose at this time, they can reasonably conclude that diabetes is present and this can be verified by various other tests. When testing for diabetes, even if more frequent measures are made, the GTT ends at two hours which is far too short when looking for hypoglycaemia.

In hypoglycaemia, however, a single test after two hours is useless because it tells us nothing about any variations that take place. I normally test every half hour for two hours, and then hourly for the next four hours. I believe that five hours is the minimum acceptable testing period, but that six hours is preferable, because sudden changes do quite frequently occur after five hours. Sometimes, I monitor for eight hours.

I also encourage patients to take a blood sample for testing whenever they feel that their symptoms are particularly trying or painful. If these moments coincide with low blood glucose, it is an important pointer to the presence of reactive hypoglycaemia. There is nothing wrong with testing on the half hour and the hour, but it is a tidiness that nature does not observe. The glucose level can plummet and return to its former level even within a period of thirty minutes.

During the GTT, I ask the patient to keep a detailed list of symptoms experienced, including the exact time when they occur. If symptoms coincide with a change in blood glucose, it may be just as important an indicator as the absolute blood glucose levels.

A Simple Way to Test   In the past, the GTT was nearly always carried out by a pathologist, who measured the glucose levels in a sample of blood taken by intravenous injection. But to draw blood in this way eight and more times in six hours is unacceptable for many patients, and fortunately it is no longer necessary. It does, however, allow insulin levels to be measured.

Technology has given us a simple means of measuring blood glucose levels by taking just a drop of blood from a prick in a finger. The blood is placed on a test strip and a chemical reaction occurs, which causes a colour change in the strip. This colour is then measured in a special machine.

The test takes only about two minutes from start to finish so that the results are virtually immediate, and it involves minimal discomfort for the patient. As the machine is simple to operate and relatively inexpensive, the tests may be carried out even by patients themselves and certainly by any doctor. It is a very efficient way of monitoring blood glucose levels and many diabetics now have their own machines to check their levels and so their insulin requirements.

It is a test, however, that *must* be carried out carefully or spurious results may occur. Pathologists tend not to accept the results of the machines. Regardless of this, and even if there is some degree of inaccuracy, the convenience and ready availability far outweigh the frequent impossibility of a pathologist or his technician being present for a continuing period of six hours, or even being conveniently there when symptoms occur, to say nothing of the expense. In any case, no single blood glucose measurement, by whatever method, diagnoses hypoglycaemia.

It is unarguable that the GTT itself is open to criticism, in that it is an artificial laboratory-type test. No-one normally eats glucose as a food, except occasionally as a drink (sugar, the main culprit, is a disaccharide — two simple sugars, glucose and fructose), any more than in real life patients sit at rest for six hours straight.

The ideal GTT would be for the patient to eat, for example, a normal breakfast and then monitor the blood glucose over the next six hours as he or she goes about normal daily activities — rushing to work, coping with the stress of work, doing the housework and so on. Then the blood glucose should be monitored and linked with the progression of the symptoms. Unfortunately this isn't usually done, but it would seem to be the best approach to sort out the difficult cases.

The Importance of the Patient's History   The history that is taken from every patient at an early consultation is very important, not only in determining whether we should carry out a GTT, but in correctly reading the curve on the graph. Again, neither the curve nor the history can be relied on in isolation.

When we are deciding whether the GTT is warranted (and it usually is in cases of food intolerance), we look at the pattern of the patient's life. If the history shows, for example, that she is waking up at 2 a.m. to raid the fridge, or is generally suffering from insomnia and not functioning properly during the day until she has had food, or gets cranky and suffers headaches if her meals are late, then we always suspect hypoglycaemia and test for it.

They may be symptoms of food intolerance without any involvement with sugar, but the odds are strong that hypoglycaemia on its own, coinciding with the food intolerance, is implicated. On the other hand midafternoon drowsiness — a very common symptom of low blood glucose — without other symptoms, may not be significant.

One note of caution needs to be sounded. There are some drugs that can add to the stress that is always present to some degree during a GTT. As these include certain common drugs, such as aspirin, a number of hormones, diuretics and some oral contraceptives, and as there can on rare occasions be quite severe reactions, it is important that the GTT be conducted either by a doctor or at least with the specific approval of a doctor. In the days when a pathologist was needed to carry out a GTT, a doctor was invariably involved, but with the availability today of the finger-prick procedures, many people can carry out their own GTTs.

A few doctors insist on the GTT being carried out late in

the morning or in the afternoon, rather than first thing in the morning, which is the usual practice because of the sheer time that is needed to complete a six-hour test. There is some evidence that patients may show an abnormal reaction to a glucose challenge early in the morning, but be entirely normal if they are challenged at noon or in the afternoon; and these doctors claim that the later reading is the correct one.

The rationale for this is that our remote ancestors, whose food adaptation we have inherited, never had a heavy breakfast because they first had to go out and catch it or pick it off the bushes, which took several hours. Early humans, therefore, consumed most of their food late in the morning or in the early afternoon. In the twentieth century, we are still maladapted to eating breakfasts rich in sugar. Therefore, the argument goes, the GTT ought to be carried out in the late morning or early afternoon if we want a true picture.

Whatever the logic of this, most doctors would find it quite impossible to fit all their GTTs into this restricted period. My own view is that if a patient shows signs and symptoms of severe hypoglycaemia in the morning after an all-night fast, then he is suffering from hypoglycaemia and needs to be treated accordingly, whatever the time of day.

TREATING HYPOGLYCAEMIA ■

As the cause of reactive hypoglycaemia is faulty eating in most cases, the solution is in our own hands. The important thing is to avoid the foods that send the sugar straight into the bloodstream and to wean the pancreas off its maladaptive habit of releasing excessive amounts of insulin into the blood. What we need, therefore, is a diet low in sugar, low in simple carbohydrate (which the body can convert rapidly into glucose), and high in foods that do not trigger the pancreas to react in this inappropriate way.

There is no cure for hypoglycaemia in the sense that we can come up with a magic formula that will allow refined carbohydrates to be eaten with impunity for the rest of a patient's life without any further risk of hypoglycaemia developing. For some people this means excluding concentrated, refined carbohydrates for life, as far as that is possible and practical. If the symptoms have been severe, most would think that it is a very fair price to pay.

Paradoxically I have found that both high-fat, high-protein, as well as low-fat, low-protein diets work effectively in over-coming hypoglycaemia, provided of course that they both ex-clude refined carbohydrate, and particularly sugar. I lean towards the low-fat, low-protein diet, because the alternative is bad news in the long term for the arteries. While a high-fat, high-protein diet may sort out the problems of the hypoglycaemia, it may well be adding greatly to the risk of something more serious and life-threatening developing. The low-fat, low-protein diet needs to be followed for life.

The Pritikin program and its variants, particularly the Ross Horne and McDougall plans, work very well with hypoglycaemic patients (see Chapter 17). All place great importance on exercise as well as diet.

Although I prefer the low-fat, low-protein diet, I should qualify that slightly because there seems to be no doubt that a high-fat, high-protein diet gives the most rapid initial results. What is essential to remember, however, is that as soon as the hypoglycaemia is under control, the fat content should be pro-gressively reduced to low levels as Pritikin recommends. Although the diet may eventually include unlimited amounts of complex carbohydrate, simple carbohydrate, or sugar, is almost always banned for life.

A low-fat, low-protein diet, or one that is basically made up of complex carbohydrates, is likely to have good results except that initially it is slower. For those who want to build up their carbohydrate intake gradually, first from 5 to 12 per cent, then to more than 12 per cent, Appendix XI lists common foods by their carbohydrate content.

The correct diet involves not only a change in the foods that are eaten, but also in eating times. Hypoglycaemic patients are encouraged to have a snack an hour or so before they expect the onset of symptoms, particularly quick energy foods, though of course not refined carbohydrates or stimulants, which only enhance the swings in blood glucose levels. As the symptoms im-prove, they will find that they need fewer snacks. In particular, they should eat small meals every three hours while they are awake, rather than infrequent large amounts.

A Treatment Too Simple For Some   Many people, largely one suspects because of the cynicism of some doctors, find it diffi-cult to accept that any form of illness can be completely con-trolled (what most lay people would call cured) simply by changing the diet. Yet that is frequently the case.

I remember one woman who came to my clinic for food testing on the referral of her family doctor. Her history suggested that sugar featured excessively in her diet. We carried out a GTT, which showed that she was suffering severely from hypoglycaemia. We recommended a suitable diet without doing any further testing and then tried to discharge her.

I say "tried", because she was most indignant and objected strenuously to being sent home without the barrage of tests that she had been promised. It took much persuasion to convince her that a new diet was probably all that she needed to make a complete recovery, and so it turned out. Our customers come to doctors with very clear expectations of what we should do for them!

What people ought to be doing, of course, is avoiding both diabetes and reactive hypoglycaemia in the first place, and this can nearly always be achieved by correct diet. By the time maturity-onset diabetes manifests itself, it may be too late to reverse it, but for the hypoglycaemic, it is never too late. Management is very straightforward, even if it needs a good deal of discipline and willpower. This makes it all the more tragic that so many hundreds of thousands of people go through life suffering unnecessarily because of this insidious disease.

Nobody, being realistic, can expect to cut refined sugar completely out of the diet. Ninety-nine out of a hundred people either will not or cannot cut it out completely. If a diet is too difficult to follow, too boring or unpalatable, nobody will bother to keep to it. The aim therefore is to reduce sugar intake as far as possible, knowing that the ideal is to cut it out altogether.

Normal blood glucose levels can be maintained from natural sources through the metabolisation of the food we eat, including fats, complex carbohydrates and proteins. These are converted into glucose as the need arises.

When Sugar Isn't Sugar   Sugar is a loose word that describes many different forms of sugar. The Americans claim to be able to describe it in seventy-one different ways under their strict labelling requirements, so that potential buyers of a product are not frightened off by a high sugar content when all types are grouped as one category — "sugar".

For every kilogram of sugar that we eat as refined sugar (the concentrated extract from natural sugar that most of us recognise as sugar), we eat 2.5 kilograms in manufactured goods, most of it again refined.

The cornerstone, then, of all hypoglycaemia therapy is an individually tailored and correct diet. Obviously, if food intolerance is also involved, patients must exclude "unsafe" foods as well, even if they would normally be acceptable in a strictly hypoglycaemic diet.

Trying to treat hypoglycaemia in any other way is pointless. Treating the symptoms without getting at the underlying cause achieves nothing except making the patient even more depressed. Drugs, psychiatry, even electric shock therapy, all of which are used by some doctors, simply aim to reduce the symptoms and do nothing about the underlying cause. You cannot tranquillise hypoglycaemia into submission, shock it or punish it; and you cannot talk it away with clichés like "the symptoms are all psychosomatic", or "it's just nerves".

The treatment of hypoglycaemia is not easy and although it is a disease that cannot be "cured" in the strictest sense, it can be controlled in the great majority of cases. To deny its very existence is the cruellest of all attitudes, because not only does this add to the sufferer's woes, by leaving him believing that he is neurotic on top of everything else, and that the symptoms are somehow brought on by his own weakness as a person — the clear inference is that if he just pulled himself together, he would get well — but it is denying him relief from a disorder that is completely controllable.

HYPOGLYCIA ▮

Hypoglycia is a condition that is closely related to hypoglycaemia. It is possible for a patient to have a normal GTT, yet still suffer from all the symptoms of hypoglycaemia, and this is usually because of hypoglycia.

In hypoglycia, because of the lack of certain chemicals and vitamins, the sugar does not metabolise properly. The symptoms are very like those of hypoglycaemia, and similarly the brain and the rest of the central nervous system are the first to be affected.

Treatment normally includes supplements of B group and C vitamins, plus mineral supplements, particularly manganese and zinc. Simple carbohydrates (sugar) must be excluded with the same thoroughness as in hypoglycaemia. I suspect that hypoglycia is also caused by food intolerance, but not enough recent work has been carried out in this area to confirm this.

Doctors are very good at putting labels on people based on clusters of symptoms, and not on the cause. As a profession we are only too quick to dismiss depressed, anxious and phobic patients as neurotic, time-consuming people who ought to go home and pull themselves together and stop wasting our valuable time. As for the delusional, the hallucinating and the confused, we tag them psychotic and usually add "schizophrenic" for good measure. If patients have no idea what is wrong with them, we say their symptoms are psychosomatic or ideopathic, diagnoses based on observable behaviour or thought patterns, without defining the underlying cause. Personality disorder is another useful label.

All of these labels may be justified in some patients. The trouble is that once they have been given, they are likely to mean that those patients will be treated until the end of their lives as neurotics, psychotics, schizophrenics or whatever. They can look forward to a succession of ever more potent and potentially harmful pharmaceutical drugs.

After twenty years on this regimen, the only miracle is that some of them still have enough intelligence to put one foot in front of the other and walk. And I say this with all the experience of a physician whose practice is very much psychiatrically inclined.

WHAT CAUSES MENTAL ILLNESS?

There are many theories to account for mental illness and the greatest mistake that we can make as a profession is to accept that any one of them is right to the exclusion of all the others.

Psychiatry's strong philosophical bias resulted in the basic assumption that, almost without exception, neurotic and psychotic symptoms are caused by an assortment of conflicts, guilt, dependencies and personality immaturities, but all occurring in a

physically entirely well person, although possibly a person genetically predisposed to be mentally ill.

If the patient isn't physically well, the argument goes, *that*
is the result of the emotional disturbance and its effect on the
patient's life, or else it is entirely unrelated to it. In other words,
there is nothing "wrong" with the patient in the sense that there
is any physical illness. There may be biochemical malfunction,
which would not show up as physical disease.

In many cases, true mental illness is clearly due to unre-
solved conflicts, repressed guilt and other emotional disturbances.
Such patients need (and often respond to) skilled psychotherapy,
both analytical (going back to the original cause of the conflict)
and supportive.

Other psychological disorders are manifestly caused by
factors that are not psychological in origin, but organic. It is
equally important that doctors understand this so that they can
be highlighted for investigation. Mental illness results from
alcohol abuse, for example, Korsakov's syndrome (the main
symptoms of which are amnesia and confusion caused by a combination of alcohol and severe food deficiency), syphilis, brain
tumours (especially the slow-growing melingiomas), or the true
endocrine diseases such as thyroidism.

Similarly, infectious, toxic, hormonal, nutritional, metabolic and immunological factors can all be involved, and frequently are, in triggering mental illness. No progress will be
made in treating the symptoms unless first the underlying
organic cause is addressed and resolved.

FINDING THE RIGHT THERAPY ■

The tendency to prescribe ever more potent drugs for so many
psychological diseases and disorders is cause for great concern.
The evidence is irrefutable in many cases that the drugs not only
achieve no positive results, but leave the patient in a much worse
condition than before they were prescribed.

Yet having said that, the popular view that drug therapy in
psychological disease is wholly inappropriate, is equally wrong.
Drugs have a very important place. Antidepressants, anxiolytics
(to relieve the symptoms of anxiety), sedatives and antipsychotic
drugs play a vital role in bringing some patients back to normality. It is short-sighted to dismiss their value on the grounds
that so much other drug therapy prescribed for psychological ill-

ness is not only inappropriate but downright bad medicine.

In between those patients who are suffering from organic disease and those whose disorders are unequivocally caused by psychological factors in their lives (and who can be successfully treated by conventional psychoanalysis and the other conventional tools of the psychiatrist) is a far larger group of patients who do not respond significantly to either approach. For very many of these, the environmental approach of clinical ecology is succeeding in an often dramatic way.

Yet other patients respond well to a combination of orthodox treatment and an ecological approach. To unravel and sort out traumas in early life may take years of therapy, but I have found that many patients, who also suffer from food or chemical intolerance, respond much more quickly to such psychotherapy once the intolerance reactions have been sorted out, even when the patients have already had extensive psychotherapy.

Each day we see strong evidence that mental and emotional conditions are environmental in origin, the result of intolerance reactions to foods or chemicals, deficiencies in the body of trace elements or vitamins, or a combination of all three. Nor is it only the comparatively minor mental disorders, devastating as these can be, that are caused by environmental factors.

Cases that look like frank (unmistakable) psychosis, severe mental derangements that affect a person's whole personality and would frequently warrant hospitalisation, respond to an ecological approach. This shouldn't be surprising, when we know that foods and chemicals are capable of producing every symptom and shade of symptom that is normally described as neurotic, psychotic or schizophrenic, as well as the even greater array of common physical symptoms and illnesses that are often dismissed as psychosomatic.

GETTING OUT OF THE WOODSHED ▮

There is a clear concept in clinical ecology that there is no definite dividing line between mental and physical disease, or at most there is a very fine one. It requires a radical change of attitude for generations of doctors brought up to believe what Freud told them — that mental illness occurs only as the result of early conditioning or trauma — even though Freud himself believed that a physiological explanation would one day be found for mental illness.

As Dr Richard Mackarness nicely put it, it is a move to get away from the what-happened-in-the-woodshed school of psychiatry, which so often fails to provide any answers at all.

The idea that some foods can induce mental disease dates back a long way. In 1621, the scholar Richard Burton, in his *Anatomy of Melancholy*, one of the most remarkable books ever written, referred to it in some detail.

Timing — or mistiming — played a considerable part in delaying the introduction of clinical ecology into psychiatry. Dr Theron Randolph first reported a cause-and-effect relationship between food and chemicals and psychiatric symptoms in the 1950s. Unfortunately for the next two generations of mentally ill patients, it was also just the time that modern psychopharmacology was expanding and the market was bombarded with the phenothiazine tranquillisers. Drug therapy was all the vogue.

In consequence, many psychiatrists, in addition to searching for some emotional scarring in their patients' childhoods, took to the prescription pad and tried to treat chronic depressions, for example, with pharmaceuticals, when their only cause was an overgenerous serving of cheddar cheese.

It wasn't always quite so blatant, of course, but psychiatrists and physicians certainly were not in the mood to turn their backs on new wonder drugs in favour of a change in their patients' eating habits.

Sociologically, it is probably even more important that we explore the link between the environment and mental illness than the association between foods, chemicals and the physical symptoms and disorders of intolerance, at least from the point of view of the patient. It is one of the cruelties of our age that the mentally ill (which all too often means only that in somebody else's perception they are different) must still bear the shameful stigma of being insane or abnormal.

It is time for some new development in psychiatry. There has been no important advance since the introduction of the antidepressant and antipsychotic drugs in the 1950s — a long time for any discipline to go without making any significant progress in its field. This failure to advance could well be redressed by clinical ecology, which is successfully treating many thousands of psychiatric patients who previously resisted all conventional therapy.

There have been many "new" antidepressant and antipsychotic drugs since the 1950s that do work, but the search still goes on for that most elusive of goals, a drug that achieves all that the best of the available ones can offer, without a single undesirable side effect. At present, we seem to be as far away as ever from achieving it.

SUCCEEDING WHERE OTHERS FAIL ■

What we see in ecological illness is the reaction to foods or chemicals that can excite or inhibit any tissue or organ in the body and produce any of the symptoms that those tissues or organs are capable of demonstrating. It is no different when that organ is the brain, which, like any other organ, is just a mass of cells. Like the heart, liver or kidneys, the brain works by the interaction of biochemical molecules, and the biochemistry of those cells can go wrong, no matter which organ is involved.

The fact that we have not yet been able to explain how these biochemical events can trigger so many non-material reactions (like fear and love, laughter and sadness) is no reason for deluding ourselves into thinking that brain cells and heart cells are somehow not made of the same stuff.

The point that I make continually about mental illness is that even though an ecological approach is not achieving anything like a 100 per cent success rate, it is still proving very successful in many situations where conventional therapy has failed.

In the case of the schizophrenic syndrome, for example, the success rate may be no higher than between 15 and 20 per cent. Nevertheless, given that the prognosis for schizophrenics without the aid of clinical ecology is a life sentence, surely it ought to be axiomatic that they should be given the chance to respond, knowing that one in six of them is likely to be helped significantly.

At the worst it involves two weeks of testing after a five-day fast, which is beneficial in its own right and which has no risk whatever attached to it. (Fasting and testing of anyone who is mentally ill must be carried out under the close supervision of a doctor or trained staff.)

To deny this to the mentally ill is to use the same argument that some cynics use against clinical ecology, that the high success rate is nothing more than a placebo effect. Apart from the fact that this is demonstrably nonsense, what does if matter? If a third of all those patients who fail to respond to hospitalisation, drug therapy and interminable visits to specialists and other doctors over years get better after taking a two cent pill or because they want to please their new doctor, what progress we have made! Because it responds to a placebo, an illness is no less an illness.

GETTING OFF THE CONSULTATION TREADMILL ■

No doctor who has adopted an ecological approach in his practice should deny that there probably is a bias in the patients he sees and treats successfully. We tend to see those people who have not done well with conventional therapy, with drugs and psychotherapy (and there are some patients who do very well with these) or who are unwilling to accept the side effects of drugs, or to resign themselves to a life that is not totally free of symptoms.

In consequence, they keep looking and they are often the patients who insist on going to multiple doctors and having multiple investigations. It is not always the doctor who insists on the patient climbing on to the treadmill of endless tests and consultations when initial tests have proved negative. It is sometimes the patients themselves who demand this. If the doctor disagrees with their attitude it makes it all the more likely that he will eventually brand them neurotic for not listening to him.

Among the patients who make their way to the clinical ecologist's rooms, there is certainly a disproportionate number of these people, whose quest for a cure and persistence lead them to try anything. Because conventional therapy has been unsuccessful, it increases the likelihood that there is an environmental factor involved, which we are able to identify and overcome.

But, having conceded our bias, it is right to say that depression, hallucination, hyperactivity, schizophrenic syndrome, aggression, fearfulness and anxiety all frequently respond when they are viewed and treated as environmental illnesses — the result not of some horrific experience in childhood, but perhaps of eating some common food too often, or of sharing a house with a gas stove or urea formaldehyde insulation.

ECOLOGICALLY TRIGGERED MENTAL ILLNESS ■

It is impossible to make any hard and fast distinction, but we often see that the true psychological patients, whose illnessses are not (or at least not entirely) triggered by food or chemicals, complain mainly of emotional difficulties in relation to particular types of life situation. They do not suffer from a multitude of physical symptoms in addition to the mental symptoms, which are often very varied.

Often these patients relate their present difficulties, which brought them to the surgery, to earlier experiences, and they have clear ideas about the kind of psychological help they believe will be beneficial. They tend to view *themselves* as having psychological problems — they are afraid to go out in public because of their agoraphobia, for example, or they fear men because of some childhood assault.

But the mentally ill patient whose disorder is caused by an ecological factor, complains predominantly of episodic or chronic symptoms, which cannot readily be construed in psychological terms. While the psychological patient's panic attacks are clearly situational — the trigger can be as varied as examinations, going out, authority, or mice — ecological patients' symptoms come on out of the blue, for no obvious psychological reason.

Although they are often worse in their severity, there is no systematic and predictable relationship with any obvious precipitant.

By contrast with psychological patients, the ecological patients are often riddled with bodily symptoms and disorders as well, most of which they have been told are psychosomatic and the result of, say, their anxiety. It is perfectly true that anxiety can be accompanied by, or cause, symptoms in any organ of the body: every organ that has an autonomic nerve supply (and every organ does) can be involved. But often the cause is ecological.

It is a real skill to identify symptoms that arise from anxiety and distinguish them from identical symptoms that are independent of the anxiety.

With ecological patients, we do not accept that the problem is a panic attack or depersonalisation, or whatever label is hung on them, but rather we recognise the symptoms as being the outward manifestation of some environmental sensitivity. These patients have not *learned* to behave in maladaptive ways — they are experiencing these abnormal states because of something they have eaten, drunk, breathed in or touched, which their systems cannot tolerate.

What they want — and what they nearly always know they want, often in spite of years of denial and even ridicule by their doctors — is help in getting rid of their symptoms.

I used to be surprised at the number of patients who

claimed that they had suspected for many years that an environmental factor might be responsible, often with no information to think this possible, let alone any way of proving it. I am no longer surprised because so often I see their instinct being proved right. Doctors are *not* always right: doctors do *not* always know best: and doctors *do* make mistakes.

TREATING PSYCHIATRIC PATIENTS ■

The detailed history that is taken from all our patients gives a lot of clues as to the likely cause of the problem. As in every case, the first priority is to rule out any organic cause before any attempt is made to treat the illness and the symptoms by an ecological approach. Experience, coupled with the knowledge of the therapy that has already been attempted and, of course, the history, will guide us to the approach that looks most promising.

With psychiatric patients, ecological treatment, whether by avoidance or neutralising drops, is never done in isolation. It must be combined with the appropriate psychotherapy, if that is considered relevant, or with any other conventional psychiatric or psychological therapy. To a greater extent than with patients whose symptoms are purely physical, there may by now be genuine psychological problems to be cleared up, even though the specific cause of the symptoms is a number of foods. These psychological problems exist not because of the intolerance, but as the result of the patient's inappropriate treatment by a variety of experts over months and years, and particularly because of the side effects of the drugs that invariably have been prescribed and consumed over long periods of time.

If you put a patient on to a regimen of potent drugs with instructions that he is to keep taking them forever, or at least until they are replaced by another, usually more potent drug, then you are bestowing on that person all the potential side effects (and none of these are pleasant) without achieving a scintilla of good.

The most relevant and the most forgotten fact in health care is that it is not drugs that cure people, but the body's own curative mechanism. There is no known connection between drugs and the disease process itself, a fact that leaves many lay people bewildered.

All that drugs do is aid the body in its natural task. Either they kill off bacteria so that the immune system can get on with the job of restoring full health, or they play a holding role until the real cause of the disease can be identified and hopefully removed.

IMPROVING THE QUALITY OF LIFE ▊

The principle behind the ecological treatment of psychological illness and symptoms is exactly the same as in the treatment of physical disorders. Each one of us is a unique individual, with special biochemical needs, and we must be treated that way. We are not simply a conglomeration of cells whose needs can all be met in an identical, regimented way by some notional minimum daily allowance of proteins, nutrients and vitamins.

The kind of food we eat, the physical and emotional stress we are exposed to, the environment where we live and work, our unique inherited individual characteristics and the exercise we take all add up to the kind of person we are, the health we can expect to enjoy and the way we ought to be treated when that health, be it physical or mental, breaks down.

Giving patients advice on how to live with their symptoms hardly matches up to the value of therapy that removes those symptoms. Clinical ecology removes the symptoms of many of the mentally ill patients treated. Even those whose illness is not mainly environmental are likely to benefit if there is some intolerance present — and many do display environmental symptoms in addition to their disease state. By removing these symptoms, we can do a great deal to improve their life quality as well, as we have seen, and this adds to the effectiveness of other more orthodox treatment.

There is a real problem with mental illness. Even though it is properly the province of the psychiatrist and there is a large number of well-qualified psychiatrists in Australia, many people are reluctant to go to them. On the other hand, if everyone who needed this kind of specialised help accepted a referral to a psychiatrist, psychiatrists would not be able to cope with the numbers.

Either way, the overworked general practitioner can expect to have to deal with many of these patients himself. If he has little idea how the symptoms arose in the first place, he is facing a near impossible task. It is no wonder that so many family doctors — unaware of what they are looking at, or even what they should be looking for, and often suspecting that the whole thing is a put-on — fall back on the vast array of drugs that the pharmaceutical companies not only offer them, but through their representatives bring great pressure on the doctor to prescribe.

All too often, they are drugs that help the doctor's workload, but do much worse than nothing for the patient.

Clinical ecology in no way attempts to usurp the role of the psychiatrist, indeed it ought to be a routine part of the psychiatrist's armoury. For the first time, however, it offers a very real and valuable aid to the family doctor in dealing with what previously appeared to be an impossible challenge.

I have no doubt that clinical ecology will make a very significant difference to psychiatry in the future, perhaps even more radical than its role in physical illness.

ANXIETY ■

Anxiety is the most common psychiatric complaint. In the medical sense, it occurs when the input to the brain and the central nervous system from the outside world through the senses, and from our inner world through memories, feelings, health and so on, fails to be adequately integrated. It is not sorted out, slotted in, interpreted and made to relate to everything else that goes on in our surroundings.

Anxiety is not a disease state, not a genetic, biochemical state, in the same way as, say, schizophrenia. It is expressed through the autonomic nervous system and particularly the sympathetic nervous system. (The autonomic nervous system is the part of the nervous system that controls and regulates the internal organs without any conscious recognition or effort on our part. The sympathetic nervous system is a part of this and connects the internal organs to the brain.)

Anxiety can affect every organ. Its symptoms, apart from an anxious feeling, can include anything from sweaty palms, palpitations and diarrhoea, to shakes, nervousness and feelings of panic and claustrophobia. It is a very common symptom of ecological illness and frequently responds well to an ecological approach.

DEPRESSION ■

Depression is probably the next most common psychiatric complaint after anxiety. It too is not necessarily an illness, but is associated with many mental and physical disorders. It follows no regular course and has no particular or specific outcome. It may be fleeting or permanent, mild or severe, acute or chronic. It is marked by sadness, inactivity and self-deprecation and it has rightly and without exaggeration been described as a living hell for millions of people. It can destroy its victims' lives and not infrequently it ends in suicide.

Although it is usually found in the middle-aged or the elderly, it can also affect patients who are fairly young. It is often believed to be the result of unhappy events in the life of the patient, such as a death, retirement or a move to a new home far from old friends. My own experience is that, while such events in life may contribute to the problem, mild depression or brain fag usually precedes them and provides the underlying mechanism for the development of the actual crisis.

Most often, depression is the result not of some traumatic life event, but the much more prosaic end product of lifelong addiction or intolerance to foods, drinks or environmental chemicals. It is, in other words, a true ecological illness in many patients and the first line of attack ought to be an ecological one.

A Difficult Disorder to Treat Like all psychological illnesses, it is easier and certainly much less time-consuming, to treat the symptoms instead of looking for the cause, particularly in something as subjective as depression. The truth is that few medical problems respond as badly to orthodox treatment as depression.

Methods of treatment tend to come and go according to the vogue of the moment — drugs, electro-shock therapy, insulin treatment and psychotherapy have all been tried with various unsatisfactory degrees of success. All these therapies were aimed at treating the symptoms instead of the cause, and perhaps one of the reasons why the ecological approach is relatively so successful is that it concentrates on discovering the cause.

Depression is often the sequel not only to mild depression or brain fag, but to prolonged periods of illness. There may be a psychological reaction to an illness. In some illnesses, such as viral flu, depression is part of the illness ("post-flu blues"); or it may be due to a depressed immune system leading to food intolerance reactions.

A distressing form of depression is the disease known as manic-depressive psychosis. In this disease, the patient alternates between depression and withdrawal at one extreme, and an abnormal stimulatory state, or mania, at the other. He swings dizzyingly from high to low and back, the extremes +4 and −4 in the pendulum of addiction (see Fig. 2, p. 58).

Two Revealing Studies The ecological treatment of depression relies on much more than simply identifying the offending foods or chemicals and then avoiding them. An interesting example of how just one aspect of this treatment can improve the prognosis is provided by two studies into the effects of exercise as a part of therapy.

In a British study, reported in the British Medical Journal, two groups of patients, who were age, sex and disease-severity matched, were randomly placed into two treatment groups. The first group was treated conventionally with psychotherapy and with drugs to counter the depression; the second spent the same amount of time with the therapist, but the drugs were replaced by an exercise program. The second group did better than those being treated with drugs.

In the second study, two psychologists at the University of Kansas, Lisa McCann and David S. Holmes, approached the problem from a slightly different direction. Forty-three depressed women were randomly placed into three groups. The first group was treated with aerobic and strenuous exercise. The second was given a placebo therapy, in which the women were told that studies had shown that relaxation with very mild exercise was beneficial in overcoming stress — in fact all that they did was relax. The third group received no treatment at all and was told that, for the moment, there was no room for them in the study.

It was a very small study, but the findings showed that the patients in the group who were doing the vigorous aerobic exercise fared much better than those in the other two groups. The exercise substantially reduced the incidence of depression and was better than relaxation, which in turn was better than doing nothing at all.

There are a number of interesting implications in these studies, even though the explanation is still unclear. The findings are certainly specific enough to encourage anyone suffering from depression to join an aerobics class. Indeed one of the recommendations that I make to anyone wanting a healthier, calmer life is to become involved in aerobics, an exercise developed to increase the efficiency of the body's intake of oxygen.

In general terms, people do less well with fasting and food testing in depression than in most other psychological illnesses, possibly because it is such a complex aetiological disease and can be triggered by so many factors both within and outside their own bodies. Those patients with reactive depression (caused by outside factors such as a death or failure, for example) do least well, as one might expect, and counselling is more appropriate; and the ecological approach is usually not the treatment of choice when the depression is a part of some other illness in which intolerance does not appear to be involved.

A good diet, meaning one that is low in refined carbohydrate in particular — unprocessed, unrefined and as near to living as possible, always helps recovery from any disease.

SCHIZOPHRENIA ■

Schizophrenia and the schizophrenic syndrome are probably the mental illnesses that are most quoted by clinical ecologists as responding to an ecological approach when almost all else fails.

Schizophrenia is a very distressing and very serious problem — for the unfortunate patients who are its victims, for their immediate families and for society. One estimate has put the incidence of schizophrenia in Western society at one in one hundred. This would mean that in Australia at present there are about 150,000 schizophrenics, condemned to a life without virtually any hope of ever again being normal, even though remission does occur for a time. A sad number of them commit suicide each year.

Most tragic is that even though people of all ages are at risk, it affects mainly young people in their late teens and early twenties. In a 1985 editorial the *Medical Journal of Australia* rightly described schizophrenia as "a national tragedy", striking as it does the young from adolescence onwards and resulting in the suicide within five years of diagnosis of a "horrifying" number of patients.

I refer to the schizophrenic syndrome, rather than to a single disease, because there is a wide spectrum of symptoms. Its early name was *dementia praecox*, which means literally "early insanity". When that name was considered to be too restrictive, it was changed to schizophrenia, meaning "splitting of the mind". Neither word is satisfactory for describing the numerous patterns of disturbances that mark the disease.

It is not so much a single illness as a group of severe mental disorders, sharing disturbances in feeling, thought and relationships with the outside world. It is very complex. To give an idea of how much confusion there still is about schizophrenia, psychiatrists still debate the question of whether there are one, two, or even four different forms of the disease.

Those who advocate two, for example, maintain that there is "process" or "nuclear" schizophrenia on the one hand, characterised by a lengthy deterioration in behaviour brought on by some organic factor; and "reactive" schizophrenia, which is precipitated by some event in a person's life and is characterised by a relatively minor thought disorder. Their prognosis for the first form is very poor, but for the second much better.

Other psychiatrists maintain that there are four quite different types of schizophrenia, differing only in the severity and form of the symptoms. These range from the mildest form, which is marked by a gradual reduction in external relationships and interests and an inability to feel any kind of deep emotion for anything, coupled with a gradual withdrawal and increasingly simple forms of behaviour; to the fourth and most extreme type, characterised mainly by illogical, unreasonable thinking, usually with delusions of persecution and grandeur, and often accompanied by hallucinations. Hearing voices and believing that they are real are common symptoms of all types of schizophrenia, and so is a thought disorder characterised by an impairment in the use of abstract concepts. Concepts such as good and bad, beautiful and ugly lose their meaning and the whole system, as we understand it, gets blurred.

The disease often strikes young people in their late teens when the pressure of study and exams, for example, mounts on them. Typically, these patients "bomb out" after a year of university. Although some improve spontaneously and some improve radically, even totally — usually after they have been treated from an ecological angle — the majority do not improve at all. Unless an ecological approach succeeds, the prognosis is nearly always a life sentence, which is why the results that clinical ecologists are achieving are so exciting and important.

How Often Do We Succeed?   It needs to be said from the outset that clinical ecology does not have a solution for all, nor at present even for the majority of schizophrenic patients. It helps perhaps one in six to a significant degree, but that is 15 or 16 per cent of schizophrenics who before usually had no hope of even the mildest recovery.

When we are successful, the schizophrenic syndrome (and indeed most mental illness) does not invariably, or even usually, disappear with no other treatment but a change of diet or environment. Sometimes there is immediate and enormous improvement, but nearly always additional therapy is needed, whether conventional psychotherapy, drug therapy, hypnotherapy or some other treatment, to relieve and reverse many of the learned maladaptations that are almost always present after any lengthy mental illness. We rarely see the "blinding light" instantaneous recoveries that are so dramatic in food and chemical intolerance, when physical symptoms disappear after a food or chemical is removed from the patient's environment.

Dr William Philpott, author of two important books on clinical ecology and medical director of the Institute for Bio-Ecological Medicine in St Petersburg, Florida, was one of the first to establish that schizophrenia — or at least certain patients with this diagnosis (not everyone branded a schizophrenic has schizophrenia) — as well as most other psychotic states and many so-called psychosomatic reactions, can be proved to be reactions to frequently used foods and chemicals.

Philpott had become consultant to a boarding school for youths with learning, emotional and social disorders. Many of them verged on the schizophrenic or were frankly schizophrenic. He carried out two double-blind studies and compared the relative effects of various food extracts and water. The results were highly significant. In a high percentage of cases, he was able to make the major symptoms disappear or to diminish to such an extent that they were entirely manageable. As soon as test meals of the "unsafe" foods were given again, the symptoms promptly reappeared.

American allergist Dr Marshall Mandell, with an enormous practice of mentally ill patients and an almost missionary enthusiasm for clinical ecology, claims even more startling results from his own studies. He believes that at least half of all the patients in mental hospitals in America suffer from what he calls "cerebral allergies": they are in the state that they are in because of intolerance to a food or a chemical.

Among the schizophrenic patients he tested, 92 per cent of one group of fifty-three suffered psychiatric symptoms after eating a certain food: 64 per cent reacted to wheat, 52 per cent to corn and 50 per cent to cow's milk — three of the mainstays of any Western diet. Interestingly, but not surprisingly, 75 per cent responded badly to cigarette smoke.

Another psychiatrist wrote of the schizophrenics he had treated:

> *Over the years, I have accumulated a number of failures, patients who have not responded permanently to any treatment I have given them. Over the past four months, I have treated about sixty of these failures with a four-day fast. Over forty were normal by the fifth morning. When the offending food was given to them, they promptly relapsed. They are now well as long as they keep away from the offending foods and most do not require any medication at all.*

Out of his responding groups, 75 per cent were unable to tolerate dairy products, and two of these were intolerant of both beef and milk. These two were chronic, relapsing schizophrenics, who had been ill for more than twenty years with at least twenty admissions to mental hospitals or psychiatric wards. Both recovered completely and remained well, as long as they avoided beef and dairy products.

The Importance of Early Treatment   The best results from an ecological approach come when we can begin treating the patient within five years of the original diagnosis of schizophrenic syndrome. The longer the syndrome lasts after that, the more ingrained the learned behaviour, in particular, becomes, and the poorer the results that we can achieve, although that certainly doesn't mean invariable failure.

I have a patient, a man who is presently 44, who has had schizophrenic syndrome for fourteen years. We identified his food intolerances and altered his diet. Although now — a few years later — he still requires moderate drug therapy, he is so much better, provided that he stays on that diet, that he is employable. That is a major achievement.

These abnormal patterns of behaviour have frequently become so ingrained that they continue to exert a powerful influence on patients, even when the primary cause of the illness has been overcome. Time and again, we help schizophrenic syndrome victims to get well on an ecological program, only to see them slip off their strict exclusion diets when they go home. Inevitably they become psychotic again and each time this happens it is more difficult to relieve their symptoms.

Frankly, this can be so frustrating that some doctors refuse even to begin treating schizophrenics unless there is someone who will help the patients maintain their diet for a lengthy period once they get home.

In my own experience, the success rate in the treatment of schizophrenic syndrome, no matter what methods are adopted, falls somewhere between complete recovery and abject failure. There is nearly always *some* benefit, and sometimes there is permanent benefit and complete control; but it is rare to have total relief of all symptoms in the short term.

In spite of that, there are some stunning successes that are elating for doctors and patients alike. It is very moving to see a person who thought that he or she was mad and at the very end of their tether, lose their symptoms simply by leaving certain foods out of their diet, or by avoiding certain outgassing chemicals. To realise that after all those years of misery, they are not mad at all, but only intolerant of some food, is like having heavy shackles cut away.

Two cases from my own files and a very strange one from the United States will help to illustrate the gravity of this disease and the problems we are up against when we try to treat it.

A Life Sentence to Illness   Ben was 22 when he was referred to me by a very eminent psychiatrist, who also held a chair of psychiatry. This doctor was moving to another university and, like all good specialists, he tried to place his patients with other doctors before he left.

Ben had suffered a breakdown five years before, when he was 17, after which he was unable to cope with anything. He developed panic feelings, loss of control, hallucinations and delusions, and a diagnosis of schizophrenic syndrome was quite properly made.

He was treated, like most schizophrenics, with phenothiazines and made modest improvement. In spite of this, of the five years before he came to me, he had spent three and a half in hospital; and the eight months immediately prior to his coming he had spent in bed. He had been given psychotherapy and electric shock therapy.

As well as his mental symptoms, Ben also suffered from migraine and was hypochondriacal, constantly concerned about his health and the possibility of having a heart attack. Panic attacks were so severe that they sometimes prevented him from leaving the house or the hospital ward. This was his condition when he first came to me and indeed I was so concerned that I immediately hospitalised him.

Because of the standing of the doctor who had referred him, I did not at first question the drug therapy that he had prescribed, which included very powerful tranquillisers, even though these left Ben very dopey.

The hospital had an active therapy program, but he was quite unable to take part in it because he was now spending about twenty hours a day in bed. After three months, his only notice-able improvement was that his time in bed reduced to between sixteen and eighteen hours a day. He was still suffering from his delusional thought patterns, hallucinations and very alarming sensations of animals and insects crawling on his skin. It was clear that Ben was either to be condemned to a lifetime of a semi-moribund existence, supported, if that is the right word, by his drugs; or we had to try to find some other solution.

Looking for some ecological explanation, we fasted Ben and by the end of the fifth day we could see real improvement. He felt better, he was more alert (we had suspended the drugs while he was being fasted and challenged), he got up earlier and spent less time in bed and, most importantly, most of his delusions and his sensory hallucinations about the creepy-crawlies had disappeared.

In spite of this obvious improvement, however, he was still far from well. I extended the fast for ten days, allowing him a mono-exclusion diet of brown rice for the last four days. By the end of the tenth day, he was essentially entirely normal and the effect on the staff and the other patients was extraordinary and inspirational.

The food testing showed that Ben was reacting adversely to coffee in particular and to all cow's milk products; to potatoes, bananas and tomatoes; and to sugar and refined carbohydrates in the form of hypoglycaemia. His glucose tolerance curve was typi-cally abnormal for a schizophrenic. A high percentage of schizophrenics, about 70 per cent, have abnormal GTTs.

Because he had been ill for so long, in fact since he was 17, Ben had not completed any formal education and, as soon as he left hospital, he began a work-training program for the disabled. At the end of his course, they found him a job, where he stayed for eight years, performing so well that he was promoted to be

the company's state manager. After that he took another significant step and with the blessing of his firm set up his own business, which prospered.

I have now followed Ben up for more than ten years and he
continues to be well. After all this time he still has to avoid most
of the foods to which he reacted badly when we first began testing
him, particularly milk and coffee. During that time he has discovered a few other foods that cause reactions and have had to be
excluded from his diet.

There was just one recent episode that reinforced the fact
that strict dietary control is a lifetime requirement for many
patients. Ben had felt so well for so long that he abandoned his
diet and began drinking coffee and eating sugar freely. He had
never lost his craving. He also stopped his regular exercise. The
symptoms gradually and subtly returned and he reached a crisis
where he was not able to cope in his own business. At that point,
he rather sheepishly came back to see me.

The symptoms included the old phobias and, although no
frank psychosis was present, there was definite paranoia. I am
sure that before long the full-blown schizophrenic syndrome
would have recurred. As it was, we were able to bring him back
to good health quickly, and he rapidly improved when he corrected his diet and restarted his exercise program.

It seems hard to imagine that all that stood between Ben
and a life sentence to the kind of existence that he was living
before he came to me was coffee, milk, potatoes, bananas,
tomatoes and sugar. What price a banana!

A Spoonful of Sugar   Another patient of mine, 32-year-
old David, was grievously affected by sugar in every form. Normally sugar, apart from the symptoms of hypoglycaemia, is not a
food that many people react to in food intolerance; but in David's
case a ripe banana or a spoonful of sugar in his coffee was disastrous.

When he arrived in my rooms, he had already been on the
medical merry-go-round for a long time and had been diagnosed
as a paranoid schizophrenic when he was 17. Some of his delusions were very odd.

He believed, for instance, that masturbation controlled the
flow of traffic, and that if he waved an arm he would influence
radio announcers. He was also troubled by what he perceived as
exaggerated movements by other people. If anyone so much as

turned their head or held their head in a particular position, he interpreted it as meaning that they were threatening and trying to overwhelm him.

Whatever the symptoms of the moment, they were much worse after he had consumed sugar in any form. His life was much happier after we had designed a diet that was safe for him. Perhaps because fifteen years had passed since he was first diagnosed, or simply because many cases of schizophrenic syndrome fail to respond to any kind of therapy, he never made a full recovery.

Ten years afterwards, he is leading a contented life. He is involved in youth work and very effectively helping disturbed teenagers who run into trouble. Just occasionally his schizophrenic syndrome (though neither of us ever uses that label) returns, and he heads for the security of the hospital for a few days. It is a very cheap price for giving this gentle, kind man a life that was completely out of the question when attempts were being made to treat him in a conventional way. He would certainly have been chronically institutionalised. He continues to need ongoing supportive psychotherapy.

Have Wine, Shoot Twelve The third case is very bizarre and was reported by an American, Dr Alexander Schauss. Schauss's research is meticulous; he is the director of the American Institute for Bio-Social Research at Tacoma, Washington, where he has facilities and funding that are the envy of his peers around the world.

His primary focus has been on basic research into the chemistry and physiological make-up of the mentally ill. He has been a consultant to numerous governments and private industries on matters pertaining to environmental and biochemical factors that affect behaviour. Some of his most controversial work has been into the relationship between diet and violence, and he has studied thousands of prisoners in US gaols to make his point that a great deal of violence is the result of faulty diet. He has a very large following and, to be entirely unbiased, a much smaller number of detractors who seem to be critical of almost everything he does, despite his impeccable research.

It is worth noting this, because it is largely Schauss's acceptance that the case is genuine that makes it important; and if it is genuine, then the implications for any others affected in the same way are fascinating.

An American millionaire bought a penthouse in a new con-dominium. It was not long before it was apparent that there was clearly something seriously wrong with this building. During the next two or three years, most of the original residents moved away, complaining of symptoms that left them feeling weak and ill, and suffering from a host of other problems that they had never experienced in their lives before.

The millionaire, however, did not move and he was still there when the authorities finally closed the building down. They had found so much poisonous outgassing into the air-condition-ing from the synthetic gas used to run the system that it was breaking down people's immune systems.

Whether that was the beginning of this man's troubles, as seemed likely because he had never consciously had any intoler-ance problems before, or whether it was simply a stage in a pro-cess that had been going on for years, is not clear. What is certain is that shortly after he moved out of the penthouse, he was drink-ing a glass of red wine at his club when he suddenly drew a gun and shot a dozen people — not killing them, but in most cases just shooting them in the legs.

He was a crack marksman so there was no question that he had tried to kill them and had simply missed. He had never been a violent man in his whole life, and his story was that he thought these people were coming to get him and he fired in self-defence. He had intended only to stop them. It was such an improbable story that it made sense only if one accepted that he had suddenly gone mad.

But why? No-one had provoked him, nothing untoward of any kind had happened in the bar before the incident.

A Deadly Little Grape   It was obviously going to be a very hard story to sell to a jury and he was clearly heading for a very long stay in a prison or a mental institution. His one hope lay in proving that something he had eaten or something in his environment had made him act in a way that was totally outside his control. He would probably never even have thought of this had he not remembered the stories of broken-down immune sys-tems in his condominium. Perhaps he too was a victim of the gas.

He went to Schauss after hearing of his extensive research into foods and crime. Though sceptical, Schauss was interested enough to take him on as a client/patient on condition that his findings would be made available to both the prosecution and the defence, no matter what they were. The man agreed.

Schauss believed that there was probably some other factor as well as the gas, even if the gas had weakened the immune system initially. What he found, after a series of double-blind studies and cross-over tests, using numerous fake wines with different constituents (so that statistically the results could not possibly be fabricated) was that the red wine that the man had been drinking had turned him into a dangerous paranoid schizophrenic.

Schauss was able to reduce him to this state at will by giving him the correct wine. But that was only the beginning. Schauss also found that it was not simply that particular brand of wine (a Californian wine) that was the cause of the reaction, because it did not always produce the symptoms. Indeed for a while this made Schauss suspect that he was being used in a very clever ploy. The violent reaction was caused by one particular type of grape which went into that one particular brand of wine. Only when those grapes from that particular vineyard were used did the man become schizophrenic!

Probably before his immune system was weakened by the escaping gas in the condominium, he would have been able to consume the grapes with impunity. Why only that one kind of grape produced the violence is a matter of individual susceptibility.

At the time of writing, the trial has still to take place, but whatever the verdict, it raises some most alarming questions. How much of the wanton violence in our society today is caused by food or chemical intolerance? And if it is true — and I have no doubt that it is — that something as basic as grapes can make a man shoot twelve people, what action do you take? To what extent can you leave a person free, however blameless they may be in law because they were not responsible for their actions, when there must be a risk of recurrence if he should accidentally eat or drink that food again? There is no question of arguing that he is insane, except possibly for that moment when all the ingredients for violence come together to produce that disastrous reaction.

This is not a doctor's dilemma, but as the role of food and drink in acts of violence becomes clearer, it is a problem that sooner or later society is going to have to address. Fortunately the extreme violence of this case is rare. Or we think it is.

35 Post-Infection Fatigue Syndrome or Myalgic Encephalomyelitis

This is a disorder that causes much confusion among the medical profession and much distress to its victims. The fact that it is much rarer than hypoglycaemia in no way makes it more tolerable for those who suffer from it. Nor does the fact that, just as with hypoglycaemia, there are still many doctors who have come to the conclusion that it really doesn't exist at all (usually because they were not taught about it at medical school).

It has been given a number of names, which is yet another cause of confusion. Its most common name, which was used for a time, is myalgic encephalomyelitis, or the ME syndrome. It then passed through a phase of being known as post-viral syndrome, or PVS, and has now emerged with the present preferred name of Post-Infection Fatigue syndrome.

Until recently, it is doubtful if more than one in a thousand people had ever heard of the condition, although reports in the media are rapidly changing that. Post-Infection Fatigue syndrome (PIFS) is apt. Its symptoms include muscle pain with inflammation of both the spinal cord and the brain (the meaning of myalgic encephalomyelitis), and it can reduce otherwise healthy and strong men and women to a state where even walking down the garden path to the letter box can force them into bed for three or four days. I have had a patient so weak that he could hardly find the strength to open his eyes; and others who were forced to sit on the floor at the supermarket while the staff brought them their groceries. Two have come to me in wheelchairs.

Yet so little is known about this disorder that there is even argument as to whether it is a disease at all. My own belief — and some researchers dispute this — is that it is not a disease in the conventional sense, but rather a syndrome, or collection of symptoms that occur at the same time.

A DISEASE WITH MANY NAMES ▮

The first known outbreak was in Los Angeles in 1934, but at that time, it was not even given a name. Then, in 1950, there was an outbreak in Iceland and it became known as Iceland disease. In 1951, there was a small outbreak in Adelaide, South Australia; and in 1955 it reappeared in London at the Royal Free Hospital.

About 300 doctors and nurses went down with a strange and debilitating disease, for which no cause was ever discovered. Some specialists suspected that it might have been a case of mass hysteria, because although some of the symptoms were physical, such as fatigue, muscular weakness and pain, others, including depression, anxiety, occasional delusions and an inability to concentrate, suggested that there might be a psychological origin. After this experience, it was given the name Royal Free disease.

Gradually, other diseases and syndromes that had been known by different names, such as Tapanui flu in New Zealand, were recognised as being PIFS/ME. In very recent years, it re-emerged yet again, this time in Sydney, as myalgic encephalomyelitis, or ME.

I believe that the best name is post-infection fatigue syndrome, which acknowledges the two factors that seem to be common to all cases, that it is caused by, or at least follows, an infection and leaves the patient fatigued. At the same time, this name avoids being specific about the symptoms, of which sixty-four have now been identified. Some or all of the symptoms can be present at one time, and it is this fact more than anything else that causes some doctors so much difficulty in grasping the reality of PIFS/ME.

One of the most common complaints from PIFS/ME sufferers is that their doctors accuse them of being neurotic and worse. "Malingerers" is how many patients believe their doctors view them.

The law of parsimony, which we were taught at medical school and which attempts to ascribe a single cause to a single problem, could not be more inappropriate when dealing with PIFS/ME. An ME society was established in Australia in 1980 as a self-help organisation to help sufferers and their families, and to try to educate doctors and others about the reality of the disease. Few organisations can have more justification for existing.

TESTING A FAMILY'S PATIENCE ■

The most prominent features of PIFS/ME are profound lethargy and a very abnormal tendency to become exhausted after even the simplest exercise. Muscle pain and weakness, headache, fluctuating impairment of concentration and mental processes, disturbed balance, hearing and vision and disturbed sleep patterns are all commonly encountered, as are problems with the bladder and bowel, and the upper respiratory system.

Some people are so badly affected by fatigue and muscle pain that they are confined to a wheelchair, and emotional problems and mood swings are the rule rather than the exception. The impact can be quite devastating, and some PIFS/ME victims have taken their own lives because of their overwhelming depression. The impact on their families is almost as devastating. When people who were previously fit, healthy and full of life suddenly get hit with an illness that puts them totally out of action, sometimes for months on end, it can test the patience and loyalty of any family to the limit.

The course of PIFS/ME is variable and it can take any one of three likely forms. The most common pattern is that the symptoms last for anything from six months to three years and then spontaneously get better. Symptoms lasting for less than six months would not qualify for a diagnosis of PIFS/ME: these symptoms are so common even three and four months after a viral illness that they are accepted as a normal consequence of a virus infection.

Alternatively, there is a pattern that can best be described as a relapsing course, where patients are quite well for months but then suffer an illness or a virus, or encounter some other stress, and relapse. It is little wonder that this form of PIFS/ME is so often looked upon as psychosomatic: the patient is subjected to stress and immediately crumbles and disintegrates.

The third possibility is that the patient is constantly ill and doesn't get better. For these people life can be hell.

At any of these levels of the illness, the degree of physical incapacity varies greatly from patient to patient and from day to day, even from morning to afternoon in the same patient. Many patients function normally until about 10 a.m., and then suddenly weaken to the point where opening a door is too difficult for them.

PIFS/ME affects people of all ages and both sexes, but typically those between their twenties and forties. Initially the onset may be gradual, or it may come without warning after, say, a gastrointestinal or upper respiratory tract infection. Some of the indicators that an attack is coming on in many sufferers are sore eyes and an exceptionally pale face, often accompanied by severe abdominal pains.

THE ELUSIVE JIGSAW ■

Many theories have tried to explain PIFS/ME, but the pieces of the jigsaw still tantalisingly refuse to come together to give a clear picture. Studies, particularly in England, have shown abnormalities of the muscles and in the functioning of the immune system, with increased signs of exposure to a virus, particularly one called Coxsackie B. More recent studies, particularly in Australia under Professor Denis Wakefield and Professor C.R. Broughton and their colleagues, implicate a virus from the herpes family, so that now we have the underlying concept that PIFS/ME is some form of a prolonged reaction to a virus and hence the name post-viral syndrome.

Most of the symptoms do affect the nervous system and the muscles and PIFS/ME does seem to be triggered by a virus, or at least frequently follows one.

Hypersensitivity to chemicals and intolerance to many foods are also usually encountered in PIFS/ME sufferers, which brings it within the area of concern of the clinical ecologist. So many cases respond to control of food and chemical sensitivities that ecological factors cannot be discounted as a primary cause.

One discovery that may be significant is that many patients respond beneficially to an antifungal regime, suggesting that for some reason, their natural immunity to *Candida albicans* has been weakened. Again, this is an ecological problem in most cases. This may well be due to the antibiotic treatment given to so many PIFS/ME sufferers, especially at the onset of the illness or infection. As we have seen in Chapter 30, antibiotics are a primary cause of *Candida albicans* getting out of control.

Possibly of interest as well was the discovery of raised serum bilirubin in a patient who had been referred to me with a diagnosis of PIFS/ME. Bilirubin is a breakdown product of the red blood cells and is responsible, for example, for the yellow colouring in jaundice. In this boy, who had been a PIFS/ME sufferer for three years, and subsequently in several other PIFS/ME patients, including a father and his two teenage sons, I found the same abnormally raised bilirubin, but no other abnormality in liver function. (Normally raised bilirubin reflects liver disease or blockage in the bile outflow from the liver, often caused by gallstones or hepatitis.)

This condition is known as Gilbert's disease and the symptoms typically include tiredness, lethargy and a tendency for it to come in episodes, with periods of normal health in between attacks — all familiar to PIFS/ME sufferers.

It may be that I have picked up so many of these cases of Gilbert's disease, which are normally rare, simply because the chronicity of their symptoms has led them to seek help by way of a fasting and food-testing approach. Fasting in Gilbert's disease can lead to a significant rise in bilirubin (which may have been only slightly elevated initially) and so lead to the diagnosis. On the other hand, it might be a complete red herring. Whichever the case, it has interesting aspects that will turn it into another small piece of this very complicated and curious jigsaw.

One of the oddities of Gilbert's disease, incidentally, is that those suffering from it ought to avoid certain medications, which worsen their condition, even though normally they would have no such effect. Many PIFS/ME sufferers also complain that the medications prescribed for them seem only to make things worse.

Although there is no specific treatment that can be recommended, there are things that can be done to make the lives of PIFS/ME sufferers more comfortable. Adequate rest is the first essential, as is ensuring that they keep within their physical limitations. Forcing themselves to keep going at their previous levels of activity is a recipe for disaster.

Identifying and then avoiding unsafe foods and chemicals gives excellent results in some patients, though not in all, so it must be attempted. Troublesome foods need to be removed from the diet. I advise PIFS/ME patients to go on a rotation diet, whether food intolerance has been established or not. Intolerance is so common — I am tempted to say that it is invariably present — that a rotation diet is the safest protection against other intolerances and addictions developing. If chemicals cannot be removed from the patient's environment, desensitising drops will probably keep the problem under control. Cigarette smoke seems to be extremely distressing to PIFS/ME sufferers.

As a general rule, bland rather than spicy foods seem to be better tolerated.

Perhaps the most valuable advice we can give to any PIFS/ME victim is to find a physician who is sympathetic to their predicament, and will give them the time and the patience to explore any avenue with them that offers the hope of providing some of the answers to this most perplexing, personal and distressing disorder.

GAMMA-GLOBULIN ■

The benefit of gamma-globulin, administered as a high-dose, intermittent, intravenous infusion, is being investigated by Professor Wakefield and his co-workers, and a double-blind study has been conducted. At the time of writing, the results are not available, but some patients who have been treated with the same approach, though not in the trial, have received worthwhile benefit from it.

I have found that some of my own patients benefit, too, from small doses of gamma-globulin given weekly by intramuscular injection — not only with PIFS/ME, but with food and chemical insensitivities in general.

A worldwide survey carried out by Weight Watchers found that Australia is the fourth most obese nation on earth. Obesity, defined as anything more than 10 per cent (15 per cent by some definitions) above recommended weight-for-age, often accompanies food intolerance and hypoglycaemia. With the rare exceptions of people who have a hypothalamic problem, obesity is always caused by eating more food than can be converted to energy.

There is no surer way of gaining weight than by eating foods that are refined, like sugar or fat, neither of which have anything but kilojoules — they contain no vitamins, no minerals, no dietary fibre. They can be eaten in great quantities without ever leaving you feeling that you have fully satisfied your hunger.

Only countries where the diet includes refined foods have an obesity problem. Compounding the situation is the fact that these are also the countries where people indulge in the least exercise and have more sedentary professions, both very important factors.

In Britain in 1981 (and the figures are much the same in Australia), 6 per cent of the male population and 8 per cent of the women over 15 were obese. (Obesity is graded from mild to pathologic, which is double or more than double the recommended weight-for-age.) That means more than 2.8 million people in Britain were sufficiently fat for their health to be threatened.

In food intolerance, the addiction factor compels a person to eat the food that is causing the problem. If that food happens to be kilojoule-dense, as it often is with sugar and other refined carbohydrates and fatty foods, then the patient will become fat.

Hypoglycaemic patients eat, usually without understanding the reason, in order to raise their blood glucose levels, and so feel better and be able to perform better. Either way, they take in an excessive number of kilojoules and end up being obese.

NOT ALWAYS GLUTTONY |

It is important for the overweight to understand that their condition is not necessarily the result of gluttony. Indeed the whole subject of obesity is very complex and many books have been devoted to this weighty problem. The causes of obesity are many and varied, but if food addiction is at the root of the problem, people who are obese are virtually unable to help themselves. They must have the help that clinical ecology in particular can offer.

Worse than the prospect of all those fat adults in Australia is the number of children who are being stuffed with food by their parents (usually themselves fat), or who are allowed to eat sweets and useless sugary food, as well as excessively fatty food.

Fat is kilojoule-dense, producing double the kilojoules per gram compared to carbohydrate or protein. In the typical Western diet 40-45 per cent of kilojoules are derived from fat and this is the big problem, as well as the consumption of refined carbohydrate and particularly refined sugar.

The risk of being obese is far too well documented to ignore. The likelihood of contracting a host of often killing degenerative diseases is substantially increased by being fat. Cerebro-vascular disease, coronary disease, vascular disorders, cancer, gallstones, hernia, diabetes, high blood pressure, arthritis and varicose veins are among the major diseases that lie in wait for those who care too little about their health and weight.

Then there is the psychological trauma of being fat. The cruelty of "You're fat! We don't want to play with you. You're disgusting!" has haunted many obese people for years after it was first hurled at them in the school playground. The prejudice never goes away. It is there at almost every stage of life from school, through to job interviews and social status. It is one of the last great prejudices in our society.

RECOGNISE OBESITY EARLY ■

It is very important to catch the problem at the first opportunity, because mild obesity is much easier to treat than gross obesity; and prevention of gross obesity is much better than being killed.

Unfortunately, people who are only mildly obese don't usually go to their doctor complaining that they are too fat. The doctor has no opportunity to caution them and advise them on the selection of an appropriate diet, even if he knows nothing of food intolerance and ecological illnesses. This is the time when it would be relatively easy to change their eating habits.

Seeking medical advice is important because it is all too easy to take the opposite path and avoid eating altogether. This even more distressing road leads to anorexia nervosa, which is increasing in an alarming way in Australian women and probably throughout the Western world. It is a complex problem.

Once the cause has been identified and the offending foods that produce the addiction have been removed from the diet, counselling is usually still required to bring down the weight to an acceptable level and to continue on a correct diet, which may need to be modified from time to time. Aerobic exercise and a carefully designed diet are an essential part of the treatment.

The act of abandoning fattening food is not in itself any guarantee that the weight will come down to an acceptable level. It has often been remarked that some fat people really don't eat any more than anyone else: they are just paying the price for over-eating or gluttony in the past and lack the expert help they need to bring down their weight by themselves.

In Appendix X, there is a list of desirable weights for adults, which I find most acceptable. Various authorities approach the question from different points of view, but this list is based on the weights that are associated with the lowest mortality rate. The concept is that your weight at 25 is the weight you should maintain unchanged for the rest of your life, because this has been shown to be associated with the lowest mortality — and that is what maintaining the ideal weight is all about.

APPENDIX I

NOTES ON FOOD-TESTING FORMS

The following notes are to assist patients in filling out food-testing forms. There is one form for each food and it is from the information on the form that a final decision will be made regarding the "safe" or "unsafe" nature of the food.

Time of Measurements

Control: just before starting to eat.
Measurements then taken at $\frac{1}{4}$, $\frac{1}{2}$, 1, 2, 3, 4 hours after the first mouthful.
Aim to complete eating within the first quarter hour.

Time

Taken from the start of eating.

Pulse

1. Always take when seated and allow at least 2 minutes to elapse after sitting down.
2. Count zero for the first beat at the start of counting, i.e. 0, 1, 2, 3, 4, . . .
3. Count for exactly 60 seconds. This gives the number of beats per minute. This is preferable, since it minimises error.
   OR
   Count for exactly 30 seconds and multiply by two to give number of beats per minute.
   DO NOT count for shorter periods of time.
4. If in doubt or unsure, ask a member of staff to check.
5. Breathe normally during the period of counting. Holding the breath or overbreathing (hyperventilating) can alter the pulse rate.

Blood Glucose

Measured by staff — please present yourself at the control, at times of 1 hour, 3 hours and 4 hours after first mouthful.
mEq = milliEquivalents per litre
mg% = milligrams per cent

Symptoms

As felt and experienced by the patient, i.e. subjective. This section is to be filled out by the patient.

List up to eight symptoms from the symptom list.
Grade as follows:

    0 absent, leave blank.
    + just recognisable, i.e. very mild.
  ++ mild.
 +++ moderate.
++++ a strong, positive reaction.

Observations

As seen by and noted by staff or relatives, i.e. objective.
This section is to be filled in by a staff member.
Up to four observations to be listed and graded as for symptoms.

Comments

Write out everything that may be relevant to the way you feel and what you are experiencing. For example, 10.30 a.m. — out walking, 11.25 a.m. — sitting in the sun, 12.40 p.m. — upsetting phone call, etc.

Writing

Write "normally" for how you feel at the time.
Write three lines on any topic or subject.
OR
Write your full name, address, telephone number and signature.
Try NOT to copy the style of what you have already written.

Assessment

Make a decision as to whether YOU think the food is "safe" or "unsafe". A staff member will do the same. The final decision is made by the doctor.
(SS = subjective symptoms; OS = observed signs; BG = blood glucose; P = pulse; W = writing.)

APPENDIX II

FOOD QUESTIONNAIRE

FOOD	TO BE TESTED	SAFE	UNSAFE	EATEN DAILY	WEEKLY	MONTHLY	NOT EATEN DUE TO SUSPECTED REACTION (*Give details*)
Alcohol	☐	☐	☐	☐	☐	☐	
Almond	☐	☐	☐	☐	☐	☐	
Apple	☐	☐	☐	☐	☐	☐	
Apricot	☐	☐	☐	☐	☐	☐	
Artichoke Globe	☐	☐	☐	☐	☐	☐	
Jerusalem	☐	☐	☐	☐	☐	☐	
Avocado	☐	☐	☐	☐	☐	☐	
Bacon	☐	☐	☐	☐	☐	☐	
Banana	☐	☐	☐	☐	☐	☐	
Barley	☐	☐	☐	☐	☐	☐	
Beans	☐	☐	☐	☐	☐	☐	
Beef	☐	☐	☐	☐	☐	☐	
Beets	☐	☐	☐	☐	☐	☐	
Berries, e.g. Black	☐	☐	☐	☐	☐	☐	
Black sauce	☐	☐	☐	☐	☐	☐	
Brazil nuts	☐	☐	☐	☐	☐	☐	
Bread (brand =)	☐	☐	☐	☐	☐	☐	
Broccoli	☐	☐	☐	☐	☐	☐	
Brussels sprouts	☐	☐	☐	☐	☐	☐	
Buckwheat	☐	☐	☐	☐	☐	☐	
Butter	☐	☐	☐	☐	☐	☐	
Buttermilk	☐	☐	☐	☐	☐	☐	
Cabbage	☐	☐	☐	☐	☐	☐	
Capsicum, red & green	☐	☐	☐	☐	☐	☐	
Carob	☐	☐	☐	☐	☐	☐	
Carrot	☐	☐	☐	☐	☐	☐	
Cashews	☐	☐	☐	☐	☐	☐	
Cauliflower	☐	☐	☐	☐	☐	☐	

FOOD	TO BE TESTED	SAFE	UNSAFE	EATEN DAILY	WEEKLY	MONTHLY	NOT EATEN DUE TO SUSPECTED REACTION (*Give details*)
Celery	☐	☐	☐	☐	☐	☐	
Cheeses	☐	☐	☐	☐	☐	☐	
Cherries	☐	☐	☐	☐	☐	☐	
Chestnuts	☐	☐	☐	☐	☐	☐	
Chewing gum	☐	☐	☐	☐	☐	☐	
Chicken	☐	☐	☐	☐	☐	☐	
Chocolate	☐	☐	☐	☐	☐	☐	
Cocoa	☐	☐	☐	☐	☐	☐	
Coconut	☐	☐	☐	☐	☐	☐	
Coffee	☐	☐	☐	☐	☐	☐	
Corn (including oil)	☐	☐	☐	☐	☐	☐	
Crab	☐	☐	☐	☐	☐	☐	
Cranberries	☐	☐	☐	☐	☐	☐	
Cream	☐	☐	☐	☐	☐	☐	
Cucumbers	☐	☐	☐	☐	☐	☐	
Cumquats	☐	☐	☐	☐	☐	☐	
Currants	☐	☐	☐	☐	☐	☐	
Dandelion	☐	☐	☐	☐	☐	☐	
Dates	☐	☐	☐	☐	☐	☐	
Devon	☐	☐	☐	☐	☐	☐	
Eggs	☐	☐	☐	☐	☐	☐	
Eggplant	☐	☐	☐	☐	☐	☐	
Endive	☐	☐	☐	☐	☐	☐	
Figs	☐	☐	☐	☐	☐	☐	
Fish white	☐	☐	☐	☐	☐	☐	
red (salmon)	☐	☐	☐	☐	☐	☐	
salt water	☐	☐	☐	☐	☐	☐	
fresh water	☐	☐	☐	☐	☐	☐	
Fruit juice (list)	☐	☐	☐	☐	☐	☐	
Garlic	☐	☐	☐	☐	☐	☐	
Gooseberries	☐	☐	☐	☐	☐	☐	

FOOD	TO BE TESTED	SAFE	UNSAFE	EATEN DAILY	WEEKLY	MONTHLY	NOT EATEN DUE TO SUSPECTED REACTION (*Give details*)
Grapefruit	☐	☐	☐	☐	☐	☐	
Grapes	☐	☐	☐	☐	☐	☐	
Guava	☐	☐	☐	☐	☐	☐	
Ham	☐	☐	☐	☐	☐	☐	
Hazelnuts	☐	☐	☐	☐	☐	☐	
Honey	☐	☐	☐	☐	☐	☐	
Horseradish	☐	☐	☐	☐	☐	☐	
Kale	☐	☐	☐	☐	☐	☐	
Kohlrabi	☐	☐	☐	☐	☐	☐	
Lamb	☐	☐	☐	☐	☐	☐	
Lemon	☐	☐	☐	☐	☐	☐	
Lentils	☐	☐	☐	☐	☐	☐	
Lettuce	☐	☐	☐	☐	☐	☐	
Lime	☐	☐	☐	☐	☐	☐	
Lobster	☐	☐	☐	☐	☐	☐	
Malt	☐	☐	☐	☐	☐	☐	
Mandarin	☐	☐	☐	☐	☐	☐	
Mango	☐	☐	☐	☐	☐	☐	
Margarine	☐	☐	☐	☐	☐	☐	
Marrow	☐	☐	☐	☐	☐	☐	
Melon	☐	☐	☐	☐	☐	☐	
Milk cow's	☐	☐	☐	☐	☐	☐	
goat's	☐	☐	☐	☐	☐	☐	
Millet	☐	☐	☐	☐	☐	☐	
Molasses	☐	☐	☐	☐	☐	☐	
Monosodium glutamate	☐	☐	☐	☐	☐	☐	
Mushrooms	☐	☐	☐	☐	☐	☐	
Mustard greens	☐	☐	☐	☐	☐	☐	
Nectarine	☐	☐	☐	☐	☐	☐	
Oats	☐	☐	☐	☐	☐	☐	
Onion	☐	☐	☐	☐	☐	☐	

FOOD	TO BE TESTED	SAFE	UNSAFE	EATEN DAILY	WEEKLY	MONTHLY	NOT EATEN DUE TO SUSPECTED REACTION (*Give details*)
Orange	☐	☐	☐	☐	☐	☐	
Oysters	☐	☐	☐	☐	☐	☐	
Papaya (Pawpaw)	☐	☐	☐	☐	☐	☐	
Parsley	☐	☐	☐	☐	☐	☐	
Parsnip	☐	☐	☐	☐	☐	☐	
Peach	☐	☐	☐	☐	☐	☐	
Peanut	☐	☐	☐	☐	☐	☐	
Pear	☐	☐	☐	☐	☐	☐	
Peas	☐	☐	☐	☐	☐	☐	
Pecans	☐	☐	☐	☐	☐	☐	
Pepper	☐	☐	☐	☐	☐	☐	
Persimmon	☐	☐	☐	☐	☐	☐	
Pineapple	☐	☐	☐	☐	☐	☐	
Plum	☐	☐	☐	☐	☐	☐	
Pork	☐	☐	☐	☐	☐	☐	
Potato	☐	☐	☐	☐	☐	☐	
Prawns	☐	☐	☐	☐	☐	☐	
Pumpkin	☐	☐	☐	☐	☐	☐	
Radish	☐	☐	☐	☐	☐	☐	
Raisins	☐	☐	☐	☐	☐	☐	
Raspberries	☐	☐	☐	☐	☐	☐	
Rice	☐	☐	☐	☐	☐	☐	
Rye	☐	☐	☐	☐	☐	☐	
Salad dressing	☐	☐	☐	☐	☐	☐	
Salami	☐	☐	☐	☐	☐	☐	
Sauerkraut	☐	☐	☐	☐	☐	☐	
Sausages	☐	☐	☐	☐	☐	☐	
Sesame	☐	☐	☐	☐	☐	☐	
Shellfish	☐	☐	☐	☐	☐	☐	
Soft drinks normal	☐	☐	☐	☐	☐	☐	
"low cal" drinks	☐	☐	☐	☐	☐	☐	

FOOD	TO BE TESTED	SAFE	UNSAFE	EATEN DAILY	WEEKLY	MONTHLY	NOT EATEN DUE TO SUSPECTED REACTION (*Give details*)
Soy	☐	☐	☐	☐	☐	☐	
Spinach	☐	☐	☐	☐	☐	☐	
Squash (incl. zucchini)	☐	☐	☐	☐	☐	☐	
Strawberry	☐	☐	☐	☐	☐	☐	
Sugar	☐	☐	☐	☐	☐	☐	
Sunflower	☐	☐	☐	☐	☐	☐	
Tea	☐	☐	☐	☐	☐	☐	
Tomato	☐	☐	☐	☐	☐	☐	
Turnip	☐	☐	☐	☐	☐	☐	
Walnuts	☐	☐	☐	☐	☐	☐	
Watermelon	☐	☐	☐	☐	☐	☐	
Wheat	☐	☐	☐	☐	☐	☐	
Yoghurt	☐	☐	☐	☐	☐	☐	
Other products	☐	☐	☐	☐	☐	☐	

APPENDIX III

CHEMICAL QUESTIONNAIRE
What is your reaction to the following? (**Tick one**.)

Like   *Neutral*   *Dislike*   *Made sick*

Coal, oil, gas and combustion products

Like	Neutral	Dislike	Made sick	
☐	☐	☐	☐	Massive outdoor exposures to coal smoke
☐	☐	☐	☐	Smoke from coal-burning stoves, furnaces or fireplaces.
☐	☐	☐	☐	Odours of natural gas fields
☐	☐	☐	☐	Odours of escaping utility gas
☐	☐	☐	☐	Odours of burning utility gas
☐	☐	☐	☐	Odours of petrol
☐	☐	☐	☐	Garage fumes and odours
☐	☐	☐	☐	Automotive or motor-boat exhausts
☐	☐	☐	☐	Odour of naphtha, cleaning fluids or lighter fluids
☐	☐	☐	☐	Odour of recently cleaned clothing, upholstery or rugs
☐	☐	☐	☐	Odour of naphtha-containing soaps
☐	☐	☐	☐	Odour of nail polish or nail polish remover
☐	☐	☐	☐	Odour of brass, metal or shoe polishes
☐	☐	☐	☐	Odour of fresh newspapers
☐	☐	☐	☐	Odour of kerosene
☐	☐	☐	☐	Odour of kerosene or fuel-oil burning lamps or stoves

Rubber

Like	Neutral	Dislike	Made sick	
☐	☐	☐	☐	Odour of rubber or contact with rubber gloves, elastic in clothing, girdles, brassieres, garters etc.
☐	☐	☐	☐	Odour of sponge-rubber bedding, rug pads, typewriter pads
☐	☐	☐	☐	Odour of rubber-based paint
☐	☐	☐	☐	Odour of rubber tyres, automotive accessories
☐	☐	☐	☐	Odour of rubber-backed rugs and carpets
☐	☐	☐	☐	Fumes of burning rubber

Plastics, synthetic textiles, finishes and adhesives

Like	Neutral	Dislike	Made sick	
☐	☐	☐	☐	Odour of or contact with plastic upholstery, tablecloths, book covers, pillow covers, shoe bags, handbags

Like	*Neutral*	*Dislike*	*Made sick*	
☐	☐	☐	☐	Odour of plastic folding doors or interiors of cars
☐	☐	☐	☐	Odour of or contact with plastic spectacle frames, dentures
☐	☐	☐	☐	Odour of plastic products in department or specialty stores
☐	☐	☐	☐	Nylon stockings or pantihose and other nylon clothes
☐	☐	☐	☐	Dacron or orlon clothing or upholstery
☐	☐	☐	☐	Rayon or cellulose acetate clothing or upholstery
☐	☐	☐	☐	Odour of or contact with adhesive tape
☐	☐	☐	☐	Odour of plastic cements

Alcohols, glycols, aldehydes, esters and derived substances

☐	☐	☐	☐	Odour of rubbing alcohol
☐	☐	☐	☐	Alcohols or glycols as contained in medications
☐	☐	☐	☐	Odour of varnish, laquer or shellac
☐	☐	☐	☐	Odour of aftershave, hair tonic, hair oil
☐	☐	☐	☐	Odour of paint or varnish thinned with mineral solvents
☐	☐	☐	☐	Odour of banana oil
☐	☐	☐	☐	Odour of scented soap and shampoo
☐	☐	☐	☐	Odour of perfumes and colognes
☐	☐	☐	☐	Odour of hair spray and other hair dressings
☐	☐	☐	☐	Fumes from burning incense
☐	☐	☐	☐	Odour of kerosene or fuel-oil burning space heaters or furnaces
☐	☐	☐	☐	Diesel engine fumes from trains, buses, trucks or boats
☐	☐	☐	☐	Lubricating greases or crude oil
☐	☐	☐	☐	Fumes from burning an excessive amount of oil
☐	☐	☐	☐	Fumes from burning greasy rags
☐	☐	☐	☐	Odours of smudge pots as road markers

Mineral oil, vaseline, waxes and combustion products

☐	☐	☐	☐	Mineral oil as contained in hand lotions and medications
☐	☐	☐	☐	Mineral oil as a laxative
☐	☐	☐	☐	Cold cream, face or foundation cream
☐	☐	☐	☐	Vaseline, petroleum jelly or petrolatum-containing ointments
☐	☐	☐	☐	Odours of floor, furniture or bowling alley wax

Like	Neutral	Dislike	Made sick	
☐	☐	☐	☐	Odours of glass wax or similar glass cleaners
☐	☐	☐	☐	Fumes from burning wax candles
☐	☐	☐	☐	Odours from dry garbage incinerators

Asphalts, tars, resins and dyes

Like	Neutral	Dislike	Made sick	
☐	☐	☐	☐	Fumes from tarring roofs and roads
☐	☐	☐	☐	Bitumen pavements in hot weather
☐	☐	☐	☐	Tar-containing soaps, shampoos and ointments
☐	☐	☐	☐	Odours of inks, carbon paper, typewriter ribbons and stencils
☐	☐	☐	☐	Dyes in clothing and shoes
☐	☐	☐	☐	Dyes in cosmetics (lipstick, mascara, rouge powder etc.)

Disinfectants, deodorants and detergents

Like	Neutral	Dislike	Made sick	
☐	☐	☐	☐	Odour of public or household disinfectants and deodorants
☐	☐	☐	☐	Odour of phenol (carbolic acid) or lysol
☐	☐	☐	☐	Phenol-containing lotions or ointments
☐	☐	☐	☐	Injectable materials containing phenol as a preservative
☐	☐	☐	☐	Fumes from burning creosote-treated wood (railway sleepers)
☐	☐	☐	☐	Household detergents

Miscellaneous

Like	Neutral	Dislike	Made sick	
☐	☐	☐	☐	Air-conditioning
☐	☐	☐	☐	Ammonia fumes
☐	☐	☐	☐	Odour of mothballs
☐	☐	☐	☐	Odour of insect-repellant candles
☐	☐	☐	☐	Odour of termite extermination treatment
☐	☐	☐	☐	Odour of DDT-containing insecticide sprays
☐	☐	☐	☐	Odour of chlordane, lindane, parathion, dieldrin and other insecticide sprays
☐	☐	☐	☐	Odour of fruit and vegetable sections in supermarkets
☐	☐	☐	☐	Odour of chlorinated water
☐	☐	☐	☐	Fumes of chlorine gas
☐	☐	☐	☐	Odour of hypochlorite bleaches
☐	☐	☐	☐	Fumes from sulphur-processing plants
☐	☐	☐	☐	Fumes of sulphur dioxide

Like	Neutral	Dislike	Made sick	

Pine

Like	Neutral	Dislike	Made sick	
☐	☐	☐	☐	Odour of Christmas trees and other indoor evergreen decorations
☐	☐	☐	☐	Odour of knotty pine interiors
☐	☐	☐	☐	Odour of cedar-scented furniture polish
☐	☐	☐	☐	Odour from sanding or working with pine or cedar
☐	☐	☐	☐	Odour of pine-scented household deodorants
☐	☐	☐	☐	Odour of pine-scented bath oils, shampoos, soaps
☐	☐	☐	☐	Odour of turpentine or turpentine-containing paint
☐	☐	☐	☐	Fumes from burning pine cones or wood

APPENDIX IV

HUMAN ECOLOGY AND SUSCEPTIBILITY TO THE CHEMICAL ENVIRONMENT QUESTIONNAIRE

This questionnaire is adapted from Theron G. Randolph.

Chemical Additives and Contaminants of Air, Food, Water, Drugs and Cosmetics

Personal and residential details

DATE _____ NAME _____
ADDRESS _____
_____ SEX _____ AGE _____
OCCUPATION _____ WORK ADDRESS _____

Please circle or tick the appropriate answer to the following:

Education
☐ Primary
   1 2 3 4 5 6
☐ High
   7 8 9 10 11 12
☐ College/university
☐ Graduate

Marital Status
☐ Single
☐ Married
☐ Widowed
☐ Separated
☐ Divorced

Work Region
☐ City
☐ Suburban
☐ Small town
☐ Rural

Distance to Work _____
   Travel by:
☐ Car
☐ Bus
☐ Train
☐ Walking
☐ Other _____

Home Type
☐ Single house
☐ Double house
☐ Apartment/unit
☐ Hotel
☐ Other _____

If Multiple Dwelling
☐ What floor? _____
☐ How long lived there _____

Region
☐ City residential
☐ City industrial
☐ Suburban
☐ Small town
☐ Rural

Garage
☐ In separate unattached building
☐ With inside passageway between house
   and garage
☐ In basement of house

HEATING AND VENTILATION OF HOME

Type
☐ Electric
☐ Hot-water or steam
☐ Warm-air (ducted)
☐ Space heaters
☐ Fireplaces

Storage Location
☐ Basement
☐ Main floor
☐ Utility room
☐ Open or closed

Kitchen Exhaust Fan
☐ Yes
☐ No

Kitchen Door Usually Left
☐ Open
☐ Closed

Fuel
☐ Electric
☐ Gas
☐ Oil
☐ Coal
☐ Wood
☐ Kerosene
☐ Other _____

Air-conditioning
☐ Window units
☐ Central system
☐ Filters—oiled or unoiled
☐ Electrostatic
☐ Activated carbon

UTILITIES

Stove
☐ Electric
☐ Gas
☐ Oil
☐ Other
   Age _____

Refrigerator
☐ Electric
☐ Gas
☐ Other
   Age _____

Food Storage
☐ Glass
☐ Enamel
☐ Plastic
☐ Other _____

Deep Freeze
☐ Electric
☐ Gas
   Age _____

Clothes Dryer
☐ Electric
☐ Gas
   Age _____

Water Heater
☐ Electric
☐ Gas
☐ Part of storage
   Age _____

FURNISHINGS AND HOUSEHOLD MAINTENANCE

Upholstery Coverings
☐ Synthetic
☐ Plastic
☐ Linen
☐ Cotton
☐ Silk
☐ Wool

Padding
☐ Cotton
☐ Hair
☐ Rubber
☐ Other _____

Mattresses
☐ Cotton
☐ Rubber
☐ Plastic
☐ Other _____

Pillows
☐ Feather
☐ Rubber
☐ Kapok
☐ Dacron
☐ Plastic

Rugs
☐ Wool
☐ Cotton
☐ Synthetic
☐ Natural fibre
☐ Rubber or plastic-backed

Curtains
☐ Cotton
☐ Linen
☐ Plastic
☐ Synthetic
☐ Silk
☐ Wool

Laundry
☐ Soap
☐ Bleaches
☐ Ammonia
☐ Detergents

Furniture Polish
☐ Yes
☐ No

Floor Wax
☐ Yes
☐ No

Cleansers
☐ Detergents
☐ Soap
☐ Scouring powder with bleach
☐ Ammonia

Deodorants and Disinfectants
☐ Air wick
☐ Lysol
☐ Pine
☐ Others _____

GENERAL

Insect Control
☐ Sprays
☐ Mothballs
☐ Moth crystals
☐ Exterminators

Ability to Detect Leaking Gas
☐ Acute
☐ Normal or average
☐ Poor or absent

When Wind is Blowing from Industrial Area Do Symptoms
☐ Increase
☐ Remain same

Drinking Water
☐ Spring or well
☐ Softened
☐ Chlorinated
☐ Fluoridated

Sense of Smell
☐ Very acute
☐ Normal
☐ Poor
☐ Absent

FOOD TESTING

NAME: _____ FOOD: _____
DATE: _____ PREPARATION: _____ AMOUNT: _____

		CON-TROL	¼ Hr	½ Hr	1 Hr	2 Hr	3 Hr	4 Hr
TIME:								
PULSE:								
BLOOD	mEq							
GLUCOSE:	mg%							
SYMPTOMS:								
1.								
2.								
3.								
4.								
5.								
6.								
7.								
8.								
OBSERVATIONS:								
1.								
2.								
3.								
4.								

COMMENTS:

WRITING:
CONTROL: 1 HOUR:

½ HOUR: 3 HOURS:

ASSESSMENT: SELF: SAFE ☐ UNSAFE ☐   SAFE ☐ SS OS BG P W
STAFF—INITIALS: SAFE ☐ UNSAFE ☐   UNSAFE ☐

APPENDIX V

FOOD FAMILIES

PLANTS

Algae
Irish moss, agar-agar, kelp
Apple
apple, pear, quince,
crab-apple, loquat, rosehips,
cider vinegar, cider, pectin
Arrowroot
dasheen, poi, taro root

Banana
banana, plantain
Birch
hazelnuts, oil of birch, filberts
Blueberry (heath)
blueberry, huckleberry,
cranberry
Buckwheat
buckwheat, rhubarb, garden
sorrel

Cactus
prickly pear, tequila
Cashew
cashew nut, pistachio nut,
mango
Citrus
orange, lemon, grapefruit,
mandarin, tangerine,
cumquat, lime, citron,
angostura bitters
Cola nut
chocolate (cocoa), cola

Fungi
mushroom, yeast (brewers and
bakers), truffles, antibiotics,

inhalant moulds are related to
yeast

Ginger
ginger, turmeric, cardamon,
East Indian arrowroot
Gooseberry
gooseberry, currant (red and
black)
Goosefoot
silver beet, spinach, sugar
beet, swiss chard, lambs
quarters
Gourd
Chinese preserving melon,
cucumber, gherkin,
muskmelon, cantaloupe or
rockmelon, honeydew melon,
Persian melon, pumpkin
squash: acorn, buttercup,
butternut, Boston marrow,
golden nugget, Hubbard
varieties, spaghetti marrow,
zucchini (courgettes)
watermelon
Grapes
grapes, raisins, sultanas,
currants, cream of tartar, wine
vinegar, wine, brandy,
champagne
Grasses
barley, bamboo shoots, corn,
lemon grass, millet, oats, rice,
rye, sorghum, sugar cane,
triticale, wheat, wild rice

Honeysuckle
elderberry

Iris
saffron

Laurel
avocado, cinnamon, bay leaves,
sassafras, cassia bark, camphor
Legumes
peas (green, field, black-eyed,
snow)
beans (navy, lima, mung,
pinto, string)
soy beans, lentils, licorice,
carob, chick peas, peanuts,
tamarind, fenugreek, alfalfa,
clover, coffee beans
Lily
onion, garlic, asparagus,
chives, leek, sarsparilla,
shallots, aloe-vera

Madder
coffee
Mallow
okra, cottonseed, maple
syrup / sugar
Mint
peppermint, sage, thyme,
spearmint, oregano, basil,
rosemary, marjoram, apple
mint, bergamot, lavender,
lemon balm, pennyroyal mint,
winter and summer savory
Morning glory
sweet potato
Mulberry
fig, hop, mulberry, breadfruit

Mustard
broccoli, brussels sprouts,
cabbage, cauliflower, Chinese
cabbage, collards, curly cress,
horseradish, kale, kohl rabi,
mustard greens, mustard seed,
radish, swede, turnip,
watercress
Myrtle
clove, guava, allspice,
eucalyptus

Nightshade
tomato, potato, eggplant,
tobacco, tree tomato, pepper
— capsicum (red, green bell
and chilli), cayenne, paprika,
pimento (not black or white
pepper)
Nutmeg
nutmeg, mace

Oak
chestnuts

Palm
coconut, date, sago
Parsley
parsley, carrot, parsnip, celery,
celeriac, anise, dill, fennel,
cumin, angelica, coriander,
caraway, lovage, chervil
Pawpaw
pawpaw, papaya, papain
Plum
almond, plum (prune), peach,
apricot, cherry, nectarine,
persimmon

Rose
strawberry, blackberry,
raspberry, loganberry,
youngberry, boysenberry,
dewberry

Soapberry
lychee nuts

Spurge
kassava meal, tapioca

Sunflower
lettuce, endive, chicory,
sunflower, tarragon, artichoke
(globe and Jerusalem),
dandelion, sesame,
chamomile, escarole, safflower

Walnut
walnut, pecan, hicory,
butternut (not pumpkin)

PLANTS WITHOUT RELATIVES

Black and white pepper, brazil
nut, coffee, olive, pineapple,
tapioca, tea, vanilla, maple,
poppyseed, wintergreen,
pomegranate, sweet potato,
hazelnut, kiwi fruit

ANIMAL PRODUCTS

Milk, beef, lamb, rabbit, pork
(ham, bacon etc.), venison

POULTRY AND GAME

Chicken, duck, turkey, goose,
grouse, partridge, pheasant,
quail, pigeon, eggs

FISH

Clupeiformes
pilchard, sprats, anchovy,
herring, whitebait

Glaxiiformes
minnows, native trout,
mountain trout

Scopeliformes
lantern fish
Siluroidiformes
catfish
Anguilliformes
eel
Beloniformes
flying fish, garfish
Macruriformes
blue grenadier, whiptail
Gadiformes
codfish
Pleuronectiformes
flounder, sole
Zenformes
dory
Beryciformes
red snapper, redfish (nannygai)
Mugiliformes
mullet, snook
Perciformes (Perch-like)
    Trichiuroidei: barracuda,
      hake, gemfish
    Stromateoidei: trevalla,
      sea bream
    Cottoidei: flathead,
      latchet, gurnard

Ophidioidei: ling
Percoidei:trevally,
   kingfish, tailor,
   morwong (silver
   bream), whiting,
   mullet, mulloway,
   snapper, black bream,
   ruff, luderick (black
   fish), perch,
   Australian salmon,
   trumpeter,
   barramundi,
   stargazer, hapuka,
   Murray cod
Labriformes
parrot fish, rainbow fish, blue
groper
Salmoniformes
trout, salmon
Cypriniformes
carp
Tetraodontiformes
    Balistoidei: leatherjacket
    Scrombroideo: mackerel,
      tuna
Rajiformes
skate

APPENDIX VI

HEADACHES AND MIGRAINE

The following is a list of foods to be eliminated from the diet of patients suffering from migraine and headache. Those with asterisks (*) have been shown to be more common in causing migraine when specifically tested in clinical trials.

*Alcoholic beverages, especially red wine and beer

Avocados

Bananas

*Beef

Broad beans

Cheese — mainly strong and ripened varieties (Cream cheese and cottage cheese are permitted.)

Chicken livers

*Chocolate and any product containing cocoa and cocoa bean, e.g. cola drinks (Carob is permitted.)

Citrus fruits

*Coffee (as a beverage and added to any other food)

*Corn

Cream — sour

*Eggs

Herrings

Hot dogs

*Milk

Monosodium glutamate (large amounts), e.g. in Chinese food

Nuts (mainly peanuts)

Onions

*Oranges

Pork

Protein extracts (yeast) — Marmite, Vegemite etc.

Raisins

Sausages — (fermented: Bologna, salami, pepperoni etc.)

*Sugar

*Tea

Vinegar

*Wheat — especially hot fresh (white) bread

Yeast

Yoghurt

It is best to avoid processed, refined, preserved, artificially flavoured and artificially coloured foods, if possible and practicable.

Other common precipitating factors include:

Oral contraceptive steroids

Smoking (tobacco) — even when the smoking is done by others

Household gas, industrial fumes, petrochemical fumes and similar

APPENDIX VII

PRODUCTS TO BE AVOIDED BY COELIAC DISEASE PATIENTS

The following is a list of prescribed drugs that contain gluten and must be avoided by those suffering from gluten sensitivity/coeliac disease. Few lists illustrate more vividly the near impossible task facing the ordinary person who is trying to avoid a substance that is responsible for his or her intolerance.

KEY TO MANUFACTURERS' CODES

BN Bayer Pharmaceutical Company
CG CIBA-Geigy Australia Ltd
CI Cilag
ES Essex Laboratories Pty Ltd
ET Ethnor Pty Ltd
FA F.H. Faulding & Co. Ltd
FM Fawns & McAllan
GL Glaxo Australia Pty Ltd
GP G.P. Laboratories
JP Janssen Pharmaceutica Pty Ltd
MB May & Baker Australia Pty Ltd
NS Nicholas Kiwi Pacific Pty Ltd
PD Parke Davis Pty Ltd
PT Protea Pharmaceuticals

RC Reckitt & Colman Pharm. Division
RK Riker Laboratories Aust. Pty Ltd
RS A.H. Robins Pty Ltd
ROS Rosken
RL Roussel Pharmaceuticals Pty Ltd
SH Schering Pty Ltd
SE Servier Laboratories (Aust.) Pty Ltd
SI Sigma Pharmaceuticals Pty Ltd
US U.S.V. Australia Pty Ltd
WW William R. Warner
WP Weddel Pharmaceuticals

Allbee with C tablets **(RS)**
Allergex tablets **(PT)**
Almacarb tablets **(GL)**
Altor-Vite tablets **(NS)**
Ambilhar tablets 100 mg and 500 mg **(CG)**
Amitrip, Amitrip M tablets **(PT)**
Amizide tablets **(PT)**
Ammonium chloride tablets 500 mg **(FM)**
Ancolan tablets **(GL)**
Andrumin tablets 50 mg **(CI)**
Antabuse tablets 250 mg and 500 mg **(CI)**
Anti-Naus tablets **(PT)**

Antipres, Antipres M tables **(PT)**
Anti-Spas tablets **(PT)**
Antrenyl tablets 5 mg **(CG)**
Apresoline tablets 25 mg and 50 mg **(CG)**
Ascorb tablets **(PT)**
Ascotin tablets (discontinued) **(FA)**
Aspirin tablets 300 mg **(BN)**
Aspirin tablets 300 mg **(FA)**
Aspirin tablets 300 mg **(FM)**
Aspirin tablets soluble **(FA)**
Aspirin/paracetamol/codeine tablets **(FM)**
Aspro Regular tablets **(NS)**
Avomine tablets 25 mg **(MB)**

Benzide, Benzide M tablets (PT)
Benzotran tablets (PT)
Betamin tablets 50 mg and 100 mg (US)
Bex tablets (NS)
Biquinate tablets 300 mg (US)
Brondecon-PD tablets (PD)
Butalgin tablets 100 mg (FM)
Butazone tablets (PT)

Calcium lactate tablets 300 mg (SI)
Calmazine tablets (PT)
Calvita tablets (NS)
Cantil tablets 25 mg (SI)
Captol tablets (PT)
Cardinol tablets (PT)
Ceetamol tablets (PT)
Cellulone tablets (PT)
Chendol capsules (WP)
Chlorquin tablets (PT)
Choledyl tablets 100 mg and 200 mg (WW)
Cilicaine VK tablets 250 mg (SI)
Codalgin tablets (FM)
Codate tablets 30 mg (US)
Codeine phosphate tablets 30 mg (FM)
Codeine phosphate tablets 30 mg (FA)
Codiphen tablets (GP)
Codis tablets (RC)
Colgout tablets (PT)
Coloxyl tablets 50 mg and 120 mg (FM)
Combantrin tablets 125 mg and 250 mg (GP)
Convuline tablets (PT)
Cortate tablets (PT)
Cyclidox tablets (PT)

Deltasolone tablets 5 mg (US)
Deltasone tablets 5 mg (US)
Demazin repetabs (ES)
Dexamphetamine sulphate tablets 5 mg (SI)

Dexmethsone tablets (PT)
Diamicron tablets 80 mg (SE)
Diastatin oral tablets (GP)
Diatol tablets (PT)
Digestif Rennie (NS)
Dilosyn tablets (GL)
Dimetane tablets 4 mg (RS)
Dipramol tablets (PT)
Disipal tablets (RK)
Disprin tablets and capsules (RC)
Diuret tablets (PT)
Diurone tablets 500 mg (US)
Donnatab tablets (RS)
Dorbanate tablets (RK)
Dormicum tablets (PT)
Doryx capsules 50 mg and 100 mg (FA)
Doxin tablets 100 mg (GP)
Drixora repetabs (ES)

E-Mycin capsules (PT)
Ensalate tablets 600 mg (RC)
Ephedrine tablets 30 mg (SI)
Epilim tablets 200 mg (RC)
Esidrex tablets 25 mg and 50 mg (CG)
Estigyn tablets (GL)

Fabahistin Plus tablets (BN)
Fabahistin tablets 50 mg (BN)
Falcopen VK tablets (discontinued) (FA)
Fedrine tablets 15 mg, 30 mg, 60 mg (US)
Fenamine Slow tablets 75 mg (FM)
Fenamine tablets 10 mg and 50 mg (FM)
Fibre Trim (RL)
Fibyrax (RL)
Flagyl tablets 200 mg (MB)
Folic acid tablets 5 mg (SI)
Folic acid tablets (PT)
Folicid tablets 5 mg (US)

Granocol (SH)

Grisovin tablets (GL)

Hi-Fluor tablets (PT)
Histalert tablets 2.5 mg (RK)
Hycodin tablets (discontinued) (FA)
Hysone tablets (PT)

Imiprin tablets (PT)
Inflam tablets (PT)
Ismelin tablets 10 mg and 25 mg
    (CG)
Isoniazid tablets 50 mg and 100 mg
    (FM)

K-Thrombin tablets 10 mg (FM)
Kwells (NS)

Lioresal tablets 10 mg and 25 mg
    (CG)
Lithicarb tablets (PT)

Mandelamine tablets 250 mg and
    500 mg (WW)
Metamide tablets (PT)
Methoprim tablets (PT)
Methyltestosterone tablets 5 mg and
    25 mg (CI)
Meth-Zine tablets (PT)
Midone tablets (PT)
Multi B Forte tablets (GP)
Multi B tablets (GP)
Myoquin tablets 300 mg (FM)

Nardil tablets (WW)
Natrilix tablets 2.5 mg (SE)
Navidrex tablets 0.5 mg (CG)
Nefrolan tablets 10 mg and 25 mg
    (MB)
Neosulf tablets (PT)
Neulactil tablets 2.5 mg and 10 mg
    (MB)
Nicotinic acid tablets 50 mg (SI)
Nikacid tablets 25 mg, 50 mg,
    100 mg (US)

Orap tablets 2 mg (JP)

Orpadrex tablets (PT)

Pacedol tablets (PT)
Palfium tablets (FA)
Panafcort tablets (PT)
Panafcortelone tablets (PT)
Pancrease capsules (CI)
Panquil tablets (ROS)
Paracetamol tablets (FA)
Paradex tablets (PT)
Parmol tablets 500 mg (US)
Pensig capsules 250 mg (SI)
Pentobarbitone sodium capsules (PT)
Pentobarbitone sodium tablets (PT)
Pethidine tablets 50 mg (SI)
Phenobarbitone tablets 30 mg (SI)
Phthazol tablets 500 mg (US)
Piptal tablets 5 mg (SI)
Piriton tablets (GL)
Polaramine repetabs 6 mg (ES)
Ponderax tablets 20 mg and 40 mg
    (SE)
Priscol tablets 25 mg (CG)
Procid tablets (PT)
Progout tablets (PT)
Promide tablets (PT)
Pro-Pam tablets (PT)
Propylthiouracil tablets 50 mg (CI)
Protran tablets (PT)
P.V.O. tablets 250 mg (FM)
Pydox tablets (PT)
Pyridium tablets (WW)
Pyridoxine tablets 25 mg and 100 mg
    (FM)
Pyroxin tablets 25 mg and 100 mg
    (US)

Quinate tablets 300 mg (US)
Quinidine sulphate tablets (PT)
Quinidis tablets 200 mg (US)
Quinine bisulphate tablets (PT)
Quinine sulphate tablets (PT)
Quitaxon tablets 10 mg and 25 mg
    (RC)

Redu-Pres, Redu-Pres M tablets **(PT)**
Respolin tablets **(RK)**
Rheumacin capsules **(PT)**
Rhusal tablets **(GP)**
Ritalin tablets 10 mg **(CG)**
Rondomycin capsules 300 mg **(WW)**

Salicylamide tablets **(PT)**
Saroten tablets 25 mg **(NS)**
S-Dimidine tablets **(PT)**
Senokot tablets **(RC)**
Serpasil tablets 0.25 mg **(CG)**
S-Methizole tablets **(PT)**
Solcode tablets **(RC)**
Solone tablets 5 mg and 25 mg **(FM)**
Solprin tablets 300 mg and 650 mg
    (RC)
Sonabarb tablets **(PT)**
Sonalgin tablets **(MB)**
Sone tablets 5 mg and 25 mg **(FM)**
Soneryl tablets 100 mg **(MB)**
Spirotone tablets **(PT)**
Stemetil tablets 5 mg and 25 mg
    (MB)
Sulfazole tablets **(PT)**
Supres, Supres M tablets **(PT)**
Surmontil tablets 10 mg and 25 mg
    (MB)

Tab-Vita B Group Forte **(NS)**
Testomet tablets **(PT)**
Thalazole tablets 500 mg **(MB)**
Thiamine tablets 50 mg and 100 mg
    (FM)
Trandate tablets **(GL)**
Trasicor tablets 20 mg, 40 mg,
    80 mg **(CG)**
Trichozole tablets **(PT)**

Uremide tablets **(PT)**
Urid tablets **(PT)**
Urimor tablets **(PT)**

Vallergan tablets 10 mg **(MB)**
Ventolin tablets **(GL)**
Veracolate tablets **(WW)**
Visceralgin tablets 50 mg **(FM)**
Vitamin A tablets 50 000 units **(CI)**
Vitamin B Group Forte tablets **(FM)**
Vitamin B1 tablets **(PT)**
Vitaminorum tablets **(FM)**

Zincaps capsules **(PT)**
Zoline tablets **(PT)**

APPENDIX VIII

IDENTIFYING FOOD ADDITIVES

An asterisk (*) denotes additives proved or strongly suspected to have adverse reactions on humans.

No.	Food Additive

Colours
100	Curcumin
101	Riboflavin
102*	Tartrazine
107*	Yellow 2G
110*	Sunset yellow FCF
120*	Cochineal, carminic acid
122*	Carmoisine
123*	Amaranth
124*	Brilliant scarlet 4R
127*	Erythrosine
132*	Indigo carmine
133*	Brilliant blue FCF
140	Chlorophylls
142	Green S
150*	Caramel
151*	Brilliant black BN
153*	Carbo medicinalis vegetalis (charcoal)
155*	Chocolate brown HT
160	Carotenoids
160(a)	Carotene, alpha-, beta-, gamma-
160(b)	Annatto (bixin, norbixin)
160(e)	Beta-apo-8′ carotenal
160(f)	Ethyl ester of beta-apo-8′ carotenoic acid
161	Xanthophylls
161(g)	Canthaxanthine
162	Beetroot red, betanin
163	Anthocyanins

Mineral salt (misc. functions)
170	Calcium carbonate
171	Titanium dioxide
172	Iron oxides and hydroxides

No.	Food Additive

Preservative
200*	Sorbic acid
201	Sodium sorbate
202	Potassium sorbate
203	Calcium sorbate
210*	Benzoic acid
211*	Sodium benzoate
212*	Potassium benzoate
213*	Calcium benzoate
220*	Sulphur dioxide
221*	Sodium sulphite
222*	Sodium bisulphite
223*	Sodium metabisulphite
224*	Potassium metabisulphite
234	Nisin

Miscellaneous functions
249*	Potassium nitrite
250*	Sodium nitrite
251*	Sodium nitrate
252*	Potassium nitrate

Food acid
260	Acetic acid
261*	Potassium acetate
262*	Sodium acetate
263	Calcium acetate
270*	Lactic acid

Preservative
280	Propionic acid
281*	Sodium propionate
282	Calcium propionate
283	Potassium propionate

No.	Food Additive

Miscellaneous functions
290* Carbon dioxide

Food acid
296 Malic acid
297 Fumaric acid

Anti-oxidant
300 Ascorbic acid
301 Sodium ascorbate
306 Tocopherol-rich extracts of natural origin
307 Synthetic alpha-tocopherol
308 Synthetic gamma-tocopherol
309 Synthetic delta-tocopherol
310* Propyl gallate
311* Octyl gallate
312* Dodecyl gallate
320* Butylated hydroxy-anisole (BHA)
321* Butylated hydroxy-toluene (BHT)

Miscellaneous functions
322 Lecithins

Food acid
325* Sodium lactate
326 Potassium lactate
327 Calcium lactate
330* Citric acid
331 Sodium citrate
332 Potassium citrate
333 Calcium citrate
334 Tartaric acid
335 Sodium tartrate
336 Potassium tartrate
337 Sodium potassium tartrate

No.	Food Additive

Mineral salt
339 Sodium orthophosphates
340 Potassium ortho-phosphates
341 Calcium orthophosphates

Food acid
350 Sodium malate
351 Potassium malate
352 Calcium malate
353 Metatartaric acid
354 Calcium tartrate

Miscellaneous functions
355 Adipic acid
363 Succinic acid

Food acid
380 Tri-ammonium citrate

Vegetable gum
400 Alginic acid
401 Sodium alginate
402 Potassium alginate
403 Ammonium alginate
404 Calcium alginate
405 Propylene glycol alginate
406* Agar
407* Carrageenan
410 Locust bean gum
412* Guar gum
413 Tragacanth
414* Acacia
415 Xanthan gum
416 Karaya gum

Humectant
420* Sorbitol

Miscellaneous functions
421* Mannitol

No.	Food Additive

Humectant
422* Glycerol

Emulsifier
433 Polyoxyethylene (20) sorbitan mono-oleate
435* Polyoxyethylene (20) sorbitan mono-stearate
436* Polyoxyethylene (20) sorbitan tristearate

Vegetable gum
440(a) Pectin

Emulsifier
442 Ammonium phosphatides

Mineral salt
450* Sodium and potassium polyphosphates

Vegetable gum
460 Microcrystalline cellulose, powdered cellulose
461 Methylcellulose
464 Hydroxypropyl-methylcellulose
465 Ethylmethylcellulose
466* Carboxymethyl-cellulose

Fat components
471 Mono- and diglycerides of fatty acids

Emulsifier
472(e) Mono and diacetyl-tartaric acid esters of mono- and diglycerides of fatty acids
473 Sucrose esters of fatty acids
475 Polyglycerol esters of fatty acids

No.	Food Additive

476 Polyglycerol polyric-inoleate
481 Sodium stearoyl-2-lactylate
482 Calcium stearoyl-2-lactylate
491 Sorbitan monostearate

Mineral salt
500* Sodium carbonate
501 Potassium carbonate
503* Ammonium carbonate
504 Magnesium carbonate

Miscellaneous functions
508* Potassium chloride

Mineral salt
509 Calcium chloride
529 Calcium oxide

Anti-caking agent
536 Potassium ferro-cyanide

Miscellaneous functions
541 Sodium aluminium phosphate

Anti-caking agent
551 Silicon dioxide

Miscellaneous functions
553(b) Talc
554 Sodium aluminium silicate
558 Bentonite
559 Kaolins
570 Stearic acid
572 Magnesium stearate
575 Glucono delta-lactone
621 Monosodium glutamate

No.	Food Additive	No.	Food Additive
627	Sodium guanylate	905*	Paraffins
631*	Sodium inosinate	909	Stearic acid
637	Ethyl maltol	920	L-Cysteine and its
900	Dimethylpoly-siloxane		hydrochlorides
901	Beeswaxes	924*	Potassium bromate
903	Carnauba wax	925*	Chlorine
904	Shellac	926*	Chlorine dioxide

Information courtesy NSW and Commonwealth Health Departments

APPENDIX IX

SALICYLATE CONTENT OF VARIOUS FOODS

NEGLIGIBLE SALICYLATE CONTENT
(≤0.1 MG SALICYLATE PER 100 G FOOD)

Fruit
Golden Delicious apple
Letona apricot nectar
Banana
Packham pears (no skin)
Plum (Kelsey green)
Letona Bartlett pears (canned)
Letona peach nectar
Pomegranate
Tamarillo
Pawpaw

Vegetables
Bamboo shoots (Sunshine canned)
Beans
  blackeye (dried)
  borlotti
  brown
  lima
  mung
  soya
  soya grits
Bean sprouts
Brussels sprouts
Cabbage, green and red
Celery
Chives
Choko (Chayote)
Horseradish (canned)
Leek
Lentil (brown and red)
Lettuce
Peas
  chickpeas (dried)
  green
  greensplit (dried)
  yellowsplit (dried)
Potato (peeled)
Shallots
Swede
Tomato juice (Goulburn Valley)

Condiments
Garlic (bulbs)
Parsley (leaves)
Saffron (powder)
Soy sauce
Tandori (powder)
Vinegar (malt)

Drinks
Aktavite
Coffee (dandelion, Andronicus
    instant, Harris instant I and II,
    Moccona decaffeinated,
    Nescafé decaffeinated)
Camomile tea
Ecco
Milo
Ovaltine

Cereals
Arrowroot
Barley (unpearled)
Buckwheat
Millet
Oats
Rice
Rye

Nuts and seeds
Cashew nuts
Poppy seed

Sugars
Carob powder
Cocoa powder
Golden syrup (CSR)
Maple syrup (Camp)

Dairy products
Cheese (blue vein, camembert,
   cheddar, cottage, mozzarella,
   tasty cheddar)
Milk (fresh full cream)
Yoghurt (full cream)

Meat, fish, eggs
Beef
Chicken
Egg, white
Egg, yolk
Kidney
Lamb
Liver
Oyster
Pork
Prawn
Salmon
Scallop
Tripe
Tuna

Alcoholic drinks
Gin (Gilbeys)
Vodka (Smirnoff)
Wine, dry white (McWilliams)
Whisky (Johnnie Walker)

LOW SALICYLATE CONTENT
(0.1–0.5 MG SALICYLATE PER 100 G FOOD)

Fruit
Apple (Red Delicious)
Apple juice (Mountain Maid)
Cherry (Morello sour, canned)
Custard apple
Figs
Grapes, S & W seedless (canned)
Grapes, Sanitarium light juice
Grapefruit juice (Berri)
Kiwi fruit
Lemon
Loquat
Lychee (canned)
Mango
Nectarine
Orange juice (Berri)
Passionfruit
Persimmon
Pineapple juice (Golden Circle)
Plum (blood, red)
Rhubarb
Watermelon

Vegetables
Asparagus
Asparagus (Triangle spears)
Beans, green French
Beetroot (Golden Circle)
Carrot
Cauliflower
Eggplant (peeled)
Marrow (Cucurbita pepo)
Mushroom
Olive (black, Kraft, canned)
Onion
Parsnip
Pimentos (Arson sweet red,
   canned)
Potato white (unpeeled)
Pumpkin
Spinach (frozen)
Sweetcorn
Sweetcorn (canned)
Sweet potato, white
Tomato
Tomato juice (Heinz, Letona)

Tomato paste (Tom Piper)
Tomato soup (PMU)
Turnip

Condiments
Bonox, liquid extract
Coriander, fresh leaves
Tabasco sauce (McIllhenny)

Drinks
Cereal coffee (Bambu, Reform)
Coca-Cola
Coffee (Bushells Instant, Bushells
    Turkish style, Gibsons Instant,
    Harris Mocha Kenya, Robert
    Timms instant)
Herbal tea (fruit, rose hip, Golden
    Days decaffeinated)

Cereals
Maize (meal)

Nuts and seeds
Brazil nuts

Coconut (desiccated)
Hazelnuts
Macadamia nuts
Peanut butter (Sanitarium)
Pecan nuts
Sesame seed
Sunflower seed
Walnuts

Sugars
Molasses (CSR)

Confectionery
Caramel (Pascall Cream)

Alcoholic Drinks
Beer
Brandy (Hennessy)
Cider (apple)
Claret (McWilliams Reserve)
Sherry (Mildara Supreme Dry,
    Penfolds Royal Reserve)
Dry Vermouth (Buton)
Rosé (Kaiser Stuhl)

MEDIUM SALICYLATE CONTENT
(0.5–1.0 MG SALICYLATE PER 100 G FOOD)

Fruit
Apples (Granny Smith)
Apples (Ardmona)
Figs (Calamata string, dried)
Cherry (sweet)
Grapes (Red malaita)
Grape juice (Berri dark)
Grapefruit
Mandarin
Mulberry
Peach
Peach (Letona)
Tangelo

Vegetables
Alfalfa
Beans (broad)

Broccoli
Eggplant
Okra (Zanae, canned)
Peppers (green chilli)
Peppers (yellow-green chilli)
Spinach
Squash (baby)
Tomato (Letona)
Tomato paste (Campbells)
Tomato soup (Heinz, Kia-Ora)
Tomato sauce (Fountain, PMU)
Watercress

Condiments
Fennel (powder)
Marmite (Sanitarium)
Vegemite (Kraft)

Drinks

Coffee (International Roast,
   Maxwell House Instant,
   Moccona Instant, Nescafé
   Instant)

Nuts

Pine
Pistachio

Confectionery

Peppermints (Allens Strong Mint)

Alcoholic drinks

Liqueurs (Cointreau)
Sherry (Lindemans Royal Reserve)
Spirits (Bundaberg Rum)
Wines, Riesling (Lindemans)
   Cabernet Sauvignon
   (McWilliams) Claret
   (McWilliams Private Bin)
   Traminer Riesling (Penfolds)
   Rhine Riesling (Seaview)

---

*HIGH SALICYLATE CONTENT
(>1.0 MG SALICYLATE PER 100 G FOOD; FOODS
WITH SALICYLATE CONTENT >5.0 MG PER 100 G ARE MARKED*)*

Fruit

Plum (SPC, dark red)
Prunes (Letona)
Raspberries (fresh/frozen)
Strawberry fresh
Youngberry (canned)

Vegetables

Chicory
*Cucumber (Aristocrat canned
   gherkin)
Endive
Mushroom (champignon canned)
Olive (green, Kraft canned)
Peppers (red chili)
Peppers (sweet green capsicum)
Radish (red, small)
Tomato paste (Leggo)
Tomato sauce (Heinz, IXL,
   Rosella)
Zucchini

Condiments

*Allspice powder
*Aniseed powder
 Bay leaves
 Basil

*Canella powder
*Cardamon powder
 Caraway powder
*Cayenne powder
*Celery powder
 Chilli flakes/powder
*Cinnamon powder
*Cloves (whole)
*Cumin powder
*Curry powder
*Dill (fresh and powder)
*Fenugreek powder
*Five spice powder
*Garam masala powder
 Ginger root (fresh)
*Mace powder
*Mint (fresh)
*Mixed herbs (leaves, dry)
*Mustard powder
 Nutmeg powder
*Oregano powder
*Paprika hot powder
*Paprika sweet powder
*Pepper black powder
 Pepper white powder
 Pimento powder

*Rosemary powder
*Sage leaves
*Tarragon powder
*Tumeric powder
*Thyme powder
Vanilla essence
*Vinegar (white)
Worcestershire sauce

Drinks
Cereal coffee (Nature's Cuppa)
Herbal Tea (Peppermint)
Teas (all varieties, bags and leaves)

Nuts and seeds
Almonds
Peanuts (unshelled)

Water chestnut (Socomin, canned)
Honey (all)

Confectionery
*Liquorice (Barratts Giant)
*Peppermints
Allens Kool Mints
Minties
Allens Steamrollers

Alcoholic drinks
Liqueurs, Benedictine
Liqueurs, Drambuie
Port (McWilliams Royal Reserve)
Rum (Captain Morgan)

APPENDIX X

DESIRABLE WEIGHTS OF ADULTS[a]

Desirable weight in kilograms and pounds (in indoor clothing), ages 25 and over

Height (in shoes)			Small frame		Medium frame		Large frame	
cm	ft	in	kg	lb	kg	lb	kg	lb
MEN								
157.5	5	2	50.8–54.4	112–120	53.5–58.5	118–129	57.2–64	126–141
160	5	3	52.2–55.8	115–123	54.9–60.3	121–133	58.5–65.3	129–144
162.6	5	4	53.5–57.2	118–126	56.2–61.7	124–136	59.9–67.1	132–148
165.1	5	5	54.9–58.5	121–129	57.6–63	127–139	61.2–68.9	135–152
167.6	5	6	56.2–60.3	124–133	59 –64.9	130–143	62.6–70.8	138–156
170.2	5	7	58.1–62.1	128–137	60.8–66.7	134–147	64.4–73	142–161
172.7	5	8	59.9–64	132–141	62.6–68.9	138–152	66.7–75.3	147–166
175.3	5	9	61.7–65.8	136–145	64.4–70.8	142–156	68.5–77.1	151–170
177.8	5	10	63.5–68	140–150	66.2–72.6	146–160	70.3–78.9	155–174
180.3	5	11	65.3–69.9	144–154	68 –74.8	150–165	72.1–81.2	159–179
182.9	6	0	67.1–71.7	148–158	69.9–77.1	154–170	74.4–83.5	164–184
185.4	6	1	68.9–73.5	152–162	71.1–79.4	158–175	76.2–85.7	168–189
188	6	2	70.8–75.7	156–167	73.5–81.6	162–180	78.5–88	173–194
190.5	6	3	72.6–77.6	160–171	75.7–83.5	167–185	80.7–90.3	178–199
193	6	4	74.4–79.4	164–175	78.1–86.2	172–190	82.7–92.5	182–204
WOMEN								
147.3	4	10	41.7–44.5	92– 98	43.5–48.5	96–107	47.2–54	104–119
149.9	4	11	42.6–45.8	94–101	44.5–49.9	98–110	48.1–55.3	106–122
152.4	5	0	43.5–47.2	96–104	45.8–51.3	101–113	49.4–56.7	109–125
154.9	5	1	44.9–48.5	99–107	47.2–52.6	104–116	50.8–58.1	112–128
157.5	5	2	46.3–49.9	102–110	48.5–54	107–119	52.2–59.4	115–131
160	5	3	47.6–51.3	105–113	49.9–55.3	110–122	53.5–60.8	118–134
162.6	5	4	49 –52.6	108–116	51.3–57.2	113–126	54.9–62.6	121–138
165.1	5	5	50.3–54	111–119	52.6–59	116–130	56.7–64.4	125–142
167.6	5	6	51.7–55.8	114–123	54.4–61.2	120–135	58.5–66.2	129–146
170.2	5	7	53.5–57.6	118–127	56.2–63	124–139	60.3–68	133–150
172.7	5	8	55.3–59.4	122–131	58.1–64.9	128–143	62.1–69.9	137–154
175.3	5	9	57.2–61.2	126–135	59.9–66.7	132–147	64 –71.7	141–158
177.8	5	10	59 –63.5	130–140	61.7–68.5	136–151	65.8–73.9	145–163
180.3	5	11	60.8–65.3	134–144	63.5–70.3	140–155	67.6–76.2	149–168
182.9	6	0	62.6–67	138–148	65.3–72.1	144–159	69.4–78.5	153–173

[a]Weights of insured persons in the United States associated with lowest mortality (*Statist. Bull. Metrop. Life Insur. Co.*, 40, Nov.–Dec. 1959).

APPENDIX XI

NATURAL CARBOHYDRATE IN FOODS
(as a percentage)

Containing approximately 5% or less

Asparagus, raw 5.0

Asparagus, cooked 3.6

Broccoli, raw 5.9

Broccoli, cooked 4.5

Butter, salted and unsalted 0.4

Cabbage, raw 5.4

Caulifower, cooked 4.1

Celery, raw 3.9

Cheese, blue 2.0

       cheddar 2.1

       cottage 2.9

       Swiss 1.7

Cucumbers 3.4

Eggs, whole, cooked 0.9

Eggs, yolks, raw 0.6

Eggplant, cooked 4.1

Lettuce 3.0

Milk, cow's, whole 4.9

Milk, skim 5.1

Mushrooms, raw 3.6

Peppers, green, raw 4.8

Radishes, raw 3.6

Spinach, cooked 3.6

Squash, cooked 3.1

Tomatoes, ripe, raw 4.7

Tomato juice, tinned 4.3

Soybeans, sprouted, raw 5.3

Watercress, raw 3.0

Yoghurt, whole milk 4.9

Yoghurt, skim milk 5.2

Zucchini, raw 4.2

Zucchini, cooked 3.1

All meats, except sausages, camp pie, tinned corned beef 0.0

All poultry 0.0

All fish 0.0

All fats and oils 0.0

Approximately 5% to 12%

Apple juice, tinned or bottled 11.9

Apricots, raw 12.8

Artichokes, cooked 9.6

Avocados, raw 6.3

Beans, mung, sprouted, raw 10.6

Beets, red, raw 9.9

Brazil nuts 10.9

Brussels sprouts, cooked 6.4

Cabbage, red, raw 6.9

Carrots, raw 9.7

Gooseberries, raw 9.7

Grapefruit 10.6

Grapefruit juice 9.2

Melon, cantaloupe 7.5

Melon, honeydew 7.7

Oatmeal or rolled oats, cooked 9.7

Onions 8.7

Oranges, peeled 12.2
Orange juice 10.0
Papaya 10.0
Parsley 8.5
Peas, raw from pod 12.0
Peas, green cooked 12.1
Peaches, raw 9.7

Peppers, red, raw 7.1
Pumpkin, raw 6.5
Soybeans, cooked 10.8
Strawberries 8.4
Turnips, raw 6.6
Watermelon 6.4

Approximately 13% and over

Apples, fresh 14.5
Apricots, dried 66.5
Apricots, raw 12.8
Artichokes, Jerusalem, raw 26.7
Bananas, raw 22.2
Beans, white and red, cooked 21.4
Beans, lima, cooked 25.6
Blackberries 12.9
Blueberries 15.3
Carob flour 80.7
Cashew nuts 29.3
Cherries 17.4
Coconut, dried 23.0
Corn, cooked on the cob 21.0
Currants, black, raw 13.1
Dates 72.9
Figs, raw 20.3
Figs, dried 69.1
Hazelnuts 16.7
Garlic, raw 15.7
Guavas, raw 15.0
Honey 82.3

Mangos 16.8
Milk, dry, whole 38.2
Peanuts 18.6
Pears 15.3
Pineapple 13.7
Pineapple, juice, tinned, unsweetened 13.5
Plums 19.7
Potatoes, baked in skins 21.0
Potatoes, boiled in skins 17.1
Raspberries 15.7
Rice, brown, cooked 15.5
Rye, wholegrain 73.4
Rye, flour, dark 68.1
Wheatbran 11.9
Wheatgerm, raw 46.7

Alcoholic beverages

Except for fortified wines, most alcoholic beverages are low in carbohydrate. Typically, beer contains 4.8%, wine between 0.2% and 8.0%, and port 14.0%.

Index